H. Remschmidt · H. van Engeland (Eds.) **Child and Adolescent Psychiatry in Europe**

H. Remschmidt
H. van Engeland
Editors

Child and Adolescent Psychiatry in Europe

Historical Development
Current Situation
Future Perspectives

STEINKOPFF
DARMSTADT

Springer

Editors' addresses:

Prof. Dr. Dr. H. Remschmidt
Univ.-Klinik für Psychiatrie und Psychotherapie
des Kindes- und Jugendalters
Klinikum der Philipps-Universität
D-35033 Marburg
Germany

Prof. Dr. H. van Engeland
Department of Child & Adolescent Psychiatry
University Hospital Utrecht
P.O. Box 85500
NL-3508 GA Utrecht
The Netherlands

Die Deutsche Bibliothek – CIP-Einheitsaufnahme

Child and adolescent psychiatry in Europe / H. Remschmidt ; H. van Engeland ed. – Darmstadt : Steinkopff ; New York : Springer, 1999

ISBN-13: 978-3-642-96005-5 e-ISBN-13: 978-3-642-96003-1
DOI: 10.1007/978-3-642-96003-1

Softcover reprint of the hardcover 1st edition 1999

Medical Editors: Sabine Ibkendanz, Beate Rühlemann – English Editor: Mary Gossen
Production: Heinz J. Schäfer
Cover Design: Erich Kirchner, Heidelberg
Typesetting: Typoservice, Griesheim
Printed on acid-free paper

Preface

The intention of this book is to provide an overview of child and adolescent psychiatry in Europe, focusing on the historical development, current situation, and future perspectives of the specialty.

Child and adolescent psychiatry is now acknowledged as a medical specialty or subspecialty in almost all European countries. Also, the number of child psychiatrists has increased dramatically over the last decade. However, there are still enormous differences from country to country, not only with regard to the number of specialists, but also with regard to the extent and nature of services provided and their diagnostic and therapeutic orientation. Furthermore, important differences exist in the training curricula for child and adolescent psychiatry within medicine and other professional fields, both inside and outside the universities, and in the image and importance of this discipline to the public.

This diversity is also reflected in the reports on the historical development, current situation and future perspectives of child and adolescent psychiatry in 31 European countries, all following the same structure in order to facilitate comparability. This structure comprises (1) the historical development and the current situation, (2) classification systems and diagnostic and therapeutic methods, (3) structure and organization of services, (4) cooperation with other medical and non-medical disciplines, (5) training and continuing medical education, (6) research, and (7) future perspectives.

After the fall of the iron curtain, the situation of states in Eastern Europe has changed remarkably. This has also influenced the development and structure of child and adolescent psychiatry in Eastern European countries. We have tried to include as many of these countries as possible.

We hope that this volume whose publication date coincides with the 11th International Congress of the European Society for Child and Adolescent Psychiatry (ESCAP) will support the aims of this society laid down in the ESCAP constitution:

- to foster the European tradition of child and adolescent psychiatry,
- to facilitate and extend the bonds between physicians practising child and adolescent psychiatry in European countries,
- to spread the results of research and experience in this branch of medicine by publishing reports and organizing scientific conferences and meetings, and
- to collaborate with international organizations with the same or related aims.

Accordingly, we hope that this volume will make a substantial contribution to the development of an empirically based child and adolescent psychiatry in Europe and facilitate cooperation between countries.

Our thanks and appreciation go to our colleagues for their enthusiasm in writing about their countries, to the staff of Steinkopff Publishers and – last but not least – to Dipl.-Psych. Johanna Schneider, Dr. Peter M. Wehmeier, Dipl.-Psych. Monika Becker, and Dr. Helen Crimlisk, who carried out the editorial work with great prudence.

Helmut Remschmidt
President of ESCAP

Herman van Engeland
Past President of ESCAP

Contents

Authors' addresses

Prof. Dr. Dr. Meglena Achkova
Alexandrovska University Hospital
1 Georgi Sofiisky Str.
BG-1431 Sofia
Bulgaria

Prof. Dr. Dieter Bürgin
Kinder- und jugendpsychiatrische
Universitätsklinik u. -poliklinik
Schaffheuserrheinweg 55
CH-4058 Basel
Switzerland

Prof. Dr. Ernesto Caffo
Clinica Psichiatrica
Cattedra di Neuropsichiatria Infantile
Via del Pozzo 71
I-41100 Modena
Italy

Prof. Dr. Herman van Engeland
Dept. of Child and Adolescent
Psychiatry
University Hospital Utrecht
P.O. Box 85500,
NL-3508 GA Utrecht
The Netherlands

Prof. Dr. Max H. Friedrich
Universitätsklinik für
Neuropsychiatrie
des Kindes- und Jugendalters
Währinger Gürtel 18-20
A-1090 Wien
Austria

Dr. Christine Frisch-Desmarez
Psychiatrie pour Enfants et
Adolescents
36 rue Tony Neumann
L-2241 Luxembourg
Luxembourg

Dr. Helga Hannesdóttir
Dept. Child and Adol. Psychiatry
Skipholti 50
IS-105 Reykjavik
Iceland

Prof. Dr. Peter Hill
Department of Psychological Medicine
Great Ormond Street
Hospital for Children
UK-London WC1N 3JH
United Kingdom

Dr. Veronika Išpanović-Radojković
Institute for Mental Health
Palmoticeva 37
YU-11000 Beograd
Serbia

Prof. Dr. Philippe Jeammet
Institut Mutualiste Montsouris
42, Bd. Jourdan
F-75014 Paris
France

Dr. Aigars Kishuro
State Mental Health Care Centre
Raina bulvaris 27
LV-1359 Riga
Latvia

Dr. Michael Levinsky
Rehabilitation Center for
Children with Disability
51, Pushkinskaya str.
UA-27001 Odessa
Ukraine

Dr. Juri Liivamägi
University of Tartu
Dept. of Cild & Adolescent Psychiatry
31 Raja Street
EE 2400 Tartu
Estonia

Dr. Eva Malá
Psychiatric Clinic
University Hospital
Vúvalu 84
CZ-Praha 5 - Motol, 150 05
Czech Republic

Prof. Dr. Jean-Paul Matot
Université libre de Bruxelles
Service de Santé Mentale
Psy Campus
50 av. F.-D. Roosevelt CP 184
B-1050 Bruxelles
Belgium

Prof. Dr. Paul McCarthy
Dept. of Child and Adolescent
Psychiatry,
St. James Hospital
James Street
IRL-Dublin 8
Ireland

Prof. Dr. Dr.Tiberiú Mircea
University of Medicine and Pharmacy
Timisoara
Str. Tarnava no. 2
RO-1900 Timisoara
Romania

Prof. Dr. Dr. Staniša Nikolić
Clinic for Psychological Medicine
Kišpatićeva 12 Rebro-KBC
RH-10000 Zagreb
Croatia

Dr. Dr. Ján Pečeňák
Department of Psychiatry
University Hospital
Mickiewiczova 13
SK-81369 Bratislava
Slovakia

Prof. Dr. José-Luis Pedreira-Massa
Child and Adolescent Psychiatry Unit
(SESPA)
E-33400 Avilés (Asturias)
Spain

Prof. Dr. Jorma Piha
University of Turku
Dept. of Child Psychiatry
SF-20520 Turku
Finland

Dr. Dr. Dainius Puras
National University Hospital
Child Development Center
Vytauto 15
2004 Vilnius
Lithuania

Prof. Dr. Dr. Helmut Remschmidt
Univ.-Klinik für Psychiatrie und
Psychotherapie
des Kindes- und Jugendalters
Klinikum der Philipps-Universität
D-35033 Marburg
Germany

Dr. Kari Schleimer
Dept. Child & Adol. Psychiatry
Malmö University Hospital
S-20502 Malmö
Sweden

Prof. Dr. Anatoly A. Severny
23,18/15 Grusinsky val.
RUS-123056 Moscow
Russia

Dr. Ingrid Spurkland
National Center for Child and Adolescent Psychiatry
Sognsvannsvn. 53-67
Postbox 26 Vinderen
N-0319 Oslo
Norway

Dr. Per Hove Thomsen
Child & Adolescent Psychiatric Hospital
Dept. of Research
Harald Selmersvej 66
DK-8240 Risskov
Denmark

Prof. Dr. Dr. Martina Tomori
University of Ljubljana
Zaloska C. 29
SLO-1105 Ljubljana
Slovenia

Prof. Dr. John Tsiantis
Athens University Medical School
Department of Child Psychiatry
Aghia Sophia Children's Hospital
Dept. of Psycholog. Pediatrics
Thivon and Levathiasstr.
GR-11527 Athens
Greece

Prof. Dr. Ágnes Vetró
Szent-Györgyi Albert Med. University
Szemmelweisz u. 6
H-6721 Szeged
Hungary

Dr. Maria José Vidigal
Clinica Infantil
Pavilhao 25
P-1700 Lisboa
Portugal

Introduction

H. Remschmidt, H. van Engeland, J. Piha

1. Historical development

The discipline of Child and Adolescent Psychiatry is now acknowledged as a medical specialty or subspecialty in almost all European countries and throughout the world. It has its roots in the neighbouring disciplines of neurology, psychiatry, pediatrics, and psychology among others. Those working in the field have learned in recent decades that interdisciplinary co-operation is an absolute necessity for scientific and clinical progress.

The historical development of the discipline of Child and Adolescent Psychiatry varies across Europe. Since the beginning of the century, however, four traditions have made substantial contributions to the current body of knowledge, as well as to the orientation of child psychiatric institutions. These traditions are still evident and influential today.

- *The neuropsychiatric tradition.* This goes back to the formerly unified disciplines of psychiatry and neurology. This tradition remains influential in Germany, and was also a significant feature in France, Italy, and in many Eastern European countries. Several scientific associations still include reference to neurology, such as the Association of Child and Adolescent Neuropsychiatry (Austria), Neuropsichiatria Infantile (Italy), and the Developmental Age Neurology and Psychiatry (Serbia). This tradition has more recently been extended in some countries to embrace substantial contributions from neuropsychology.
- *The remedial clinical tradition (heilpädagogisch-klinische Tradition).* This movement started in Austria and Switzerland, promoted by Hans Asperger in Austria and Paul Moor in Switzerland. The approach was later continued as the so-called psychosomatic tradition in pediatrics and still plays a major role in childrens' hospitals with departments of child psychosomatics.
- *The psychodynamic-psychoanalytic tradition.* This tradition evolved mainly in Western Europe and was developed from the work of Sigmund Freud, Anna Freud, Alfred Adler, Melanie Klein, René Spitz, and other pioneers of psychoanalytic work with children.
- *The empirical, epidemiological, and statistical tradition.* This has emerged over recent years in a number of European countries, with a strong focus in England, Scandinavia, Germany, and Switzerland. It has been strongly influenced by Michael Rutter's work in England and also from research impulses from the United States.

It is important to realize that these traditions of research and clinical practice did not evolve successively, but rather, simultaneously. There has, however, been a swing in recent years toward the empirical approach, particularly focusing on the biological aspects of child and adolescent psychiatry.

All countries in Europe have set up national organizations, although these have different orientations and functions. In most countries, those working with children and adolescents are represented by one body. An exception is Finland, where the associations for adolescent psychiatry and child psychiatry exist as separate entities.

The first symposium of European child psychiatrists took place October 30–31, 1954 in Magglingen/Switzerland. At this meeting, the first attempts were made to establish a unifying scientific association. The official foundation of the *Union of European Pedopsychiatrists* occurred in 1960 at the first European congress in Paris. Further congresses were held in Rome (1963), Wiesbaden (1967), Stockholm (1971), Vienna (1975), Madrid (1979), Lausanne (1983), Varna (1987), London (1991), Utrecht (1995), and Hamburg (1999). The name of the society was changed following a decision at the congress in Madrid from the *Union of European Pedopsychiatrists (UEP)* to the *European Society for Child and Adolescent Psychiatry (ESCAP).*

The history of Child and Adolescent Psychiatry in the different countries is described in the following chapters, all of which start with a historical perspective.

2. Current situation

The number of child psychiatrists has dramatically increased over the last decade in nearly all European countries. The current situation in the 31 European countries described is shown in Table 1, which shows data on the professional and scientific organizations, the departments of child psychiatry, the number of child psychiatrists, and population data for each country. It can be seen that there is a long tradition of Child and Adolescent Psychiatry beginning in France (1937) and Germany (1940). As far as the number of university departments is concerned, France also holds the top position (n = 33), followed by Germany (n = 26) and Italy (n = 24).

Provision of services varies widely across Europe. This is also demonstrated in Table 1, which shows the ratio of child and adolescent psychiatrists to the population under the age of 20 years. Using this as a measure of services, the best provision is to be found in Switzerland (1: 5,300), followed by Finland (1: 6,600), France (1: 7,500), and Sweden (1: 7,700). It is also interesting to note that the proportion of the population under 20 also varies widely across Europe, the lowest rate being found in Italy (20 %) and Germany (21 %), and the highest rate in Ireland and Iceland (both 31 %), Slovakia (29 %), and Serbia (28 %).

The data in this table must be considered approximate and provisional. It has proved difficult to obtain reliable, comparable information about services and departments. Despite some reservations about the quality of the data, we still felt it was important and illuminating to include it here, as it reveals large differences in service organization and provision. Further details, including the special needs and problems of individual countries are elaborated upon in the specific chapters of this book. The prevailing impression is of considerable heterogeneity, with able 1. Survey of the current situation of CAP in 31 European Countries

Country	Name of associat.	Year of foundat.	University departm. in CP	Other departm. in CP	MD in CP	Population (in 1,000's)[1]	Persons < 20 y (in 1,000's)[1]	Persons < 20 years (%)	Pers. < 20 y per MD in CP
1 Austria	CANP[2]	1974	1	8	65	8,134	1,859	23	28,600
2 Belgium	CAP	1961/76	4 (2/2)	19	300	10,175	2,385	23	8,000
3 Bulgaria	CAP	1993	3 (0 chair)	9	46	8,240	1,939	23.5	42,000
4 Croatia	CAP	1990	3	3	35	4,672	1,125	24	32,000
5 Czech Rep.	CAP[4]	1960	4 (0 chair)	13	116	10,286	2,524	24,5	21,700
6 Denmark	CAP[4]	1953	4 (1 chair)	12	141	5,334	1,263	23.6	9,000
7 Estonia	CAP[4]	1973	1	2	20	1,421	372	26	18,600
8 Finland	CP	1956	5	19 child 15 ado	196	5,149	1,286	25	6,600
9 France	CP	1937	33	120	2,000	58,805	15,010	25.5	7,500
10 Germany	CAPP	1940	26	145	781	82,079	17,323	21	22,000
11 Greece	CP	1983	3	22[6]	160	10,662	2,477	23	15,500
12 Hungary	CAP	1990	1	7	55	10,208	2,499	24.5	45,000
13 Iceland	CP	1980	1 (0 chair)	0	10	271	085	31	8,500
14 Ireland	CAP	1983	2	12	36	3,619	1,135	31	31,500
15 Italy	CNP	1959	24	15	1,200	56,783	11,297	20	9,400
16 Latvia	CAP[4]	1950	1	3	26	2,385	614	25.7	23,600
17 Lithuania	CAP	1996	2	3	60	3,600	998	27.7	16,600
18 Luxembourg	–	–	0	1	4	425	101	23.7	25,000
19 Netherlands	CAP	1948	7	19	257	15,731	3,800	24	14,800
20 Norway	CAP	1957	4	60	130	4,420	1,130	25.5	8,700
21 Portugal	CAP	1989	0	3	99	9,928	2,412	24	24,300
22 Romania	CANP	1992	3	10	200	22,396	6,023	26.9	30,000
23 Russia	CAPP[3]	1992	0	99	1,300	146,861	40,326	27.5	31,000
24 Serbia	CAP, DANP[7]	1979	4	14 outpatient	57	10,526	2,957	28	51,800
25 Slovakia	CAP	1971	3 (0 chair)	5	113	5,393	1,575	29	14,000
26 Slovenia	CP	1979	2	12 outpatient	24	1,972	475	24	19,800
27 Spain	CAP	1978	1	17	200	39,134	8,739	22	43,000
28 Sweden	CAP	1956	6 (4 chairs)	24	282	8,887	2,166	24	7,700
29 Switzerland	CAPP	1957	5	11	315	7,260	1,662	23	5,300
30 Ukraine	CAP[4]	1995	1 (2)[5]	40	438	50,125	13,153	26	30,000
31 U.K.	CAP	1971	16 (18 chairs)	60	547	58,970	15,036	25.5	27,500

1 Source: International Programs Center (IPC), U.S. Census Bureau, estimates 1998; 2 CANPP: Child - Adolescent - Neurology - Psychiatry - Psychotherapy; 3 CAPP: Child, Adolescent, Psychiatrists, Psychologists; 4 Section; 5 (2) Research institutes outside universities; 6 including 15 child guidance services; 7 DANP: Developmental Age Neurology and Psychiatry (1979)

regard not only to the proportion of child psychiatrists, but also to the organisation of departments and services, the structure of institutions and the research, training and continuing medical education which occurs within them.

3. Future perspectives

The countries which make up Europe are becoming ever closer; comparison, understanding the reasons for differences and the evaluation of disparate structures is essential. The future development of the discipline of child and adolescent psychiatry has to be responsive to the changing needs of children and families. In addition, it must nurture an environment which facilitates good quality research, as well as high quality education for trainee and qualified psychiatrists and other mental health professionals.

While the chapters in this book reflect diversity rather than a homogeneous picture, it is nevertheless hoped that some goals for the future can be drawn from the data provided in this book:

- Child and Adolescent Psychiatry must be integrated into the training curricula of medical students in every university in Europe. In order to achieve this, every medical faculty should establish a department for Child and Adolescent Psychiatry.
- The training curricula for specialists in Child and Adolescent Psychiatry in Europe should be harmonized, giving trainees the opportunity to work in different countries and to exchange knowledge, as well as ideas. Within the European Union, the section of Child and Adolescent Psychiatry of the UEMS, as well as the ESCAP board, have taken the first steps in this direction. In the future, other European countries should be included in this process.
- In comparison to other specialties, research in child and adolescent psychiatric disorders and child mental health in general has not been well supported or encouraged within Europe. The 5th framework of the BIOMED program of the European Union does not contain child mental health as a major area. It is, therefore, vital that attempts be urgently made to bring these issues to the attention of the responsible bodies within Europe.
- The structure and organization of services should be based on empirical grounds, using epidemiological data and modern methods of treatment evaluation and quality assurance.
- Finally, the scientific communication within Europe should be facilitated by improving intra- and interdisciplinary communication. This can be achieved by means of scientific journals, European and international meetings and the setting up of a network of clinical studies, supported by countries both in- and outside the European Union.

In order to achieve these goals, a considerable joint effort will be required by all countries. The work involved will, however, be worthwhile, resulting not only in a good future for the discipline of Child and Adolescent Psychiatry, but also for the children and families whom we are trying to help.

Child and adolescent psychiatry in Austria

M. H. Friedrich

1. Definition, historical development, and current situation

Definition

Child and adolescent neuropsychiatry is the medical discipline which deals with all types of neurological and psychiatric phenomena, defects and variants, as well as those pertaining to biology-related development and constitution.

Historical development

Theodor Heller, whose description of "infantile dementia" which later became known as "Heller's syndrome", and was referred to as such in medical literature, started off as a teacher in Vienna. After having begun his investigations there, he continued this work at the medical pedagogic society in Munich.

The first department for medical pedagogy was established by the Nobelist, Pirquet, in 1911 at the Vienna General Hospital. He entrusted Lazar, who was open to psychoanalytic ideas and the notion of individual psychology, with the task of organizing the department. After World War I, medical pedagogy constituted a wide field of activity, so much so that after World War II a major discussion ensued as to why the pediatric clinic had a ward for medical pedagogy to deal with children suffering from nervous or psychological disorders, whereas the psychiatric clinic lacked a department of this nature. Pirquet and Wagner von Jauregg had talked about establishing a facility for treating young patients beyond the age of 14 or 15; and after World War II members of the psychiatric-neurological university clinic dealt intensively with questions relating to child psychiatry.

Austria was one of the founding members of the "World Federation of Mental Health" which was founded in 1948 in London. It was then that a concrete discussion of child psychiatric problems, with a view towards Europe as a whole, began. Associations for psychoanalysis and individual psychology had already established child guidance clinics in Vienna before World War II. They were reopened after 1945, after having been closed during the war. A typically American kind of "child guidance" movement also came into being after the war, and outpatient clinics were established. A synopsis of depth psychology, psychotherapy, and pedagogy, which had been tentative, was now realized.

In 1950/51 Hans Hoff took over as head of the psychiatric-neurological university clinic in Vienna and established a separate ward for children and adolescents.

It was opened in 1951, and in 1953 the ward became an independent department, of which the neuropsychiatrist, Walter Spiel, became the chairman. From the very start the newly created department offered school instruction and supervision. Between 1953 and 1974, the pediatric department expanded several times. Ultimately it consisted of 18 beds, a large garden, and auxiliary wards for ergotherapy and work therapy. And from 1956 on, a teacher provided instruction on a regular basis. As early as 1953 Walter Spiel, the department chairman, had already established close contact with top European child and adolescent psychiatrists. That same year the first international congress for psychic hygiene was held in Vienna. It served as an important impetus for further activities in the field. Austrian doctors were given the opportunity to pursue post-graduate studies in the United States, thanks to Rockefeller Foundation grants. As a result, the "Magglinger Group", which consisted of European child psychiatrists, came into being. The members met regularly for intensive discussions of developments in the field in an informal setting, without a formal program.

In 1958 the "International Congress for Mental Health" was held in Vienna. The main emphasis was on questions concerning refugee children in the aftermath of the Hungarian revolution which had taken place in 1956.

In 1960 the President of the United States invited Austrian child psychiatrists to attend the "Chichester Seminar", which dealt with legal, political, and scientific findings in conjunction with questions concerning children and adolescents.

From 1961 on, the field of child psychiatry became more and more established. Spiel received tenure in "psychiatry and neurology", with special emphasis on child and adolescent neuropsychiatry, the number of students in the field increased from 60 to 300, and in 1964 the university created a chair for child and adolescent psychiatry. At that time an agreement was reached between the medical pedagogy ward of the pediatric university clinic and the pediatric ward of the neuropsychiatric university clinic to work together closely. As a result, plans for a new university clinic were approved in 1967; construction began in 1971. On December 5, 1972 Walter Spiel was named professor and chairman of the department of child and adolescent neuropsychiatry. In 1974 the department moved to a new building, and in 1975 the University Clinic for Child and Adolescent Neuropsychiatry was formally inaugurated. The previous number of beds was increased from 18 to 32; this number has remained constant to this date.

The new clinic was divided into two wards with 16 beds each; there were also two outpatient facilities: one general, and one for epilepsy patients. In the course of further expansion the two wards with 16 beds each remained; the outpatient facilities were enlarged more and more, and no longer consisted solely of the two mentioned above. Instead, there was an outpatient facility for muscle disorders, one for neuropsychology, and one for testing. During this period the psychological segment of the clinic, which had always been a principle, multi-professional element right from the beginning, continued being expanded.

The structure of the department for child and adolescent neuropsychiatry in Vienna is based on a close interrelationship of psychiatry and neurology, a tightly-woven psychosocial network, and psychotherapeutic polypragmasy. There had already been a long tradition of linking neurology and psychiatry in treating adult patients when this model was applied to children and adolescents, as well. The creation of a psychosocial network was a matter of course; here was a confluence of many elements: medical pedagogy, social-psychiatric directions, the psychohygienic movement, the child guidance movement, and the classic university structure for medicine.

It was no wonder that Walter Spiel, the founder of child and adolescent neuropsychiatry in Vienna, especially furthered the interaction of the various individual schools of psychotherapy. He had learned therapeutic tolerance from his father, Oskar Spiel. It was especially during World War II that psychoanalysts and individual psychologists met at the Spiel home for discussions, thereby keeping important intellectual property alive.

Walter Spiel headed the clinic until his retirement in 1991, at which time he received emeritus status. The chair remained vacant until December 1, 1996 when Max H. Friedrich was appointed as head of the one and only university clinic for child and adolescent neuropsychiatry in Austria. In this new position Max H. Friedrich expanded on and redefined Walter Spiel's basic concepts:

- The holistic concept of child and adolescent neuropsychiatry according to somatic, intellectual, emotional, and social aspects was further expanded.
- The idea of a multi-professional network was adopted as a whole, and now encompasses 10 different professions within the framework of child and adolescent neuropsychiatry. In addition to doctors and psychologists, there are nurses, guidance counselors, social workers, ergotherapists, physiotherapists, speech therapists, special kindergarden instructors, teachers, and technical assistants.
- Since the social network is of vital importance, top priority was given to existing social contacts to the youth welfare service, schools and school psychologists, juvenile courts, and all private and public establishments concerned with youth welfare.
- The psychotherapeutic polypragmasy which Spiel had introduced became more extensive. In this manner psychoanalysis, depth psychology, group therapy, behavior therapy, music therapy, and family therapy are all linked together.

In Vienna there is, in addition to the university clinic for child and adolescent neuropsychiatry, a medical pedagogy ward which is integrated into the university pediatric clinic. The ward is run by a pediatric neuropsychiatrist. There is also a municipal pediatric neurological department which includes rehabilitation and child psychiatry. The head of this facility is also a child and adolescent neuropsychiatrist. Due to the Austrian structure with regard to child and adolescent neuropsychiatry, the head of a pediatric psychosomatic department is a pediatrician. This is the case because training in Austria consists first and foremost of training in various specialties, in series. To become a child and adolescent neuropsychiatrist the candidate must first have completed his/her training as a psychiatrist, a neurologist or as a pediatrician, after which three years of training in the field of child and adolescent neuropsychiatry is mandatory.

The Austrian structure outside of Vienna varies significantly. In most provinces, except for Carinthia, children who are psychiatric patients are mostly placed in pediatric facilities, whereas adolescent psychiatric patients are placed in the respective psychiatric departments.

The international role of Austrian child psychiatry can be documented as follows:

- At the 1971 UEP congress in Stockholm, W. Spiel was designated president of the European Union for Child Psychiatry. Poustka was named congress secretary, and Friedrich treasurer.
- In 1975 the European Child Psychiatry Congress, the topic of which was "Psychotherapy in the Field of Child Psychiatry", took place in Vienna. Friedrich became vice-president and held this position until 1991. From 1983 to 1991 he was board secretary of ESCAP.
- Spiel, Friedrich, and Berger were also members of the Colloquium Pedopsychiatricum and in 1980 organized one of the regular meetings which was held in Vienna.
- The Austro-German Child Psychiatry Congress took place in Salzburg in 1978 and in Feldkirch in 1984. On these occasions the close connection and cooperation between these two countries was clearly documented.
- Poustka, an Austrian, now holds the chair in Frankfurt, and Resch the one in Heidelberg. Friedrich was offered the chair in Hamburg which he declined. Georg Spiel was the temporary chairman of the department of child psychiatry in Berlin.

Current situation

Austria has a population of 7.87 million, of which 24.4% are children and adolescents between the age of 0 and 19.

According to a study conducted by experts in the field (psychiatrists, pediatricians, and child and adolescent neuropsychiatrists), there are 40,000 new child psychiatric cases per year.

In Austria there are 65 registered child and adolescent neuropsychiatrists, plus approximately 40 trainees.

2. Classification systems, diagnostic and therapeutic methods

Classification systems

The university clinic for child and adolescent neuropsychiatry in Vienna uses the ICD-9/ICD-10 classification system, as well as a system developed at the clinic in 1988 whereby the case history, the psychopathological status, and the neurological status are considered equally in determining the current and dynamic situation.

Diagnostic methods

The psychopathological criteria developed by Berger, Friedrich, and Schuch, as well as Scharfetter are applied in child psychiatric diagnoses, as are the ICD-9 and DSM-IV classifications.

Therapeutic methods

Austrian child psychotherapists use many different methods of therapy, including Walter Spiel's "key-lock paradigm"; all of them are individually adapted for the respective patient. In this manner, each child receives the optimal type of therapy in treating its illness. The methods applied include psychoanalytic depth psychology, individual psychology, group therapy, family therapy, and cognitive methods. Music therapy, as well as specific and pragmatic methods such as autogenic training, concentrated kinetotherapy, and Jakobsonian relaxation therapy are also used.

3. Structure and organization of services

Guidelines for services for children and adolescents with psychiatric disorders

Within the framework of the Austrian system of public hospitals, there is a university clinic for child and adolescent neuropsychiatry at the university hospital in Vienna. In Innsbruck and Graz, there are child psychiatric departments at the psychiatric university clinic and at the pediatric university clinic.

In Vienna and Klagenfurt, there are separate departments for child and adolescent psychiatry at provincial hospitals. In all other provincial capitals, child and adolescent psychiatry is integrated into either psychiatric or pediatric university clinics.

Types of services

All clinics for child and adolescent neuropsychiatry in Austria have general outpatient facilities. University clinics have additional special facilities for outpatients.

Since child and adolescent neuropsychiatry is a specialization in addition to psychiatry, neurology or pediatry, close cooperation with the respective parent disciplines is a matter of course.

Throughout the country there are various types of child guidance oriented care available through child psychiatric consultants within the framework of the youth welfare system and the school system, or, as the case in Vienna, on an independent basis.

Outpatient services

In the entire country only an extremely small percentage of outpatient care is in the hands of child psychiatrists in private practice. In Vienna there are only two child psychiatrists in private practice; both of them are registered as pediatricians within the national health insurance system. All other patients make use of public facilities.

Daypatient services

At present there are no daypatient services, since the national health insurance providers have not entered into any contracts of this nature. Especially the three university hospitals are working hard at establishing daypatient facilities.

Inpatient services

A total of 350 beds are available for patients in the area of child and adolescent neuropsychiatry in Austria. The structure regarding patients is not at all homogenous; there are neurologic, pediatric, neurologic-psychiatric, psychosomatic, slightly handicapped, and severely handicapped patients. For this reason, it is impossible to establish a key by means of which the number of beds needed per number of inhabitants can be calculated.

Complementary services and rehabilitation

The public system of youth welfare, private homes such as "SOS Kinderdorf" which have their own psychological observation wards with psychological consultants, and group homes with counselors and psychiatric consultants are closely linked together. Even though the network functions adequately, there is room for improvement.

There are very few rehabilitation centers for chronic psychiatric patients run by the individual provinces themselves.

Personnel

In general, there has been a lack of child and adolescent neuropsychiatric services in Austria. The new psychotherapy law, which was passed in 1991, and the services provided by psychotherapists are now making up for the demand.

Funding of services

In Austria, the national health insurance system pays for inpatient and outpatient care in full, if it is provided at a public hospital or other facility. If the patient goes to a psychiatrist in private practice, approximately 33 % of the fee is refunded. Simple medical diagnostic and pharmaceutical therapy is covered in full by insurance.

Long-term institutionalization is paid for within the youth welfare system, or by the parents.

Evaluation

In 1997/98 a system for evaluating all medical services provided by hospitals throughout Austria was implemented. The results of this evaluation in the area of child and adolescent neuropsychiatry are not yet available.

4. Cooperation with medical and non-medical disciplines

Thanks to the Austrian structure, psychology, neurology, and pediatrics are closely linked together as the parent disciplines of child and adolescent neuropsychology. There is even greater cooperation between clinical psychologists and clinical therapists, who work together as consultants.

5. Graduate/postgraduate training and continuing medical education

Graduate training: The role of medical faculties

The Austrian Society for Child and Adolescent Neuropsychiatry is currently in the process of creating a logbook for child and adolescent psychiatrists, in order to develop a standardized training program to be based on the main specializations and sub-disciplines in the book. The UEMS guidelines are also being taken into consideration.

An examination for a specialization in child and adolescent neuropsychiatry is not being planned, since this discipline is currently only an addition to existing specializations.

Postgraduate training, a joint effort

In addition to the basic specialization in psychiatry, neurology or pediatrics (6 years), additional specialization in child and adolescent neuropsychiatry takes two years, for pediatrics one year of psychiatry, and for psychiatry and neurology one year of pediatrics.

Continuing medical education in child and adolescent psychiatry and psychotherapy

Similar to the situation in Germany, continuing medical education is necessary, but not obligatory.

Training programs for other disciplines

Child and adolescent psychiatrists and psychotherapists work together with pediatricians, special pedagogues, medical pedagogues, teachers, nurses, and social pedagogues at seminars which are held on a regular basis.

6. Research

Research fields and strategies

Research in the field of child and adolescent psychiatry in Austria is conducted primarily in one of the following areas:

- Psychoses
- Eating disorders
- Epilepsy
- Headaches

In 1996 these four areas were established as the primary focus of research within the framework of the University Clinic for Child and Adolescent Neuropsychiatry in Vienna. This does not mean that research in other areas may not be conducted; however, because financial resources have been drastically reduced, a concentration on these areas has become necessary.

Individual special outpatient departments at the university clinic, as well as research facilities throughout Austria, have conducted research in special fields, in addition to the main areas of research listed above. This includes research in the following fields:

- Forensic child and adolescent psychiatry,
- ADHD syndrome,
- Neurological rehabilitation, including psychosocial areas,
- Psychopharmacology, and
- Social pediatrics.

Research training and career development

For this purpose young colleagues are sent to various European countries, in order to receive training and to take part in courses.

A number of Austrian colleagues participate regularly in exchange programs, with EU countries and the U.S.A. This will continue to be a focal point in the future.

Funding

The scope of Austrian research supported by the Foundation for Scientific Research is very limited. As a result, only epilepsy research is being funded on a larger scale. All other special areas of research are currently supported by very minimal funding.

7. Future perspectives

At present, the prospects for future innovations look very dim. In the next few years there will have to be structural analyses in order to find out why it is particularly the child and adolescent neuropsychiatric system in Austria which is so starved financially if it does not produce sensationalist results.

Research

In a small country, the future demands that research concentrates on focal points. One of these is continuing research on child and adolescent psychoses, as well as forensic psychiatry which is applied particularly in psychosocial innovations throughout the EU, as well as in Austria. Scientific research on anorexia nervosa and bulimia is interconnected throughout Austria, and there is a lively discussion concerning drug research. The University of Vienna is taking the initiative as an international research center and plans to create a link between medicine and other disciplines at the university.

Child and adolescent psychiatry in Belgium

J.-P. Matot, B. Verbeeck, J.-Y. Hayez

1. Definition, historical development, and current situation

Definition

It seems to us impossible to describe correctly the child and adolescent psychiatry organization without placing it in a much larger context: that of child and adolescent mental health. The latter includes professionals and institutions involved in education, social work, and law. Our description starts from the "hard core" of professionals and institutions whose mission is to diagnose and to treat psychopathological disorders among children and adolescents, but their mission is then extended to sectors in which diagnosis and treatment are of secondary importance for the benefit of other missions, such as educational, protectional, and/or legal ones.

One of Belgium's peculiarities is its threefold government: federal, communitary, and regional, and this has a considerable impact on psychiatry. The federal government remains the competent authority in regard to most matters of health, including hospital standardization and subsidizing, establishing a list of medical activities which are refunded by the social security organization (INAMI).

On the other hand, the three regions (Flanders, Wallonia and Brussels) are the competent authorities in matters that can be "personalised": so much so that mental health services are dependent on the regions for approval and for subsidizing. Finally, education and youth assistance are within the competence of the three communities (Flemish, which includes Flanders and the Flemish-speaking people of Brussels; Francophone, including Wallonia and the French-speaking people of Brussels; and the small German-speaking community in part of Wallonia).

Belgium's health care system has managed to reconcile independent practice and public institutions, as well as to make them complementary with regard to child and adolescent psychiatry; the "hard core" consists of an ambulatory network for diagnosis and care, including, on the one hand, independent child and adolescent psychiatrists and psychologists, and the mental health services on the other hand. Full-time or part-time residential structures complete this network, but there are very few of them compared to other European countries.

Historical development

Child and adolescent psychiatry in Belgium started in 1923 when the first mental health community clinics were set up under the aegis of the Belgian National

Mental Health League. At that time, the philosophy of these community clinics was to care for mentally ill people outside asylums, and they organized educational sections intended mainly for mentally retarded children. The first period of child and adolescent psychiatry, strongly influenced by the works of Piaget, was essentially geared toward the study and the evaluation of intelligence. Thus, taking care of learning problems at school and of mental retardation became the core of early pedopsychiatry, at least until World War II, and even until the early 1950s. In 1936, Doctor Dellaert founded in Antwerp an ambulatory medico-psychological service for children.

After World War II, there appeared a broadening of discipline toward other pathologies. The term "child psychiatry" first appeared in 1945, and it referred to the clinical activities of the first "medico-pedagogic" teams.

As early as 1946, through the impetus given by Doctor Jadot-Decroly, there was a new trend in the hospitals of Brussels Free University aiming at individualizing the psychological care of children. As a result, the first out-patient unit of child and adolescent psychiatry was opened in 1948 in the pediatrics department of Professor Robert Dubois in the University Hospital of Saint-Pierre in Brussels. That same year, a child mental health section was set up by Doctor Callewaert in the community clinic of the Mental Health League, and, a year later, a section for adolescents was added. Five years later, in 1954, an "out-patient unit for nervous children" was set up by Doctor Nicole Dopchie in the psychiatric department of Professor Nyssen at the University Hospital Brugmann. And so, from the start, the question arose as to whether pedopsychiatry was part of pediatrics or of psychiatry. In 1963, Doctor Dopchie was appointed head of the pedopsychiatric unit in the pediatrics department of the University Hospital Saint-Pierre.

The influence of psychoanalysis became more and more obvious in the pedopsychiatric clinic (the Belgian Society of Psychoanalysis was founded in 1946). It received even more momentum with Doctor Danielle Flagey who introduced, in Belgium, the psychoanalytic approach to children's and adolescents' treatment in a clinical perspective inspired from the one at the Paris school of child psychoanalysis, led by Serge Lebovici and René Diatkine.

At the same time, the Piaget tradition was maintained, and a clinic of mental retardation was set up by Doctor Portray in the pediatrics department of Professor Dubois.

In 1957, the Catholic University of Louvain took on Professor Pierre Fontaine as pedopsychiatrist in the pediatrics department of Professor Denys. In 1960, Doctor Fontaine opened an out-patient pedopsychiatric unit in the psychopathology department of Saint-Pierre Hospital in Leuven (Professor Rouvroy), and he himself took part in the training of assistants.

Also in 1960, the first units of residential observation and treatment were founded in Brugge and in Gent. At the same time, steps were taken in Antwerp, Kortrijk, and Leuven toward the recognition and the establishment of child and adolescent psychiatric clinics for children and adolescents, both within psychiatric and general hospitals, in order to achieve missions of diagnosis, observation, and treatment.

As early as before World War II, Professor Dellaert was teaching "De psychologie van het afwijkende kind" ("The psychology of the delinquent child") at the Catholic

University of Louvain. In 1943, professor of psychiatry Nyssen, from Gent, was the first to publish, in Flanders, a textbook called "Leerboek der psychiatrie en Heilopvoedkundige behandeling" ("Handbook of psychiatry and its application in health education"). The first specific teaching of child psychopathology took place in 1954 in the nurses' college of the Brugmann Hospital with Doctor Nicole Dopchie as lecturer. However, it was not until 1963 that a lectureship of child and adolescent psychiatry was organized at the Free University of Brussels, in the faculties of medicine and of psychology, within the framework of Professor Paul Sivadon's chair of psychiatry. The first to be in charge was Professor Nicole Dopchie, and in 1968, the lectureship became autonomous when a chair of child and adolescent psychiatry was set up at the Free University of Brussels (ULB). At the Catholic University of Louvain, a chair of child psychiatry was created in 1966 in the faculty of psychology. A set of courses in psychopathology and in children's therapy and rehabilitation were part of this chair which was first held by Professor Pierre Fontaine. In 1972, the latter introduced family therapy and systemic thinking in the university with the help of the psychologists Edith Tilmans and Bella Borwick.

At the University of Liège, on the other hand, the teaching of child and adolescent psychiatry did not gain autonomy, vis-à-vis of adult psychiatry, and this slowed down the introduction of this discipline in the region.

In fact, the development of child and adolescent psychiatry teaching at the university in the faculties of medicine and psychology was a deciding factor contributing to the expansion of the clinical field, in hospitals with pediatric services, and in specific hospitals, also in the community clinics of mental health which organized multidisciplinary teams for children and adolescents, as well as in independent practices.

There is a substantial limitation, however, due to the restricted criteria which govern the recognition of the services where future psychiatrists are able to complete their training.

These criteria include the need to have a definite number of hospital beds, a condition which is obviously not fulfilled by a large majority of child and adolescent psychiatric services.

Recent advances: Scientific and professional societies

The "Société Belge de Psychiatrie Infantile et des Disciplines Connexes – Belgische Vereniging voor Kinderpsychiatrie en verwante disciplines" was founded in 1961. It was dissolved in 1974 and replaced by two separate societies, one French-speaking, the other Flemish-speaking, but grouped together within the Belgian Federation of Regional Societies of Child Psychiatry. The two regional societies evolved in different ways: the French-speaking society maintained a purely scientific approach which called for the foundation of a professional association of French-speaking pedopsychiatrists (APPF) (Association Professionnelle des Pédopsychiatres Francophones) in 1976, while the Flemish Society favored both scientific progress and professional support.

The French-speaking society became, in 1997, the "Société Belge Francophone de Psychiatrie de l'Enfant et de l'Adolescent et des Disciplines Associées". It is a member of the European Society of Child and Adolescent Psychiatry (ESCAP) and at the moment, it has more than two hundred members, approximately a third of whom are psychiatrists and pedopsychiatrists. It is headed by a board of ten members who are elected at the general assembly for a period of two years, and they can be re-elected twice. Every year, it organizes several thematic seminars, and it publishes an internal bulletin twice a year.

The "Association Professionnelle des Pédopsychiatres Francophones", whose aim is to promote a child and adolescent psychiatry of quality, publishes a bimonthly internal bulletin. It is managed by a board whose members are elected at the general assembly. Specific documents are worked out by commissions, in particular on matters relating to the organization of action plans for prevention and care, or concerning child and adolescent psychiatric qualification.

Current situation

Since child and adolescent psychiatry is not administratively recognized in Belgium as a specialization, it is difficult to estimate the precise number of psychiatrists who have had adequate training and experience in treating children and adolescents. It is just possible to estimate their number through membership of professional and scientific associations: there are about 150 practitioners in French speaking Belgium, many of whom, however, practice child and adolescent psychiatry only part-time. As a general rule, these practitioners have attended, on average, a two or three year period of training – part-time or full-time – and of supervision in the hospital or ambulatory services of child and adolescent psychiatry during their five-year psychiatric training (one year is given to neurology or to neuro-pediatrics, and another one to adult psychiatry). Depending on the university, the study of child and adolescent psychiatry is either integrated into general psychiatry or organized separately.

The majority of French speaking child and adolescent psychiatrists have also had a psychotherapy training, mostly psychoanalytic and/or systemic, and sometimes, though rarely, rogerian or cognitive-behavioral. These types of psychotherapy training are offered by private institutions or by the universities. The number of child and adolescent psychiatrists is insufficient in Belgium. A study done by the Confederation of Mental Health Leagues estimated that, as far as the French speaking community of Belgium is concerned, a little more than 125 full-time pedopsychiatrists would be needed in order to attain the number of staff legally required in the existing ambulatory and residential institutions.

This situation will probably get worse, due to the introduction, beginning in 2004, of a numerus clausus limiting the access to medical practice and, therefore, the number of specialists.

The shortage of child and adolescent psychiatrists is worsened by the uneven geographical distribution, with a larger number of specialists practising in the big cities, particularly in Brussels, to the detriment of provincial towns and rural areas.

2. Classification systems, diagnostic and therapeutic methods

Classification systems

Classifications such as ICD 10 and especially DSM IV are not used much by clinicians in French-speaking Belgium, but more so in the Flemish-speaking region. These are indeed distant from the type of reference in French-speaking child and adolescent psychiatry, the latter being based on an understanding of the structures which underly the mental functioning of the child and of his family, referring to systemic and psychoanalytic theories. Moreover, these classifications are quite incomplete as far as the description of some pathologies is concerned, such as pre- and para-psychoses in children. As a result, a certain number of French-speaking services prefer to use the French Classification of Child and Adolescent Mental Disorders (Misès et al. 1988). However, its ponderousness prevents it from being widely used. Thus, all these international classifications are not widely used in the majority of departments, with the exception of a few residential units, and this is due to the fact that for professionals there are too many administrative constraints that are time-consuming and produce too few clinical results.

The use of the DSM IV classification is, in fact, essential only in matters relating to some articles in English speaking scientific journals. On the other hand, the DCO-3 classification, which has been assessed since 1995 in the USA and in several European countries, seems to be quite useful in helping infant clinicians make a proper diagnosis. This makes it possible to have the authorities acknowledge and recognize the specificity of such a clinic and to further its development.

Diagnostic methods

Clinic diagnoses receive many benefits from practising psychological examinations: these allow one to refine the understanding of both intellectual and instrumental disorders (relying on the tests and studies achieved by the Piaget school) as well as emotional disorders (through projective tests) and to analyze their interactions as well as to determine therapy indications. The logopedic and psychomotor evaluations are useful complements to establish the diagnosis.

The differential diagnosis of neuropediatric disorders resorts to the whole range of medical specific examination, biological and electrophysiological explorations, and to medical imaging. The examination of an infant is done with the help of the Bailey test, whereas the assessment of the abilities of the baby relies on the Brazelton scale.

Therapeutic methods

In Wallonia and Brussels, the therapy approach is often based on a psychoanalytic understanding of the child's mental functioning, taking into account the systemic dimension of family relationships. In Flanders, however, having recourse to cognitive-behavioral patterns is more frequent for diagnosis as well as for treatment. Prescribing medication is not common in Wallonia and Brussels, except in the case of some specific indications, but it is far more widespread in Flanders.

In the French-speaking community, on the other hand, careful attention is given to the institutional setting within which the methods of treating children, adolescents and the family are to be implemented. Here, the emphasis is put on flexibility and adapting the therapy to the needs of both children and parents, rather than applying rigidly any preconceived therapy program. In fact, a provisional therapy plan of action must be defined in such a way that it is shared by the child (or the adolescent), the family, and the therapist; to try and impose upon the child and the family an a priori specific treatment would be wrong and useless.

Generally speaking, the trend is to sufficiently extend the period of diagnostic investigation and to analyze thoroughly both the child and the family, so as to include an important therapy dimension. This allows one to limit the indications for individual psychotherapies for the child or the adolescent to the ones that are most likely to come to a favorable conclusion.

Another important aspect of present therapy concepts concerns the organization of cooperation within the network of professionals and institutions; this is essential particularly in the cases of heavily disturbed children and of disorganized or chaotic families.

3. Structure and organization of services

Outpatient services: Mental Health Centers

These services were officially introduced in 1975 and are made up of multidisciplinary teams which include, for a basic team of general psychiatry, at least one full-time (38 hours per week) psychiatrist, psychologist, social worker, and secretary. Some division into sectors has been foreseen under certain conditions of approval insofar as these services have to cover geographical areas of about 50,000 inhabitants. However, this sectorization is quite flexible: it is seen as a responsibility toward the needs of the population, making sure that these are answered in the best possible way, rather than an obligation on behalf of the inhabitants to consult one particular service and not another one.

These services are coordinated by the Leagues of Mental Health, one in Brussels, the other in Wallonia. They were introduced by the government as a main opportunity of action diagnosis and treatment but also for the prevention of mental health diseases. It must be said, however, that their limited number as well as staff shortages have caused this ambitious project to be hardly practicable.

This is even more true as far as child and adolescent treatment is concerned; the legislators, both in the initial Royal Order of 1975 and in the 1995 Decree, which defines the approval criteria of mental health services, did not anticipate that each SSM (Mental Health Service) would need at its disposal a specialized team for children and adolescents as well as a basic team of adult psychiatry.

At the moment, only a minority of the services in Wallonia and Brussels have such a specialized team at their disposal. It must be added that the minimum statutory number of staff in these specialized teams is less than that of adult psychiatry teams: it is reduced to a half-time psychiatrist for children and adolescents and to a three-quarter time social worker and psychologist.

In Flanders, mental health services are about to undergo a major restructuration: it includes regrouping, in function of approximately 20 geographical areas, more than 86 centers spread over the five Flemish provinces and coordinating the various functions of diagnosing and of treating within these areas. With regard to child and adolescent psychiatry, at present only 16 centers out of 86 have a full multidisciplinary team for children and adolescents, whereas others manage to organize consultations without a full specialized team at hand.

Hospital teams

Child and adolescent psychiatry is the "poor relative" of Belgian hospitals. It is practically non-existent outside university hospitals and, even there, it has very limited means at its disposal. It is essentially geared toward ambulatory treatment and, usually, its existence is closely linked to that of pediatrics.

Most of the time it is integrated into a general psychiatric service, sometimes, but rarely, into a pediatric service, and it has only a limited autonomy.

Its mission is twofold: to provide consultations for external patients and to organize "liaison" activities, i.e., diagnosis, treatment, and even prevention for inpatients in the various units of the hospital. The latter type of consultation, the most specific one, poses enormous administrative and financial problems; since such consultations are not sufficiently refunded by the social security, "liaison" child and adolescent psychiatry has proven even less profitable than adult psychiatry in hospital institutions, which in turn has slowed its development.

In Brussels, eight hospitals, of which three academic hospitals and three university hospitals, out of a total of about twenty hospital institutions, benefit from a child and adolescent psychiatric consultation. Furthermore, the actual availability of child and adolescent psychiatrists for outpatient and liaison consultation in these hospitals – all together – does not exceed 5 to 6 full-time positions. The situation is even worse in hospitals situated in provincial towns.

S.O.S. children-parents teams

These centers have to deal with physical and sexual abuse, as well as with neglect within families. Unlike mental health services, these teams are governed by the communities. On the French speaking side, they were introduced in 1985 by a Decree of the French-speaking Community of Belgium, later revised in 1998, so as to offer specific services such as diagnosis, indications, and follow-up of therapy measures aiming, among other things, at minimizing the interference of the courts in such problems. The teams were first subsidized and coordinated solely by the "Office de la Naissance et de l'Enfance (ONE)" (Birth and Child Office), but now the

Ministry of Social Affairs of the French-speaking tries to increase his direct control in the field.

The S.O.S. Children-parents teams are multidisciplinary ambulatory teams, usually but not necessarily coordinated by a child and adolescent psychiatrist. Some of the teams work in close collaboration with hospitals owning an emergency service as well as pediatric and psychiatric hospitalization, which appears to be an effective solution to the problems arising frequently from situations of crisis and emergency.

Since the teams were set up, there has been a substantial increase in the number of reportings and of situations where intervention was required, and this poses a real problem insofar as no optimal therapy follow-up can be guaranteed for all cases.

As a result, it becomes increasingly obvious that the S.O.S. children-parents teams should be seen as the core of a wider plan of action: in order to attend their missions, they should provide assistance, training, and support to non-specialized professionals, make diagnoses and set up the framework for therapy and/or protection; they should therefore have a qualified and well-trained staff who could enjoy good working conditions (for instance training and supervision); on the other hand, effective medium-term follow-ups of children and families will have to be done through a kind of relay which should preferably be provided by the mental health services, working closely with these S.O.S. teams.

Centers of functional rehabilitation (Centres de Réadaptation Fonctionnelle – CRF)

by: André Denis

The CRF are among the oldest therapy structures of ambulatory psychiatry. These were set up about half a century ago. At the beginning they concentrated on acquired handicaps linked to organic pathologies; however, since then they extended their skills, as time went by, toward adult congenital handicaps and, later, toward complex pathologies with medical, psychological, and social determining factors, coupled with some kind of disability with regard to social and/or professional integration. Thus, they are all defined according to the kind of therapy responsibility they take for handicaps and for polyhandicaps. However, CRF professionals who are on the borderline of medical and mental health areas find it difficult to have their clinical activities coincide with a strictly medical concept which covers only partially the needs of patients taken care of.

Working exclusively within their boundaries, the CRF are able to view, in a most direct approach, the patient's problems of integration and of adaptation. The teams that make up CRF, contrary to those of the mental health services, include more rehabilitation specialists (physiotherapists, psychomotor specialists, occupational therapists, nurses, social workers) than psychologists and psychiatrists.

Their therapy techniques are part of the mediation therapies but do not exclude more specific psychotherapy approaches. Their work must comply with the rule of grading: care is provided only if a prior request has been made, and it is granted for a limited period only, usually one year, but it may be renewed.

Subsidizing depends on two authorities:

- The Wallonia Agency for the Integration of Handicapped People ("Agence Wallone pour l'Intégration des Personnes Handicapées", AWIPH) takes a part of the operating costs,
- whereas the treatment of each patient taken care of is subsidized by the National Institute of Illness and Disability Insurance ("Institut National d'Assurance contre la Maladie et l'Invalidité – INAMI"), covering also some of the operating costs.

Daypatient services

Day beds in child and adolescent psychiatry

The 1976 hospitals programming set the number of day beds in child and adolescent psychiatric departments as being 0.32 per 1000 children and adolescents, i.e., about 800 day beds for all of Belgium, or, per region, 70 day beds in Brussels, 450 in Flanders, and 270 in Wallonia.

French-speaking Belgium is poorly equipped with day therapy structures for both children and adolescents. Moreover, forty percent or so of the available day beds are mostly occupied by autistic disorders.

INAMI agreements

As far as part-time residential medical care is concerned, there are few INAMI agreements and they have hardly helped developing original methods of treatment.

At the moment, some overtures seem to be taking place concerning young children, with the recent approval to have 15 day beds set up in Brussels for children showing early development disorders, combining therapy at home and a part-time stay at a day center.

Inpatient services

Beds in child and adolescent psychiatry

The 1976 hospitals organization indicated that the number of day and night beds in child and adolescent psychiatry should be 0.32 per 1000 children and adolescents (Royal Decree of 3/8/76). If we are to limit the age of adolescents to 19, this represents about 800 beds for all of Belgium, or, per region, 70 beds in Brussels, 450 in Flanders and 270 in Wallonia.

The Royal Decree of 29/3/77 mentioned furthermore that these beds, "intended for young patients requiring either urgent intervention in cases of crises, or observation or active treatment", should be organized in functional units of 6 to 10 patients; moreover, children had to be separated from adolescents. It was also specified that a functional and close link should be established with a service of pediatrics or of internal medicine, of adult psychiatry, with the mental health services, and with the institutions for handicapped people, and this cooperation should be agreed upon on paper. When this program was put into practice, it did, however, not bring about a coherent mental health network. In the Brussels region, practically all beds (60/70) are intended for adolescents with the exception of 10 beds which accommodate children from the age of three or four and adolescents for long-term treatment of psychoses. On the other hand, a certain number of beds intended for adolescents are occupied by young people aged 18 to 25 and whose problems are more of a post-adolescent nature, while there is not a single hospital unit for assessing diagnoses and for treating crises among children below the age of 13.

In the five Flemish provinces, there are 328 beds shared by 9 services; among these beds, 219 are in psychiatric hospitals and 109 in general hospitals. Two services, in Antwerp and in Leuven, have a university training function. Furthermore, only these two benefit from an interdisciplinary child and adolescent policlinic. A school of special education is annexed to these clinics. One service can accommodate 8 babies (maximum age: 12 months) with their mothers.

Beds in pediatrics

The absence of psychiatric hospitalization units for children tends to be compensated, despite important functional limitations, by the use of beds in pediatrics ; we take also advantage of the pedopsychiatric liaison activities in order to hospitalize children below the age of 13 who show acute psychiatric disorders. The advantage of this formula is to make such hospitalizations rather "common", but its limits are obvious: some children, whose symptoms proves too "noisy", cannot benefit from it, although precisely in such cases the hospitalization has the most value. The teams in charge of care do not receive specialized training to handle difficult cases; the various types of medical care, which is exclusively organized in function of somatic treatment, are ill-adapted to the needs of these young patients. In difficult situations, conflicts of competence and of responsibility arise between pediatricians and child and adolescent psychiatrists.

INAMI conventions

The "Institut National d'Assurance contre la Maladie et l'Invalidité – INAMI" (National Institute of Illness and Disability Insurance), the federal health care organization, is the competent authority to approve, referring to specific criteria, various programs aiming at rehabilitating people who suffer from medical disorders, i.e., among others, children and adolescents who suffer from psychiatric disorders.

The philosophy of these approvals is to compensate for the deficiencies in existing institutions and services, so that full medical care can be provided, mainly in institutions where only part-time treatment is given. Unlike what is practised in traditional hospital beds, the INAMI agreements allow a subsidy directly linked to the reality of the activity undertaken. However, in the absence of global political projects concerning health care planning and programming, the INAMI agreements barely cover the shortage of hospital equipment for children.

Psychiatric beds for adults

Hospitalizing children below the age of thirteen in adult psychiatric units, fortunately, only happens in quite exceptional circumstances. On the other hand, it happens that some adolescents, showing pathological signs that may prove dangerous, are hospitalized in "adult" beds, due to the absence of a psychiatric hospitalization closed-in unit for adolescents. These adolescents are often transferred to psychiatric hospitals from closed-in institutions of youth welfare (IPPJ) which prove inadequate to look after violent adolescents with psychiatric disorders.

Complementary services and rehabilitation

Psycho-medico-social centers (PMS)

PMS centers ensure a detection and a guidance to children who have difficulties in adapting at school; they have no therapy mission. In actual practice, the teams at PMS centers – which do not include any pedopsychiatric function – have to face numerous cases of children, adolescents, and families in difficulties, and without having either adequate training or adequate working facilities, they insure functions of guidance to these people, which causes a problem of relay that should be implemented between PMS centers and the therapy network. The mission at "specialized" PMS centers, on the other hand, is to guide children who have been directed to special education.

Medico-pedagogic institutes (Instituts Médico-Pédagogiques – IMP)

These institutes are intended for young people under the age of 18 suffering from a mental, physical, and/or emotional handicap. Official recognition of the handicap falls within the competence of three regional organizations.

The decision to classify IMPs in the education sector comes from their administrative and, for most of them, functional organization; it is clear, however, that these structures have a dual function: education and, at the same time, treatment. Moreover, some IMPs have developed a real therapy project, which would tend to have them classified in the health sector. So the question arises as to how to define such institutions and the children they accommodate, as a function of the concept of handicap and not that of pathology. There is, at the moment, a real danger of doing away with the therapy aspect of IMPs, and this danger becomes obvious when their pedopsychiatric function is again being questioned.

Regarding psychiatric disorders, we are mainly concerned with the IMPs which accommodate children and adolescents who are "suffering from emotional problems showing a neurotic or prepsychotic condition and requiring appropriate education" (category 14) or suffering from mental deficiency (category 11). It is regrettable, however, that the other IMP categories which accommodate children suffering from sensory, neurological, and other handicaps do not benefit from pedopsychiatric training and support.

These institutions follow a system of full-boarding or semi-boarding (from 8 to 18 hours). The number of boarding and semi-boarding beds available in category 14 varies from one province to the other: from 5 boarding beds per 1000 children between the ages of 0 and 19 in the province of Namur, to 1.2 per thousand in the province of Liège (average: 2.9 ‰); from 0.16 semi-boarding per 1000 children in French-speaking Brabant or the province of Liège, to 4 beds per 1000 children in the province of Hainaut (average: 1.95 ‰). Depending on the cases, the IMPs organize a school of special education on their premises, or they cooperate with one or several schools outside their institution.

Special education

Special education has been through an important development in Belgium. It is organized according to eight types, each coinciding with the various forms of children's handicaps. With regard to the usual pedopsychiatric practice, mainly the following types are concerned: type 1 (minor mental deficiency), type 2 (medium or serious mental deficiency, type 3 (emotional disorders), and type 8 (instrumental disorders: only in primary school with special education).

Protectional and social welfare organizations

There are a large number of them. They are run by the communities but suffer from little coordination with health and education institutions. Their characteristic is that they are often concerned about quick results assessed in terms of evident behavior. We shall limit ourselves to describe the most important ones.

Ambulatory organization

An important decree in the French-speaking community of Belgium organized in 1991 a social welfare for young people in difficulties. De facto, this decree took away from the juvenile courts their competence in matters relating to social welfare intended for "underage children in danger", which they had ruled until then, and it passed it on to the youth welfare administration.

Youth adviser (Conseiller à la Jeunesse – CAJ) and youth welfare service (Service d'Aide à la Jeunesse – SAJ)

This is the most important brainchild of the decree: children, adolescents under 18, and families in a crisis or in social difficulties may go and see these services for arbitration, support, and decisions which may lead to separation, and placement in a special institution, on a voluntary basis. Also, situations where "minor youths in danger" are involved may be submitted to the adviser through a series of professionals and services, in order to try and obtain the approval of the family to organize "voluntary aid"; failing that, the adviser may transfer the case to the juvenile magistrate who will decide which measures of "constraint aid" (article 38) should be taken: it is obvious that there is some ambiguity about the term "voluntary" aid. Moreover, youths or families who are not satisfied with the services of a SAJ may put in a complaint to the juvenile court which will give a ruling in civil court (article 37 of the decree).

Ambulatory welfare teams (Equipe d'Aide en Milieu Ouvert – AMO)

They were established by an order of the French-speaking community (21/12/1989), and usually include a coordinator, a university bachelor, one or more social workers and educators, and a secretary. They are competent to take actions of prevention, either individual or communitary, of social mediation, of stimulation toward integration. Some of them have a number of emergency beds for young people, easily accessible on demand.

Residential Organization

Institutions subsidized by the youth welfare administration in the French-speaking community (Administration de l'Aide à la Jeunesse – AAJ) and by the Flemish Fund ("Vlaams Fonds") in the Flemish community

In the French-speaking community, a large majority of the institutions mentioned in this section originate from private initiatives but are approved by the youth welfare administration. They are accessible only after a decision (to be reassessed yearly) made by the youth welfare adviser or by a juvenile magistrate, either when he or she implements constraint aid, mentioned earlier, or when he or she sends young delinquents to one of these institutions.

Institutions for minor youths

They are divided into two categories: family homes, managed by a couple having educational qualifications, able to accommodate ten children at the most (including the couple's own children), and special institutions able to accommodate about 75 beds maximum. Some of these institutions get supplementary means to accommodate difficult adolescents under the "Special projects" scheme (1987 Decree of the French-speaking community).

Emergency accommodation centers (Centres d'accueil d'urgence – CAU), first accommodation centers (Centres de Premier Accueil – CPA), observation and orientation centers (Centres d'observation et d'orientation – COO)

These institutions offer some accommodation, often in cases of family crises: CAUs offer a non-renewable accommodation for a maximum of 14 days; CPAs offer emergency accommodation for one month, renewable for two weeks; and COOs offer accommodation for a maximum duration of three months, renewable once only; all of them put special emphasis on diagnosis and reorientation.

In the Flemish community, observation and orientation centers offer accommodation for a duration of maximum two years, with a possible extension of one year.

Public welfare centers (Centres Publics d'Aide Sociale - CPAS)

Some CPAS, especially in the larger cities, have their own homes whose operating characteristics do not differ from the AAJ ones. Minor youths are admitted, in principle, on a voluntary basis negotiated with the family.

Residential institution of the birth and child office (Office de la Naissance et de l'Enfance – ONE)

Besides some medico-pedagogic institutions and a few homes that help out in social matters, ONE also subsidizes crèches and nurseries.

Juridical organization

The underlying philosophy in matters relating to the judicial organization is evolving in Belgium as well as in the other European countries. Until now, juvenile law considered young delinquents above all as youths in difficulties, requiring global aid. This position, however, tends to be modified under the pressure of "safety" concerns which have gained increasing ground in recent years.

So it evolves toward re-focusing on taking into account only the criminal act, calling for the implementation of sanctions "with educational intentions". At the same time, it leaves more room for mediation in which the specific characteristics of the various professionals and the differences of their role are often compromised. In legal procedures, on the other hand, more attention is given to what the child has to say, and he can benefit from the help of a solicitor.

Ambulatory Organization

Public prosecutor's department for youth and juvenile courts

We have already mentioned that these authorities were competent to implement constraint aid, following a request by Youth Welfare Services. They are also competent in some civil legal matters (approval of adoption; establishing family blood relationship; some kinds of litigations concerning the right to keep the children).

Their most specific competence, however, is called "protectional": they are, thus, in charge of measures to be taken in the cases of loss of parental rights and of underage delinquency (article 36.4 of the 1965 act ruling youth protection). We shall develop only this latter competence as it is the most frequent one.

When the magistrates of the public prosecutor's department for youth have to deal with complaints, they may either leave them unanswered, give a warning, preside over a mediation, or refer the matter to the juvenile magistrate. The latter initiates a preliminary investigation called "preparatory procedure" (relating to the young person's personality and to his/her life environment, but not to the actual facts) and, from then on, he can take "provisional measures" for a maximum duration of six months. He then forwards a motivated opinion to the public prosecutor who will decide, within two months, whether or not to refer the matter back, a second time, to the same magistrate for a public hearing and trial. The magistrate may then decide not to pursue the matter any further, to admonish the young person, to let him/her free under certain conditions (social conditions, therapy and compensation conditions), or to place him/her in one of the residential institutions mentioned in the previous section (usually in AAJ homes or IPPJ). In order to implement his decisions, the magistrate has to call on the director of youth welfare (Directeur de l'Aide à la Jeunesse – DAJ) and his services (Service de Protection Judiciaire – SPJ). Unless an appeal has been lodged, the juvenile magistrate remains responsible for the follow-up of the case.

The public prosecutor's department may also choose, at the same time, to refer the matter to an examining magistrate who will forward the case to the juvenile magistrate and to the board for elder teenagers with a view to remove the case from the court. The juvenile magistrate may also relinquish a case relating to an offense, committed after the age of 16, and refer it to a repressive jurisdiction for adults. However, he or she cannot do this in reference to the seriousness of the facts, but only in reference to the refusal on behalf of the young person with regard to the "educational" action taken by the court.

Director of youth welfare (DAJ) and youth protection service (SPJ)

When the measures taken by the juvenile magistrate, in matters relating to "delinquency" (article 37 of the 1965 act) or to "constraint aid" (article 38 of the 1991 decree), when such measures require resorting to institutions which depend on the youth welfare administration (Administration de l'Aide à la Jeunesse – AAJ), one calls on the director of youth welfare and his/her specific social service, the Youth Protection Service. This intermediary social authority has de facto wide powers of assessment and orientation, whereas the decisions made by the magistrate are of a general nature.

Educational orientation centers (Centres d'Orientation Educative – COE) and educational and philanthropic activities centers (Services de Prestations Educatives et Philantropiques – SPEP)

Educational orientation centers are multidisciplinary teams, made up of one coordinator having a university degree, two social workers, one psychologist, and a secretary; it has been provided for that each judiciary district should have at its disposal at least one COE which is mainly responsible for constraint aid (guidance to the young person and to her/his family, home visits, assistance and social mediation decided by the magistrate and implemented by the DAJ). COEs may also be called on by the CAJs with regard to voluntary aid, but this happens less frequently.

The educational and philanthropic activities services are also multidisciplinary teams (coordinator, criminologist, psychologist, social worker, educator, secretary). They organize and supervise the implementation, by the young person concerned, of measures including "educational and philanthropic activities" imposed by the magistrate: it concerns a certain amount of hours to be spent in "compensation jobs", which the young person has agreed to do, and which are to be done at employers' (often public services or related services) previously contacted by the SPEPs.

Specific residential organization

Public institutions for youth protection (Institutions Publiques de Protection de la Jeunesse – IPPJ)

Among the five existing institutions in the French-speaking community (there is none in the Brussels region), four are intended for boys and one for girls. Most of them are open; in this case, they operate according to a daily educational program, including resocialization, and even, to a certain extent, psychological guidance, in such a way that, more or less explicitly, the sanctions factor is not forgotten.

One of these institutions is closed-in, and two others have a closed-in area at their disposal; they are intended for youths who have committed more serious offences and who are considered dangerous, if not impossible to treat in open institutions. In fact, admissions to IPPJ are only for adolescents; nevertheless, in principle, young people under 12 may be sent there, too.

Imprisonment

Minor youths from the age of 14 who have committed serious offences may be imprisoned, in a specific area and for a maximum duration of 15 days, not as a punishment, but only when the magistrate, during his preliminary procedure, is unable to immediately place the young person in an appropriate institution. From the age of 16, the magistrate may, as we have mentioned earlier, relinquish certain cases, concerning serious offences, when she/he considers that the young person involved does not qualify for specific measures for minor youths. If, subsequently, these youths are sentenced to imprisonment by the ordinary courts, they can no longer benefit from any special protection (from the same age, minor youths who are considered by the court, as suffering from serious mental illness and as not being responsible for their actions may be admitted in adults institutions of social protection).

4. Cooperation with medical and non-medical disciplines

Cooperation with pediatrics

As mentioned earlier, some pediatric services in university hospitals have developed, within their department, a clinic of child and adolescent psychiatry, mainly for cooperation purposes; this, however, remains an exception. More often, one has to rely on the child and adolescent psychiatry units, when and if they are joined to psychiatric services, in order to assure that there is some pedo-psychiatric liaison in the pediatric hospital units of university hospitals. On the other hand, a large majority of pediatric services in non-university hospitals do not benefit from any kind of cooperation in matters regarding liaison pedopsychiatry, which results in an alarming deficiency as far as the quality of treatments is concerned.

The organization of liaison pedopsychiatry is one of the weak points of the health and prevention system in Belgium. The demands for profitability, which hospitals are subject to, and the inadequate importance given to liaison psychiatry, which penalizes in particular child and adolescent psychiatry because of the specific nature of its interventions, all these prevent medical and non-medical administrations of hospital institutions from developing, even to a minimum degree, this most essential sector of all hospital activities. In order to compensate for such deficiencies, some highly specialized pediatric units, especially in oncology and in AIDS pediatrics, usually with the help of private funds obtained from patronage, take on psychologists directly attached to the unit; thus, they make it possible to implement multidisciplinary treatments that young patients and their family need.

It would prove extremely beneficial if cooperation between child-adolescent psychiatrists and pediatricians were submitted to a dialogue and to a common reflection about educational and training courses.

It would be to the advantage of both specializations if they got to know each other better, systematically throughout theoretical courses and clinical training. The aim is not to do away with the speciality of each discipline or with the differences between them, but rather to ensure some common knowledge and experience for mutual recognition, for a better diagnosis assessment and for more precision in therapy indications.

Finally, in what concerns more specifically liaison pedopsychiatry, defining the norms of training and support in pediatric services, while including statutorily a pedopsychiatrist and a pedopsychologist, both part-time, with consequently a subsidy adjustment for these positions, this would give some impetus toward developing an integrated approach to psychosomatic pathologies and to medical psychology with children and adolescents.

Cooperation with psychiatry

Although child and adolescent psychiatry has not officially been recognized yet as a distinct specialization, in practice its identity is clearly defined and acknowledged: this is confirmed by the number of societies and of associations distinct from adult psychiatric ones.

In hospitals, child and adolescent psychiatry is often part of a psychiatric department and more rarely part of a pediatrics department. In mental health services, the child and adolescent psychiatry teams may operate as autonomous units or as an additional service to the adult patients' team. Despite it being administratively included into general psychiatry, which seems highly arguable and tends, as we see it, to ignore, in a general way, the specific status of children and adolescents in our society, despite that fact, the functional ties between general psychiatry and child and adolescent psychiatry are far from being satisfactory. As an example, let us mention the lack of specific hospitalization units, open or closed-in, for adolescents, due to the fact that psychiatric beds for adolescents are often merged into general psychiatric units, where there is little or no specific staff training or specific responsibility procedures; the absence of cooperation regarding the awareness of the consequence in terms of psychic health, are concerned, and of the mental affections of their parents who are being treated in psychiatry, has caused a prejudicial deficiency in terms of prevention, detection, and treatment.

An opportunity to have adult psychiatrists become efficiently sensitive to child psychopathology and to the problems of parenthood would certainly be to include a specific training program, both clinical and theoretical, in their degree course.

Cooperation with education

The school is a privileged partner of child and adolescent psychiatry: many psychological disorders appear through difficulties at school, in the learning area or, more widely, when problems arise related to school life integration. De facto, teachers take part in more than half of the consultations of child-adolescent psychiatry (according to the 1997 Brussels SSM statistics), either directly or, more often, by making parents aware of the problem. The same applies to the teams of psycho-medico-social centers (CPMS): these are attached to school institutions and play an important part in supporting teachers and in developing a real prevention of infant mental health at school, far beyond a mere detection of learning difficulties. It implies, of course, that a specific definition of the missions to be achieved by the centers, as well as the assignment and the training given to their staff coincide with these objectives. An ambitious policy of prevention in schools, coordinated by the CPMS and the IMS (medical school inspection) could make use of the means already existing in the mental health services and in some family planning centers.

Defining such a policy of prevention and coordinating the existing resources in order to carry it through could significantly improve this obviously most restricting factor until now: the education and training of teachers and the support given to them. Clinical experience, which has been corroborated by various surveys done in school environment, reveals indeed a persistent lack of knowledge and a persistently inadequate attitude among many teachers, with regard to certain matters relating to children's and adolescents' mental health.

The same applies to the ill-considered wait-and-see policy in nursery schools toward children who show obvious signs of progressive psychic pathologies that have not yet been diagnosed: the treatment could, thus, be delayed two to three years, and after that the seriousness of the inability to adapt to primary school requirements will no longer be possible to deny. The same goes for feelings of helplessness and the fear of it, provoked by some suicidal attitudes among adolescents and leading to an absence of reaction on behalf of the teachers with regard to pathologies; nevertheless, the dangers of these, in terms of mortality and of morbidity, would justify the implementation of well-determined initiatives (Hoyois et al. 1998).

Two other areas of cooperation between teachers and pedo-psychiatrists, and their teams, are special education and medico-pedagogic institutes. Directing children towards either one of these structures depends on a certificate issued by a registered team following a thorough diagnosis assessment.

Registered teams are either PMS Centers, mental health services, hospital pedo-psychiatric teams or S.O.S. children-parents teams. As far as IMPs are concerned, regular reassessments, made by a registered team, should enable the therapy organizations, as well as the educational and institutional ones, to become adapted to the progress of the child and the family.

In special education, specialized PMS centers are responsible for assessing and for following-up school orientation.

5. Graduate/postgraduate training and continuing medical education

Training of child and adolescent psychiatrists

Because the specialization in child and adolescent psychiatry has not been recognized in Belgium, administratively speaking, the professional training of child and adolescent psychiatrists still falls within the scope of general psychiatry specialization. This training includes a five year full-time practical training in clinical services registered by the Ministry of Health, as well as theoretical courses organized by the faculties of medicine.

Moreover, at least two scientific studies have to be done, one of which must have been published for the first time in a reputed scientific journal; the other one must have been addressed in public at a congress or at a scientific conference, either of them well-known.

Practical training must include at least two years in the services of adult psychiatry and one year in neurology or in neuro-pediatrics; another two years may be spent in the hospital or in extra-hospital services of child and adolescent psychiatry, full-time or by combining two half-times. One year of pediatrics, or even of internal medicine, could replace one year of psychiatry.

As a general rule, doctors who wish to turn to pedo-psychiatry must complete two and sometimes three years of training in places where pedo-psychiatric specialization is available, making sure, usually, that they can benefit from clinical experience with children and adolescents, both in hospitals and in extra-hospital institutions. The very limited number of registered training services in child and adolescent psychiatry has made it impossible to train a sufficient number of child and adolescent psychiatrists to fill all the positions needed, both in public services – who have called on adult psychiatrists as a result – and in independent practices. The situation may get worse in the near future as a result of the implementation in the year 2004 of a numerus clausus restricting the access to medical practices and, consequently, to specializations as well.

Training of child and adolescent psychotherapists

In Belgium, there are no regulations controlling the practice of psychotherapies; only psychotherapies conducted by psychiatrists are partially refunded by the social security organization, regardless of the number of sessions and duration of the treatment. The training of child and adolescent psychotherapists depends on the responsibility and the initiative of practitioners. This is done through various types of training offered by private and university organizations, usually for three years, in psychoanalytic specialization, and completed with individual supervisions, generally with child psychoanalysts. In the same way, practitioners who wish to turn to family therapy usually follow one of the various trainings in systemic family therapy for a duration of three years as a general rule. Training in the behavioural field also begins in this way. Admission to one of these trainings is usually subject to having previously practised in a child and adolescent clinic for at least two years and this restricts, de facto, access to such training to pedo-psychiatrists and to psychologists who have been working in clinics. Often training in systemic family therapy is far more accessible to mental health professionals.

6. Research

There is a very wide range of research areas covering various aspects such as in-depth study of child and adolescent psychopathology, including in particular the study of the impact of family functioning and the forms of transgenerational transmission. Another aspect is the research and the actions taken with the aim of assessing the effectiveness of therapy and of pathologies or in connection with well-defined family or social problematics; yet another aspect concerns the criteria required for making proper use of the existing structures of prevention and care, and their accessibility. There is also the study of the correlation between psychopathological disorders and biological variables, especially among adolescents, following the patterns of research done in adult psychiatry.

We would like to emphasize here that the main obstacle to the development of pedopsychiatric research resides in the problem of subsidizing which not only researchers have to face, but also the services that are keen to further research activities done by junior child and adolescent psychiatrists. These problems are linked at the same time to the nature of the psychopathological research done, to the poor interest in mental health research shown by public organizations, and to the absence of common interests with pharmaceutical companies.

7. Future perspectives

It can be said that, on the whole, a young discipline such as child and adolescent psychiatry, has managed in a few years to build up the conditions required for a good practice in Belgium. However, much remains to be done still in order to obtain an adequate balance between the needs in matters of care and prevention and the existing network. We are convinced that the universities, as competent authorities, should implement a series of improvements:

- The number of psychiatrists who have had an appropriate training in child and adolescent psychiatry is, at present, insufficient to answer the need for positions to be provided in public services and the needs in independent practices. It is therefore essential, bearing in mind the implementation of the numerus clausus in 2004, to try and ensure that a sufficient number of positions for specialization is set aside for psychiatry, and that, among these positions, a certain quota equivalent at least to the present opportunities is put aside for doctors who wish to specialize in child and adolescent psychiatry.
- Adult psychiatrists play an important part in directing parents and children to the appropriate category of pedo-psychiatric care. Therefore, one year of experience in child and adolescent psychiatry in the course of their five year training would appear very useful indeed.
- In the same context, a one-year training experience in child and adolescent psychiatry during the training of pediatricians would also prove highly beneficial.
- Considering the importance of general practitioners in prevention and care structures regarding child and adolescent mental health, moves should be made toward developing a specific training in child and adolescent psychiatry, because it has been far too restricted until now. A basic awareness of child psychiatry, as well as of adolescent and first age psychiatry, would ensure and enhance the quality of practice among general practitioners.
- An incidental matter that has been shelved for several years concerns the recognition of specialization or even super-specialization in child and adolescent psychiatry. It should be seriously taken into consideration in particular as far as standardization of medical training throughout Europe is concerned.

Even if the latter point could be negotiated by the universities, it nevertheless falls within the competence of their own authorities for final decision-making. Other initiatives in that matter would be welcome:

- If specialization in child and adolescent psychiatry were to be individualized, it would be highly desirable if a distinctive administrative list of general psychiatry and, on the other hand, of child and adolescent psychiatry could be established, taking into account the specific characteristics of both practices. This would make it possible to receive adequate refunds from the social security.
- Liaison pedo-psychiatry should be developed either by highlighting the list mentioned above or by integrating child and adolescent psychiatrists and psychologists into the funding of pediatric beds.

- The structures of specific care in the various categories are insufficiently developed in Belgium; they should be subjected to appropriate programming and subsidizing, and it should be essential to integrate also those structures which have an obvious therapy function, although they depend, at the moment, on authorities other than the public health: some medico-pedagogic institutes, some residential or ambulatory institutions of Youth Welfare Administration, as well as the S.O.S children teams.
- Research into child and adolescent mental health should receive more attention from organizations responsible for the principles and the financing of medical research.
- As it is the case with medical care, prevention in matters concerning child and adolescent mental health should be subjected to an in-depth study in order to set up programs which reflect a global policy in the area.

Finally, professionals and politicians as a whole should be more mindful of child and adolescent mental health; they should ensure that it is not progressively diverted towards welfare practices, or even toward control practices that are more concerned with security than with social matters. The experience these practices acquired over recent years has shown abundantly how harmful the results can be.

Acknowledgment We would like to extend our thanks to Professors Nicole Dopchie and Pierre Fontaine for their invaluable assistance in setting up this text.

Selected references

Hoyois P, Hirsch D, Matot JP (1998) Suicide et tentatives de suicide á l'adolescence. Ligue Bruxelloises pour la Santé Mentale, Bruxelles

Misès R, Fortineau J, Jeammet P, Lane IL, Mazet P, Plantade A, Quémada N (1988) Classification française des troubles menteaux de l'enfant et de l'adolescent. Psychiatrie de l'Enfant 31: 67–134

Child and adolescent psychiatry in Bulgaria

M. Achkova, N. Polnareva

1. Definition, historical development, and current situation

Definition

Child and adolescent psychiatry is a very young professional qualification in our country. It was realized as late as the 1950s that such a differentiation in the medical practice was possible and this resulted in the establishment of the first ward in child psychiatry in 1959. It was attached to the adult clinic within the psychiatric department. Other medical specialists at the medical faculty in Sofia, such as pediatricians, neurologists, and general practitioners, continued for a long time not to be interested in the psychological and psychopathological problems of children, and the adult psychiatrists are just starting to realize the importance of the child's development for the mental health of the adult.

Historical development

In this sense during the 1960s, child and adolescent psychiatry in Bulgaria remained dependent on adult psychiatry, which can be explained by the following factors.

Organizational

During that period, similarly to that in the former USSR, a broad and well-connected system of so-called dispensaries was created. They were regional psychiatric centers of the outpatient type which identified, registered, and treated patients with psychiatric problems. The whole country was divided into regions for the purposes of inpatient and outpatient care. Although extensively criticized and trying to transform themselves into regional centers for mental health, the dispensaries still remain the basic framework of our child psychiatric network.

Conceptual

Because of the dominant framework of "official" bulgarian psychiatry, psychodynamic and psychotherapy practice was denied, and the concept of the development of child psychiatry followed the philosophy and the experience of the treatment and care for adults. In this context, only serious cases of psychopathology and disability sought and received treatment and because of this the child ambulatory centers quickly lost their prestige and turned into obligatory annexes to the adult psychiatric centers.

Human resources

The hospital chief doctors themselves were not aware of the nature and specifics of the work with children, adolescents, and their families. Very often the promising specialists were oriented to adult psychiatry, and it was impossible to form multidisciplinary teams. This led to isolation of the professionals working with children and, very often, to a change in their professional choice. The absence of a professional association and a specific qualification in child psychiatry was also a problem for the formation of a professional identity and progress.

Because of all these reasons child psychiatry developed mainly in the university centers. The clinic in Sofia with 65 beds became independent in 1978 and the unit in Varna with 30 beds is still a ward in the clinic for adults. In the 1970s children and adolescents with psychoses, epilepsy, and mental deficiency were treated there, and it was during the 1980s that the interest in treating emotional and behavior disorders increased. This was inevitably accompanied by attempts for expansion of the outpatient child psychiatric care. In the course of time, the multidisciplinary teams became an obligatory requirement and the clinical child psychologists found their real place in them. This enabled the development and differentiation of the therapy. Children with mental retardation were oriented to institutions which provided long-term training and social rehabilitation. The number of requests for treatment of specific developmental disorders, child autism, and eating disorders increased. The therapeutic approaches were changing, in many institutions full-time positions for clinical psychologists were introduced. An opportunity for permanent child psychiatric consultation was created in the central counseling pediatric clinic.

Recent advances

We have to point out several important events in the development and modernizing of Bulgarian child and adolescent psychiatry in theory and practice.

Two French-Bulgarian colloquiums were arranged in 1981 and 1986 in Sofia and Paris. Bulgarian university professors and French psychiatrists with psychoanalytical orientation (Prof. S. Lebovici, Prof. R. Mises, Dr. J. Lucas et al.) took part in them.

In 1985, epidemiological research of the emotional and behavior disorders among children from 7–11 years started in cooperation with Prof. M. Rutter from London, and this research followed the pattern of the survey carried out at the Isle of Wight, UK.

The VIIIth Congress of the European Society of Child and Adolescent Psychiatry was held in Varna in 1987, and its main subject was "The Vulnerable Child".

Training in family therapy started in 1988 conducted by Swedish specialists in the area of family psychotherapy. In the spring of 1989, this training developed into the first systematic training in family therapy in our country which finished in 1993. The training was carried out by a team from Lund University, Sweden, led by Prof. M. Cederblad and finished with the graduation of 10 child psychologists and psychiatrists as family therapists. The regular and frequent contacts facilitated not only the introduction of family psychotherapy in Bulgaria but actually assisted the practice of child psychiatrists as well.

In this situation we faced the large political, social and economic changes. They took away the ideological limitations of the development of our profession but at the same time they put forward requirements for serious changes and reforms which would bring us closer to the European standards.

The experience of the following years showed that child psychiatrists were much more open and eager to applying new approaches in their everyday practice. They were spared long years of imposed conceptualization of the psychopathological phenomena without the knowledge and use of psychodynamic theories. To a great degree that was because of the lack of interest in what they were doing, which naturally led to less control of their work and ideas. That is why they were the first professionals in the field of mental health who applied the psychoanalytic models, system theories, and an orientation towards prevention in their therapeutic and teaching practice. In practice, the integration of psychotherapeutic ideas and skills in the psychiatric and psychological community started with the active participation of the specialists working in the area of child psychiatry. On the other hand, our collaboration with international centers working in the fields of genetics and neuropsychology of child psychoses, eating disorders, and addictions provided opportunities for the development of a modern understanding of biological psychiatry and revision of the past experience of primitive biological interpretations of psychopathological phenomena.

One of the most obvious results from the changes after 1989 was the opportunity for having long-term joint initiatives with European universities and associations.

Two important international projects started in 1992. The first one is called "Training of university psychiatrists and specialists, working in the area of child mental health". This program was financed by TEMPUS-Phare and the participants were Sofia Medical University, Université de la Mediteranée, Marseille, France, Université Catholique de Louvain, Belgium, and the University in Cluj-Napoka, Romania. It was a three-year project and it facilitated the systematic introduction of psychodynamic concepts, new organization of child mental health care and the stimulating introduction of the specialty of child psychiatry.

The second project which was approved for implementation in the same year was the establishment of the first multifunctional center for outpatient treatment of children and adolescents with the objective of development of outpatient university child psychiatry. It was of great importance not only for the actual work but for the introduction of the team model for work, the daycare, and ambulatory forms of treatment. The project was financed by the French Hospital Association of the Order of Malta (Association d'Oevres Hospitaliers Françaises de l'Ordre de Malte) and finished with the construction of the new child psychiatric clinic "St. Nikolas" which was officially opened in 1997.

During 1995 and 1996 another project was financed by TEMPUS: "Prevention of child mental health in child psychiatry". It was implemented by Bulgarian psychiatrists and psychologists from the two university clinics in Sofia in cooperation with three french child psychiatric clinics from Lyon, Marseille, and Paris, which are headed respectively by Prof. J. Hochman, Prof. M. Rufo, and Prof. Ph. Jeammet. The project included training for Bulgarian professionals in France and Belgium (Prof. C. Lepot-Froment) and 4 conferences were organized: Ethics and prevention in child psychiatry practice, Economics of the health care for children in the light of mental health prevention, Prevention during early childhood, Prevention during early adolescence. This project created the opportunity to research the needs of the psychiatric and psychological care in Bulgaria, of the resources for the development of the child psychiatric network, and the possibilities for the replacement of the existing consulting offices in the regional dispensaries with modern centers for diagnosis and therapy with qualified multidisciplinary staff. The results of the work were analyzed and published in a detailed report which was made available and distributed in the government and university institutions.

The association of the child psychiatrists and allied professions was established in 1991.

In 1995, child psychiatry was recognized as a profile specialty by the authorized government bodies. In 1996, the leading university professors were recognized as specialists in child psychiatry and, after passing an exam, the other university child psychiatrists received a diploma. In 1997, a training for a group of psychiatrists from different regions started and the idea was consulting teams to be formed all over the country. They are mainly in the big cities attached to the state structures and gradually the network of these centers will reach the European standards for the proportion between the number of child psychiatrists and the population. On the other hand, after a period of differentiation and search for identity, accompanied by clear separation from adult psychiatry, our collaboration with the state structures in the field of training and joint projects for a reform in psychiatric practice will gradually acquire the characteristics of a partnership based on equality.

Current situation

Having in mind the difficult circumstances of the transition period after 1989, which in Bulgaria was especially painful, some specific aspects of the situation in our country should be pointed out. A drop in the total number of the population and respectively of children, because of negative birth rate and rising death rate among children, has been seen. Deep economic and ideological crises in health care have led to minimal functioning of many of the institutions and a lack of well-prepared physicians in the private sector.

Structure of child and adolescent psychiatric care: There are 15 child psychiatrists in Sofia, there are 6 psychiatrist in the country, and 25 physicians are included in training projects. There is one inpatient unit in Sofia and one in Varna (the third largest city in Bulgaria), and each of them has 30 beds.

2. Classification systems, diagnostic and therapeutic methods

Classification systems

Since the mid 1980s, mainly for research reasons, DSM-III and DSM-III-R have been used and now DSM-IV is applied. In clinical practice ICD-10 is currently broadly used. Specific standard forms are developed mainly in the university clinics for interviewing, evaluation, and therapeutic strategies which include the children, their families, and people from their close surrounding. In everyday practice, psychodynamic and family-system models for the formulation of the individual case are used.

Diagnostic methods

A large spectrum of diagnostic procedures to study cognitive and affective development is used, and special attention is paid to the period of early development, family history and interaction, psychic trauma, and the specific coping mechanisms. An evaluation is done of the concrete social context.

By tradition we have good contacts with child neurologists, neuropsychologists, and electrophysiologists.

Therapeutic methods

The multidisciplinary treatment of children and the availability of child psychiatrists with different orientations creates the possibility even within the limits of one institution different therapeutic methods to be applied. In the late 1980s and the early 1990s, family system psychotherapy was very popular. Now because of our collaboration with the French child psychiatry, psychodynamic approaches are more and more frequently applied. Psychodrama, play therapy, art therapy, group therapy, and behavior therapy are used. Most of the children, in cases when there is a trained medical team, are included in an individually designed therapeutic plan which includes work with the parents and the people from the close surrounding of the children. Specific programs are developed – for child victims of violence, children with psychosomatic problems, infants and adolescents with maladaptation, and children with learning problems. Of course, serious disorders, mainly of adolescents, need treatment with medication, frequently in inpatient units where programs for treatment of eating disorders are also available. Since 1989 the program for rehabilitation of children with early childhood autism and Rett Syndrome, whose prototype is the program of the TEACCH Division (E. Schopler 1976), has been applied.

3. Structure and organization of services

Types of services

The country is divided into sectors and the child psychiatric services use the sectors for adults. Every big city has a child psychiatric ambulatory unit but very often the physician there works without the necessary paramedical team.

Because most of the institutions working in the area of child psychiatry are in the process of construction, we are going to explain the current structure of the university clinics. The outpatient clinic and the inpatient clinic in Sofia belonging to the same university hospital "Alexandrovska" are on separate territories which does not hamper their collaboration.

Outpatient services

The outpatient clinic includes a day-treatment center and a structure for counseling, consultation, and ambulatory treatment of children, adolescents, and their families. This dyadic form provides the opportunity for dealing with the enormous requests on the one hand and for quick referrals to a therapeutic program for day-treatment on the other hand. The restriction of the requests within the region which we are obliged to cover is not possible now, before the establishment of other similar structures in the country.

Daypatient services

The clinic "St. Nikolas" also functions in the university hospital in Sofia. "St. Nikolas" clinic offers daycare and a large number of individual and group activities. It is practically the first center of this type, and in the future it will serve as a model for establishing regional child centers for mental health in the country. Another multidisciplinary outpatient center for children and adolescents will be created at the center for mental health in Sofia.

Inpatient services

The inpatient clinic, which has 30 beds, actually provides services to half of the territory of Bulgaria. The requests come from the outpatient clinic (at weekly joint conferences) or directly from child psychiatrists or pediatricians.

Personnel

The staff in these clinics include, besides the child psychiatrists, clinical psychologists, speech therapists, nurses with special qualifications, pedagogues, and social workers. It has been suggested that the experience of the university clinics be used as a prototype for setting the norms for formation of multidisciplinary teams.

4. Cooperation with medical and non-medical disciplines

Besides our traditionally good relations with other medical specialties – neurologists, pediatricians, gynecologists, allergologists, dermatologists – our cooperation with non-medical services and specialists in prevention of child mental health is expanding and becoming more active. It is expressed in joint seminars and shared consulting. An example of such cooperation is the collaboration in the area of prevention of child violence and treatment of psychic traumatism.

5. Graduate/postgraduate training and continuing medical education

Postgraduate training in child and adolescent psychiatry requires a two-year extra training after graduation in general psychiatry. The training includes supervision of practice at the university clinics, theoretical training through participation in seminars, and independent development of a given thesis. The training is arranged in the two university child and adolescent psychiatric clinics in Sofia. The two years are divided into inpatient, day-treatment, and outpatient forms of work. The training finishes with an exam which consists of a practical and a theoretical part. A state diploma is then given to the graduate.

This is an opportunity for a continuing training of psychiatrists in the form of one-week courses on up-to-date and specialized subjects which are different every year.

6. Research

By tradition, since the 1970s, there has been serious scientific research in the area of childhood epilepsy, early psychoses, and developmental retardation. In the 1980s, the emphasis was on social psychiatry and epidemiology of emotional and behavior disorders. Research was done on depression, adolescent crises and psychoses, violence and psychic traumatism, childhood autism, and eating disorders. The interest in research of the family, evaluation of therapies, and organization of prevention of child mental health disorders has been rising recently.

7. Future perspectives

Despite the serious economic crisis in the country, the priority in the future development in child psychiatry is the development of strategies for promotion of child mental health. In terms of organization, this means restructuring and improvement of a network of child psychiatric services with multidisciplinary teams responsible for a given catchment area. In terms of training, the objective is not only post-graduate training, but also continuing medical education in child and adolescent psychiatry and psychotherapy. The association of child psychiatrists and allied professions, which at the moment has 47 members, assists actively in the organization of local and international seminars and is monitoring and developing the standards of good child psychiatric practice. The strengthening of the process of opening of child psychiatry to the community and active collaboration with specialists from medical and non-medical professions which are related to child mental health is an extremely important objective. The discussion on ethical problems related to practicing of child and adolescent psychiatry which has already started, will be permanent and will aim at the integration of different practical, theoretical, and organizational aspects in the context of a changing world.

References

Schopler E, Reichler RJ (eds) (1976) Psychopathology and child development: Research and treatment. New York: Plenum Press

Child and adolescent psychiatry in Croatia

S. Nikolić, V. Rudan, V. Vidovic

1. Definition, historical development, and current situation

Definition

Child and adolescent psychiatry is a medical psychiatric discipline that primarily takes into account the emotional and social dimensions, which differentiates it from organologic adult psychiatry in the strict sense of the term. Furthermore, it concerns a particular population of children and adolescents who are in the process of development.

Historical development

The developmental history of child psychiatry and psychotherapy in Croatia is connected with the name of Dr. Maja Beck-Dvoržak, who established the first child psychiatry service and became the teacher of all subsequent specialists. Today the work of Prof. M. Beck-Dvoržak can be followed through her scientific and professional articles, which were most frequently published in the journal Psihoterapija, of which she was one of the co-founders. In the late 1960s, an article by Prof. Maja Beck-Dvoržak entitled "Child Psychiatry in Paris" appeared in the journal Neuropsihijatrija. This work reported on training she had received in child psychiatry at the pedopsychiatric clinic of Prof. Heyer in Paris, founded in 1925, where the first cathedra in Europe for child psychiatry was established. Under Prof. Heyer and somewhat later under Prof. S. Lebovici and R. Diatkine, eminent child psychiatry experts in Paris, Dr. M. Beck-Dvoržak specialized in child psychiatry. Upon returning to Zagreb, she began to develop a service for child psychiatry and psychotherapy at the Neuropsychiatric Clinic of the Rebro Hospital and to assemble her first students and associates.

Dr. M. Beck-Dvoržak presented her concept of developmental child psychiatry and its fundamental concepts in Croatia in an article entitled "La protection de santé mentale des enfants", published in the French journal Information psychiatrique in 1969. It is also necessary to single out from her opus "On the Contribution of Psychoanalysis to Child Psychiatry", written in 1975, since Maja Beck-Dvoržak never stopped considering and developing child psychiatry in its entirety as a complete discipline that encompassed the prevention, diagnostics, treatment, and rehabilitation of the mental disorders of children and adolescents. In this article she wrote: "If we review the past, we see that the first physicians who engaged in child psychopathology during the 19th century were generally concerned with mental retardation and character disorders within the framework of delinquent behavior. They were under the powerful influence of pedagogy. Only after the insights provided by the physician and psychiatrist S. Freud, the inventor of psychanalysis, was greater interest aroused among medical professionals concerning the more discrete psychiatric symptoms in children. The discoveries by psychoanalysis in this area in no way collided with the results of other biomedical and clinical disciplines such as neurobiology, neurology, and pediatrics. Psychoanalysis demonstrated that development is not merely simple biological maturation but a process that represents the interaction of the fundamental biological traits of a child and his relation to the immediate surroundings" (p. 213–214).

With time, the Child Psychiatry and Psychotherapy Section of the Neuropsychiatric Clinic in Zagreb grew, becoming in 1969 the Department for Child and Adolescent Psychiatry and Psychotherapy, and finally the Polyclinic, which today at the Clinical Hospital Center serves as an educational and research center in child psychiatry and psychotherapy for medical students, physicians, clinical psychologists, and professionals in related disciplines.

Recent advances

Advances in child and adolescent psychiatry in the Republic of Croatia have been recently spurred by the following:

- There has been great interest in the postgraduate study of child and adolescent psychiatry, introduced at the Medical School of the University of Zagreb in 1974. This study, in the absence of postgraduate specialization in child and adolescent psychiatry, served for years not only for scientific training but also in the professional qualification of psychiatrists and graduates in other related professions: psychologists, pedagogue-rehabilitation specialists, etc.
- At the proposal of the Croatian Academy of Arts and Sciences, in 1990 Prof. S. Nikolic initiated the establishment of the Croatian Society for Infant, Child, and Adolescent Psychiatry and Psychotherapy (acronym: CROSICAP) whose members are child and adolescent psychiatrists, school physicians, pediatricians, and also specialists from related professions, psychologists, pedagogues-rehabilitation specialists, social workers, etc. Owing to the efforts of Prof. S. Nikolic, in 1994 the society became a full member of IACAPAP. In 1997, the medical section within CROSICAP, owing to joint efforts by Prof. S. Nikolic and Assist. Prof. Vlasta Rudan, the current president of CROSICAP, became a member of ESCAP.
- In 1994, the Ministry of Health approved a program for narrow specialized postgraduate study in child and adolescent psychiatry.
- At the initiative of UNICEF, Dr. Nenad Jakušic founded the Society for the Protection of Children from Abuse and Neglect in 1996.
- At the initiative of Assist. Prof. Vlasta Rudan, in 1998 the Croatian Society for Child and Adolescent Psychotherapy was established.
- War and the ensuing suffering required more detailed study of the pathogenesis and therapy of PTSD among children and adolescents, in which domestic

specialists (Assoc. Prof. Vesna Vidovic, Dr. Damir Dezan, Dr. Nenad Jakušic, Dr. Jugoslav Gojkovic) participated together with a number of experts from other countries (Holland, U.S.).

Current situation

According to the 1991 census, the number of inhabitants in the Republic of Croatia totalled 4,784,265, of whom 1,252,469 were children and adolescents under 20 years of age, representing approximately 26.2 % of the total population. Presently in the Republic of Croatia there are 35 psychiatrists engaged in child and adolescent psychiatry, in government institutions. This means that per 136,693 inhabitants or 35,784 children and adolescents below 20 years of age there is one psychiatrist engaged in child and adolescent psychiatry whose services are financed by compulsory health insurance. For now, only a few of the psychiatrists engaged in child and adolescent psychiatry are in private practice, and the fees for their services are not presently covered by health insurance. However, if we finally take the number of the 39 psychiatrists engaged in child and adolescent psychiatry, the situation will appear somewhat better, i.e., one child and adolescent psychiatrist per 122,673 inhabitants or 32,114 children and adolescents younger than 20 years of age.

At present in Croatia, child and adolescent psychiatrists are psychiatrists specialized in general psychiatry who have pursued postgraduate studies and other forms of education (university diploma courses in child psychiatry and training in child psychotherapy) through their own training analysis, consultation, and supervision of their professional work with children and adolescents who have psychiatric disturbances.

Since narrow specialization in child and adolescent psychiatry has only been approved since 1994, the Ministry of Health has only recognized such a level of competence in four psychiatrists in Croatia. However, other general psychiatrists with additional seminar training continue to work in the area of child and adolescent psychiatry. Formal recognition as specialists in child and adolescent psychiatry can be obtained by psychiatrists who complete the additional two-year postgraduate program in child and adolescent psychiatry, specified by an act of the Ministry of Health dated 1994.

The Croatian Society for Infant, Child, and Adolescent Psychiatry now numbers 112 members. The Croatian Society for Child and Adolescent Psychotherapy was established in mid 1998 and has only recently commenced operations and attracting members.

Much still needs to be done for the development of child and adolescent psychiatry in the Republic of Croatia, but without the support of government ministries and expert commissions, there will not be significant progress. One of the greatest difficulties is the distribution of child and adolescent psychiatric services and/or professional personnel. The existing facilities for child and adolescent psychiatry in Croatia are predominantly located in Zagreb, with 31 psychiatrists.

In other cities, a service for child and adolescent psychiatry has been organized in Osijek while psychiatry clinics of the medical schools in Rijeka and Split are being organized or planned. In Split, an outpatient service has been organized with only one psychiatrist for children and adolescents (there is a similar situation in Pula), while in Rijeka a department was established in mid 1998 for adolescent psychiatry with two psychiatrists who have additional training in child psychiatry. In Rijeka, only one psychiatrist has a private practice in child and adolescent psychiatry.

In addition to the cities mentioned and other cities in the Republic of Croatia such as Pula and Slavonski Brod, outpatient services are being opened for child and adolescent psychiatry. However, there are also large cities in Croatia that have not begun organizing child and adolescent psychiatric services.

There are continued attempts regarding the planning of independent specialization in child and adolescent psychiatry, to be coordinated with those from the European community, and regarding more complete epidemiological and other investigations in the domain of infant, child, and adolescent psychiatry.

2. Classification systems, diagnostic and therapeutic methods

Classification systems

In Croatia, by a decision of the Ministry of Health, the ICD-10 classification system is used in all medical fields including child and adolescent psychiatry. Some psychiatrists additionally use the DSM-IV classification system. All the medical services are required to keep medical documentation. In hospitals, documentation is more extensive and contains the most important data from the patient medical history, current disorder, multiaxial ICD-10 diagnosis, and a brief review of the therapeutic measures and recommendations. When a patient leaves the hospital, the physician is required to issue a letter of discharge containing data on the patient's disease, tests performed in the hospital, his condition at the time of discharge, recommendations for therapy or other measures proposed for the purpose of improving the health status of the patient within the framework of other institutions or the family. The letter of discharge is issued in child and adolescent psychiatry to parents or to the patient himself if he is an older adolescent, and in some rare situations it can be delivered directly to the authorized general practitioner.

Diagnostic methods

Clinical evaluation and psychological testing are the two basic diagnostic procedures in child and adolescent psychiatry, in addition to EEG, neurological examination, various laboratory tests, the most modern scanning (special imaging techniques) and/or other special techniques. Special diagnostic techniques are used in work with very small children and their mothers, family evaluations, and in the area of specific developmental disorders.

Therapeutic methods

The therapeutic approach is causal, i.e., therapy is aimed at the hypothetical or verified cause. The clinical orientation in child and adolescent psychiatry, i.e., biological versus psychodynamics, also affects the frequency of the use of psychopharmaceuticals in the sense of advantages that prescribing psychopharmaceuticals will yield in relation to psychotherapy. In Croatia, psychodynamic psychotherapy is present although it is used in an eclectic approach with the integration of various methods, most commonly psychodynamic, behavioral, and cognitive. Of group techniques, family therapy, psychoanalytic psychodrama, and group psychotherapy of children and adolescents are employed according to various theoretical approaches, depending upon the education of the therapist, the purposes for which they are used, and the therapeutic goals.

3. Structure and organization of services

Guidelines for services for children and adolescens with psychiatric disorders

The services for child and adolescent psychiatry are presently not an integral part of the services for primary medical care consisting of the family physician, pediatric service and gynecologic service. The Croatian Psychiatric Association is attempting to influence the Ministry of Health to alter this situation. The psychiatric service generally proposes overall reorganization, emphasizing that activities should be community-based. Attempts are being made to follow this model in child and adolescent psychiatry, for which services are even less adequately distributed than for adult psychiatry, and in many areas of the country still completely undeveloped. Services for children and adolescents with special needs are not distributed regionally either.

Types of services

The various types of psychiatric services for children and adolescents are not well distributed in Croatia.

Primarily, activity occurs through outpatient services for general psychiatry in health centers and through psychiatric clinics within general hospitals. Actually, only two institutions in the country (in Zagreb and Osijek) have the triad system of outpatient services, daypatient services, and inpatient services in hospital wards, and each region or at least each county seat in the country should have it.

Zagreb is an exception because it has the University Polyclinic for Child and Adolescent Psychiatry and Psychotherapy at the Rebro Hospital, the Special Psychiatric Hospital for Children and Young People, and the Center for Chronically Ill Autistic Children which is operated by a non-physician pedagogue and therefore, due to general disapproval by psychiatrists engaged in child psychopathology, has been excluded from health service.

In Osijek, in addition to the psychiatric clinic, there is a hospital ward for child psychiatry with a daypatient hospital, branch clinic, and community health services. The situations in Rijeka, Split, Pula, and Slavonski Brod were previously described.

Of the complementary services, there are various types of foster homes for abandoned and abused children as well as residential facilities for abandoned and orphaned children and for children with severe sensory or motor disabilities.

Outpatient services

In the institutions mentioned, general psychiatrists are in charge of the clinical and polyclinical activities. They sometimes refer patients for therapy to other institutions, private practitioners or to other members of their own team, depending on the indications (psychologist, special education teacher, social worker, speech pathologist, etc.). In pediatric clinics, mental health consultations are generally performed by psychologists, with or without consultation with a psychiatrist.

In Croatia, there is one psychiatrist for children and adolescents per approximately 130,000 inhabitants. In Zagreb, the largest city in Croatia with approximately one million inhabitants, there are 31 available child and adolescent psychiatrists, i.e., one psychiatrist per 32,258 inhabitants. The remaining 8 child and adolescent psychiatrists are not equally distributed throughout the rest of the Republic of Croatia.

Fundamental training in psychotherapy is part of the narrow program of specialization in child and adolescent psychotherapy. Questions concerning independent work by non-physician psychotherapists have not been completely settled although the pedopsychiatric service collaborates extensively with them.

Daypatient services

There are only two day hospitals for child psychiatry in the country. One, in Osijek, is connected with a hospital ward and the psychiatrists work together with patients from the day hospital and the hospital ward. The second, in Zagreb, is a special psychiatric hospital for children and adolescents that has a day hospital which functions independently of the hospital ward. Another day hospital is being organized at the Psychiatric Clinic in Rijeka, that will function independently of a hospital ward.

Inpatient services

As mentioned, there are only two hospital wards for the treatment of children and adolescents with psychiatric disturbances. The one with the largest number of beds (31) is located in a special psychiatric hospital for children and adolescents in Zagreb. The smaller, second one, with 10–12 beds, is located in Osijek. In Zagreb, which has approximately one million inhabitants, there are only 3.1 beds per 100,000 inhabitants, which is less than needed by the city of Zagreb and Zagreb

County, not to mention the large inflow of children and adolescent patients referred from all over Croatia. All the ward facilities are somewhat cramped and worn and should be reconstructed and modernized. This is one of the fundamental reasons that there is no rooming-in for parents. It is also not possible to separate groups of patients, who sometimes require special treatment.

Complementary services and rehabilitation

In 1995, the Assembly of the Croatian Society for Infant, Child, and Adolescent Psychiatry came to the conclusion that urgent reorganization of the psychiatric care of children and adolescents was required due to a crisis situation in the organization of pedopsychiatric activity caused by inadequate conditions, a shortage of personnel, and the repeal of the law for the co-financing of health services of the Center for Autism in Zagreb, which occurred following the direct inspection conducted by a delegation from the Republican Bureau for Health Insurance. The Center for Autism, owned and operated by the Ministry for Education and Sport, unfairly became merely an educational institution for autistic children and adolescents, functioning mostly without consulting psychiatrists. In our opinion, the Center for Autism should not be permitted to be operated as a primarily educational institution but should be reorganized within the framework of a psychiatric service.

Personnel

Personnel are still generally allocated according to the number of patients and not according to patient requirements or the time necessary to perform various tasks, although this would certainly improve the quality of service and be useful in the assessment of cost and benefits.

Funding of services

According to the Health Insurance Act, compulsory health insurance covers all the citizens of the Republic of Croatia. The insurance is based on the family unit, i.e., the policy holder and members of the immediate family. Children up to 15 years of age and women during pregnancy and delivery have unlimited health coverage. Children over 15 years of age are entitled to unlimited health care for the duration of their schooling.

Compulsory health care is financed from health insurance premiums paid by every employee and employer. The collection of funds is organized by the Croatian Bureau of Health Insurance. The bureau defines the standards and norms for all aspects of health care according to the levels and types, including child and adolescent psychiatry. Citizens can also insure themselves with entirely private or supplementary insurance, furnished by other providers.

All insured persons, including children and adolescents, enjoy the rights of compulsory health insurance in accordance with the Law, including the following:

- The right to the free choice of physician according to the place of residence. This particularly refers to the family physician, specialists for children's diseases and school medicine because of eventual house calls, treatment in the home and emergency medical assistance;
- The right to choose the polyclinic and hospital institution (in which psychiatric services for children and adolescents are mostly located);
- The right to primary health care (including a check-up by a selected physician, house calls, treatment in the home, emergency medical assistance, necessary medicines via prescription and orthopedic devices);
- The right to polyclinic consultation in health care (that encompasses all the specialties in the polyclinic medical services in diagnostics and therapy, including child and adolescent psychiatry, on the basis of physician referral and medical documentation from the selected physician);
- The right to hospital treatment in hospitals for acute and chronic diseases on the basis of physician referral and medical documentation from the selected physician, which also refers to child and adolescent psychiatry;
- All employees in government or private institutions and enterprises have the right to sick-leave compensation when prevented from working due to illness.

The Croatian Bureau of Health Insurance makes contracts with individual physicians in private practice, health care centers and hospitals regarding the providing of health care to those persons insured by the Bureau according to fixed fees.

There are very few private psychiatric services for child and adolescent psychiatry in the Republic of Croatia, so that such services are chiefly connected with the government hospitals, either university or county, as polyclinic consulting or hospital services. A relatively small number of child and adolescent psychiatrists work outside of hospitals in psychiatric clinics for children and adolescents as part of health centers, and this is in the large cities.

The Ministry of Social Welfare through the system of Social Security Insurance has assumed the responsibility for physically and severely mentally handicapped children and adolescents.

4. Cooperation with medical and non-medical disciplines

Cooperation with pediatrics

The best collaboration has been developed with neuropediatricians, not only concerning epilepsy but other disturbances and diseases of the brain, metabolic disturbances that create symptoms of CNS dysfunction, etc. However, collaboration with neuropediatricians seems better than between pediatricians and child and adolescent psychiatrists. Probably one of the reasons is that Croatian psychiatry is mostly psychodynamically oriented in the understanding of a problem and in psychotherapeutic work, while psychologists are more behavior and cognitive oriented. Most likely, communication between psychologists and pediatricians is facilitated by the concrete nature of both disciplines, orientation toward consciously easily recognizable goals and more rapid and active interventions. Psychodynamic psychiatrists, who rely more on indirect conclusions and have become accustomed to unclear and slow progress in diagnostics and therapy, are more in contact with their own feelings and physician-patient reactions. Therefore, the expectations of one and the other side are often fairly unrealistic and are not based on an understanding of the problems and possibilities of those on the other side.

Cooperation with psychiatry

All psychiatrists engaged in the mental health of children and adolescents in Croatia are actually specialists in general psychiatry, who have only had the opportunity for more narrow specialization in child and adolescent psychiatry since 1994. However, the majority of general psychiatrists engaged in child and adolescent psychiatry worked in this field prior to the approval of more narrow specialization. This common educational background and other specific historical factors have brought psychiatrists nearer to each other and simplified their collaboration. In adolescent psychiatry, there is frequent overlapping so that adolescents are often hospitalized in psychiatric wards for adults or are treated at clinics for general psychiatry. Family therapy is also where the spheres of activity and professional interests overlap.

Cooperation with doctors in private practice

According to the Health Act, the majority of family physicians will have to go into private practice. This has still not affected specialist services to the same extent, particularly not those outside of primary health care. Since very few psychiatrists engaged in child and adolescent psychiatry are in private practice, the clinical services of child and adolescent psychiatry are still very connected with the government institutions, where compulsory health insurance covers services.

Cooperation with non-medical institutions and professionals

Cooperation has been developed with school psychologists and teachers in regular and some special schools for children with severe disorders in psychophysical development. There is also good cooperation with social workers in the centers for social work, particularly in the services for juvenile delinquency, abused children with alcoholic parents, and expert witnesses for awarding the custody of minor children following divorce cases.

Cooperation between psychologists and nonmedical personnel with the psychiatric services is well established. Outside of these services, there is an unresolved question concerning the possibilities for their independent work as psychotherapists. We hope that the situation will improve for nonmedical professionals who would like to learn and work independently as psychotherapists in the private sector.

5. Graduate/postgraduate training and continuing medical education

Graduate training: The role of medical faculties

In undergraduate training, child and adolescent psychiatry does not exist as a separate subject. In the fourth-year psychiatry course during medical study, child psychiatry receives only two hours of attention, providing only the most rudimentary information on psychopathology and treatment. However, in the third-year psychological medicine course, an extensive explanation is given for the psychodynamics of personality development, i.e., the basic psychological development of the child.

For the past five years, medical students have been able to take elective courses, some covering individual chapters from child and adolescent psychiatry, which are well attended.

Postgraduate training, a joint effort

The recently passed law on the postgraduate training of physicians has established child and adolescent psychiatry as a sub-specialization lasting two years after the study of general psychiatry. It includes rotations in hospital and nonhospital wards of child and adolescent psychiatry, pediatrics, psychiatry, and specialized institutions for the care of handicapped and autistic children as well as a compulsory postgraduate course in child and adolescent psychiatry. The postgraduate course, established in 1974, is organized by the medical school in cooperation with the corresponding clinics. Before child and adolescent psychiatry was recognized as a separate specialty, many physicians were trained through this course, on-the-job experience, and under supervision. The postgraduate course, with 400 hours devoted to theoretical instruction in topics including child development, psychopathology, and treatment, places strong emphasis on research without sufficient practical instruction, which is compensated for thorough work and supervision.

The organization of the health services has produced a situation in which a number of psychiatrists with this background and without education formally approved by the Ministry of Health have been oriented toward child and adolescent psychiatry.

Continuing medical education in child and adolescent psychiatry and psychotherapy

For physicians, continuing medical education is organized via various courses in child and adolescent psychiatry. Courses on individual psychotherapeutic techniques are particularly well attended, and their programs are coordinated with the requirements and criteria of the corresponding European psychotherapeutic associations.

Training programs for other disciplines

The postgraduate course in child and adolescent psychiatry is also open to cooperating non-physician professionals, e.g., psychologists, social workers, and special education teachers, and has been well received.

Because the majority of child and adolescent psychiatrists and experts in related mental health professions serving children in Croatia are concentrated in Zagreb and some other major cities, large regions of the country do not have such experts available. Therefore, continuing education has been organized for physicians and experts from related professions in the regional health centers in Split, Rijeka, and Osijek, significantly improving the situation.

6. Research

In research, two tendencies can be observed. One is in connection with the large approved projects financed by the government, and the other is in connection with smaller research tasks conducted by individual researchers for their own needs, with no financial support from such institutions.

Research fields and strategies

Systematic epidemiologic research studies have not been undertaken until now. Our strategic goal is to conduct a research project on the present status of the psychological health of children, adolescents, and families, especially because of the need for a systematic determination of the long-term impact of the recent war on the psychological health of the young generation and the needs for the better organized care of the psychological health of children and families. Research has focused on psychological war traumas, through individual projects financed by domestic and international institutions and in cooperation with eminent foreign research centers. There have also been various research projects in connection with the psychological development and health of infants.

Research training and career development

The previously mentioned postgraduate course in child and adolescent psychiatry is largely oriented toward research and research training. No career advancement for a physician in our milieu is feasible without research trials, especially in a teaching career. After the completion of the postgraduate course and defense of the masters thesis, physicians receive the title of master of science; and after the defense of the doctoral dissertation, they can be chosen for the profession of higher education.

For career advancement in the hospital hierarchy to the highest level, the title of "primarius", it is essential to show that the physician has not only clinical but research experience also. In the field of child and adolescent psychiatry, a significant number of professionals at the large clinical centers have earned the highest scientific and professional title.

Funding

Research projects are financed by the Ministry of Science and Technology after public competition. Child and adolescent psychiatry does not receive preferential consideration, although preference would be expected due to its social significance.

7. Future perspectives

We are presently in a state of anticipation concerning the further development of child and adolescent psychiatry after we have legally obtained the possibility for subspecialization. Since such training takes a long time and will probably be financed by the health institutions that need such personnel, and the present possibilities for health care spending are inadequate, it is feared that until the economic situation improves, there will be no major changes in the development of the profession or in the area of research.

We believe that we must fight for a better position of child and adolescent psychiatry within the framework of undergraduate training at the medical schools through the forming of a separate subject of child and adolescent psychiatry. This can be a very difficult task since the general trend is to reduce the number of subjects and examinations in the curriculum.

Research

We anticipate that the priorities will be understood in the society and that we shall be able to conduct systematic research in the areas of epidemiology and early psychological development.

Training

Greater activity is anticipated in the creation of educational projects for physicians and specialists in related professions and in increasing the number of elective courses in the area of child and adolescent psychiatry for medical students.

Selected references

Beck-Dvoržak M (1958) Child Psychiatry in Paris. Neuropsihijatrija 6 (1–4): 233–239

Beck-Dvoržak M (1969) La protection de la santé mentale des enfants. L'information Psychiatrique, 45 (3): 259–264

Beck-Dvoržak M (1975) The contribution of psychoanalysis to the child psychiatry (in Croatian Language), Psihoterapija, 5 (2): 213–215

Cicchetti D, Cohen D (1995) Developmental Psychopathology, Vol. 1, 2. Wiley, New York

Lewis M (ed) (1996) Child and Adolescent Psychiatry, A Comprehensive Textbook. 2nd ed., Williams & Wilkins, Baltimore

Nikolić S (1988) Mental disorders in children and adolescents (in Croatian language), Školska knjiga

Nikolić S (1982) Child and adolescent psychiatry, Propedeutics (in Croatian language), Školska knjiga

Turek S (1997) Croatian model of the health insurance. In: Topić, E, Budak A (eds) Current Approach to the Diagnosis and a Therapy in Primary Health Care (in Croatian language), Medicinski Fakultet Sveucilista u Zagrebu i Skola narodnog zdravlja Andrija Štampar, Zagreb, pp 172–178

Young G, Ferrari P (eds) (1998) Designing Mental Health Services and Systems for Children and Adolescents: A Shrewed Investment. Brunner & Mazel, London (book series of IACAPAP)

Child and adolescent psychiatry in the Czech Republic

E. Malá

1. Definition, historical development, and current situation

Definition

The approach toward child and adolescent mental health care is of a multidisciplinary nature. One of these clinical and medical disciplines is precisely child and adolescent psychiatry, dealing with prevention, diagnostics, therapy (both pharmacotherapy and psychotherapy), and rehabilitation of mental disorders. Further, it embraces consulting, expert opinions, and research.

A human being is defined as a bio-psycho-social unit. That is why pedopsychiatry takes into account both social and medical aspects when treating adaptation and developmental disorders, dedicating special attention to evolutionary, mental, and somatic features.

Historical development

The history of mental health care dates back to the 19th century. In 1871, K. S. Amerling founded the first institute for mentally retarded children called "Ernestinum". Having both medical and pedagogical training, it was natural for Amerling to combine these two fields in his institute. Abandoned and neglected children eventually found their home. In 1911, a law was passed concerning the rights of children and duties of parents. Later on, the focus shifted to social issues and at the same time pedopsychiatrists first described the syndromes and symptoms of mental disorders.

K. Hertfort (1871–1940) became the first professor of psychopathology with early onset and the chief of the first pedopsychiatric outpatient department in Prague. Further, Hertfort opened the first genetic station and lectured widely for both medicine students and trainers. His work mainly explored differential diagnosis of mental retardation. In 1923, a former South Bohemian Jesuit's convent was turned into the first mental home for mentally ill children and adolescents. In 1924, the construction of a modern school facility with a swimming pool and a gymnasium was completed and in 1929 the construction of workshops for work-therapy was completed in Oparany. The interwar years in what was then Czechoslovakia saw an expansion of the net of pedopsychiatric outpatient departments, now professionally manned: a psychiatrist, psychologist, and a social worker (usually female). In 1947, J. Apetauer founded the first inpatient pediatric department at the psychiatric clinic in Prague. Being mainly interested in youthful criminality and forensic medicine, he was the first person to emphasise the possibility of different degree of maturity in adolescents of the same biological age.

In 1971, J. Fisher founded and opened the first psychiatric clinic in Prague. All over the Czech Republic, there was a mushrooming of outpatient departments, pedopsychiatric establishments under medical faculty hospitals, and mental homes. There was increasing cooperation with school guidance counsellors.

In 1961, a sub-department of child psychiatry was established under the Institute of Postgraduate Training (IPT) and in 1963 the first three pedopsychiatrists passed their final qualification exams.

Since 1961, 189 physicians have passed their fellowship boards and have become CAP experts, i.e., there is one pedopsychiatrist per 100,000 inhabitants. In 1998, there will be 12 pedopsychiatric inpatient establishments under clinics, hospitals, and mental homes disposing 390 beds and 4 pedopsychiatric mental homes with 368 beds.

Recent advances

Immediately after the political changes in 1989, a group of experts began working under the auspices of the Ministry of Health (MoH), and in 1990, they elaborated a draft of a new health care system. The main principles of this draft were the following:

- The new system of health care will form part of a global strategy for health regeneration and promotion.
- The state will guarantee adequate health care to all citizens.
- Health services will be provided in a competitive environment.
- Every community shall implement the principles of the state health policy in its territory.
- Every citizen will have the right to choose his physician and health care facility.
- The monopolistic position of the state health services will be abolished. The prevailing form of health care will be public health services. (Provision of health care services for the "public" was understood to be offered regardless of ownership of the health facilities, i.e., either private, communal, of church or state.)
- A basic element of public health care will be the autonomous health care facilities (with its own legal status, in contrast to the components of the former Distric Institutes of National Health – DINHs).
- Therapeutical care will particularly focus on primary health care and also on outpatient care in general.
- The health care will derive its financial means from different sources (insurance funds, state budget, community resources, enterprises, citizens, etc.).
- An obligatory health insurance will form an indispensable part of the health care system.

Current situation

Psychiatric disorders represent 2–3 % of the health problems in the Czech Republic. 10 % are children with psychic disturbances. 10 % are alcohol and drug addictions, which are on the rise. The incidence of accomplished suicides is steadily decreasing.

Psychiatry consumes 2–3 % of the total health care expenditure. Psychiatrists represent 2.8 % of total doctors. Psychiatric beds represent 12.4 % of total medical beds (11,640 psychiatric beds – 1.1 per 1,000 inhabitants). There are 11,400 psychiatric beds in mental hospitals and 10,420 beds in psychiatric departments of general hospitals. In the last 6 years, the capacity of psychiatric beds has decreased by 20 %. 33 % of the capacity of the psychiatric clinics are occupied by long-term patients (their hospitalization exceeds one year).

The long-term trend of ever decreasing birth rate (seen throughout the industrial world) has been with us since the mid 1970s and in 1997 it reached a minimum level. In the last decade, birth rate indicators were consistently below the sustainable reproduction line, despite the fact that the number of people over 60 has more than doubled since 1945, due to decrease in mortality rate (e.g., longer average life expectancy).

This section is based on an OECD study (by the Czech Association for Health Services Research) and the 1997 Czech Health Statistics Yearbook.

The health care sector still has not seen any major restructuring schemes. The government investment policy did not mend the imbalance in the structure and technical equipment of various hospitals and health establishments. Each year, the Ministry of Health calls for subsidies, but no analysis of needs, concept and – mainly – changes in financing have been carried out. Currently, a controlled restructuring of beds, hospital tenders (i.e., Ministry of Health picks hospitals worth signing an insurance agreement with), and attempts to increase the coverage of long-term care costs are now under way. The ideal reduced number of beds would be about 54,000 acute and 30,000 long-term care beds.

In pedopsychiatry, the reduction is not necessary. There are 368 beds in specialized institutes for children and 390 beds in child psychiatric departments under hospitals and mental homes.

The number of children and adolescents hospitalized with a mental disorder is approximately 12,000. (The break down according to psychiatric diagnoses is 24 % per F 20–29 and 8 % per F 30–39.) The number of children and adolescents registered for using psychoactive substances is ever rising. The 1994 figure was around 2,000, out of which 221 were children. In the age group under 15, the male-female ratio is 1.5:1 which later on goes up to 2:1.

When examining disturbing social phenomena, we rarely come to positive conclusions. With regard to suicides, however, it is safe to say that in the Czech Republic the number of suicides is gradually decreasing. The 1994 data (the latest data available) are the lowest of the last three decades. Comparing 1970 with 1994 (18 suicides per 100,000 inhabitants), there was a 30 % drop. The suicide rate in boys from 5–14 years of age is 2–3 times higher than in girls. (As opposed to other countries, in the Czech Republic there is a considerable difference in male-female suicide ratio already in such young children.) The number of suicides committed by children and adolescents (younger than 19) is 86 suicides per 100,000 inhabitants and accounts for 4.6 % of the overall number. The small increase in suicides committed by male adolescents reflects changes in the Czech drug scene. More and more adolescents are experimenting with illicit drugs and still more are becoming addicted to "hard drugs", resulting in a higher incidence of lethal intoxication. These may be considered suicides in the broader sense of the word.

2. Classification systems, diagnostic and therapeutic methods

Classification systems

In all Czech hospitals and outpatient establishments, the ICD-10 classification system is used. Insurance companies demand an ICD-10 diagnosis for each medical or psychological treatment, otherwise, they refuse to cover the bill. Nevertheless, apart from the ICD-10, the DSM-IV classification and diagnostic system is often used at university clinics and research departments. In training centers, like the IPT or Faculty Hospitals and Clinics (FHCs), the complex diagnosis is assessed according to 5 basic axes. Axis 1 represents the clinical diagnosis (in the case of a mental retardation, it is either the basic or the second diagnosis), axis 2 reflects the development of personality and its characteristics, axis 3 contains the somatic disorders affecting mental and intellectual development or directly linked to the diagnosed psychiatric disorder. Axis 4 includes psychosocial stressors, and axis 5 covers the overall adaptation potential of the patient. The diagnosis is expected to provide a clinical picture from the etiological (possibly also genetic), psychodynamic, psychosocial, therapeutic, and prognostic viewpoints.

Diagnostic methods

Pedopsychiatric and pedopsychological examination defines the intellectual and developmental level reached by the child, the interpersonal relationships, family communication patterns, and deviant forms of behavior. When suspecting an organic cause of the disease, a neurological examination, EEG recording (including sleep deprivation), CT, and sometimes even NMR or SPECT is advised. Often, a genetic, endocrinological, speech therapy, and other examinations are deemed necessary. Basic hematological and biochemical examinations are considered a matter-of-course.

Therapeutic methods

The majority of outpatient and inpatient establishments employ pharmacotherapy along with some sort of psychotherapy. A small number of establishments (mainly psychological centers) employ psychotherapy alone. Recently, we have witnessed a growing demand for child psychoanalysis, perhaps as a reaction to the suppressive approach towards dynamic psychotherapeutic methods under communism. More CAP experts are being trained in behavior-cognitive techniques. Also, several psychotherapeutic centers for family therapy have been founded.

3. Structure and organization of services

Guidelines for services for children and adolescents with psychiatric disorders

In 1998, a new concept of psychiatry is to be adopted. The basic structure of the future CAP is the following:

- Complex pedopsychiatric treatment is provided for children and adolescents younger than 18 (according to the Convention on Rights of Children, part I, p. 1, a child is any human being younger than 18) who are suffering from a mental disorder or for those in an acute, life-threatening, critical situation. The care comprises description, diagnostics, classification, treatment, rehabilitation, re-education, and prevention of mental disorders in this very age group. It explores the degree of individualization of the child, his/her family, and social background, adaptation potential and quality of mental health.
- A multidisciplinary approach is a guarantee of cooperation with other branches of medicine or other children and youth organizations and institutions.
- Approximately 19 % of the population is younger than 18. About 13 % of them are estimated to suffer from some kind of mental disorder requiring professional assistance. Special assistance is usually provided by psychiatric inpatient and outpatient establishments. There are also 154 special institutes of social youth care with 12,200 beds for children and adolescents. About 1,600 of the patients are permanently invalid and 4,200 need permanent assistance. Out of the total, 141 institutes are designed for the mentally handicapped (11,000 beds), 8 for the mentally and physically handicapped (230 beds), and 5 for the physically handicapped only (1,200 beds). These are 1993 figures. The 1997 scene is the following: institutes for physically handicapped youth – 1,082 places, institutes for physically handicapped youth suffering from a combination of handicaps – 115 places, institutes for physically and mentally handicapped youth – 678 places, institutes for mentally handicapped youth – 9,903 places.

Types of services

The Czech Republic has a satisfactory net of outpatient establishments which are gradually being privatized. There are 110 outpatient departments employing 80 CAP experts. The bed care is provided in all sorts of establishments. Altogether, there are 460 beds in the psychiatric hospital departments and 410 beds in mental homes. The bed care of children is quite satisfactory, but there is a critical gap in the care of adolescents. There are no adolescent inpatient facilities, no day and night care establishments, no crisis centers, protected workshops, temporary accommodation facilities, adolescent group homes, etc.

The Czech Republic does not have a single bed establishment for adolescents or adolescent drug users. The care of adolescent drug users younger than 15 is provided by adult drop-in centers. Having successfully handled the acute phase, the adolescents have nowhere to go. They are sent home and experience tells us that the subsequent inpatient care (which is almost never on a day-to-day basis) is badly insufficient. The indicator of drug dependency among children (under 15) is rising steadily. Child drug users are typically admitted to child anesthesiology and resuscitation departments and then sent to mental homes and psychiatric departments, where there is no innovative program to offer them.

Outpatient services

Psychiatric outpatient care of children and adolescents comprises psychiatric diagnostics and is provided in cooperation with other health and non-health establishments. Types of care included are dispensary care, complete therapy, rehabilitation, re-education, and possible re-socialization of children and adolescents. All forms of psychotherapeutic approaches, both individual and group, are employed, including parent and family therapy. There is one establishment per 100,000–150,000 inhabitants.

What is missing in the Czech Republic and what is the new concept – due in 1998 – to bring?

Mainly more forms of psychiatric outpatient care of children and adolescents are missing.

Outpatient dispensary care

The number of children and adolescents treated for a mental disorder amounts to 23,000 (of which 18,000 are children and 5,000 adolescents) or to less than 1 % of the total number of children and adolescents in the Czech Republic.

Children and adolescent crisis centers

Children and adolescent crisis centers provide pedopsychiatric care aimed at acute conditions, with a possible short-term admission to a hospital or a daycare establishment. In extreme cases, a parent may be admitted together with the patient for a couple of days. It is a first-contact establishment, which can be either on its own or combined with another bed establishment or adult crisis center offering professional pedopsychiatric care. The crisis center may include a child and adolescent telephone help line. The help line operates either 24 h a day or less and is manned by people with different professional backgrounds. There are 4–6 help lines per 100,000 inhabitants.

Daypatient services

Daycare establishments are therapeutic units offering intensive curative care impossible to provide on an outpatient basis. The emphasis is laid on psychotherapeutic, educational, re-educational, and rehabilitation programs (e.g., after-treatment of mentally ill children and adolescents, programs for children with specific learning disorders, etc.). At intervals these centers can also be used for specific work with adolescents. The daycare establishments are run either on their own (contrary to WHO recommendation) or under CAP hospital departments, mental homes or crisis centers.

Inpatient services

The organization of bed care is effective only at the regional level, i.e., covering approximately 1 million or more inhabitants.

- Regional hospitals (a region covering about 100,000 inhabitants) need small diagnostic-curative centers for pedopsychiatric patients. These centers may be combined with a pedopsychiatric outpatient establishment, a crisis center, etc. and typically have 4–8 beds located in the pediatric department. There is one diagnostic-curative center per 100,000–150,000 inhabitants.
- CAP departments exist under hospitals in a catchment area of approximately 100,000 inhabitants, providing diagnostics and treatment of disorders in children without breaking the family ties. Five beds are needed per 100,000 inhabitants. If there are more than 10 children in one department, a class must be set up, ideally led by a teacher of children with special needs. These beds may form a part of daycare establishments or crisis centers.
- CAP departments under mental homes are designed for diagnostics in cases of patients who need more than outpatient treatment, i.e., who need long-term inpatient care (up to several months). The continuity of school attendance is provided in these departments, as well as in the mental homes, and patients are being educated according to their condition. Five beds are needed per 100,000 inhabitants.
- CAP departments of psychiatric clinics provide highly professional, all-embracing, complex psychiatric care, a fusion of psychiatry, clinical science, and education in medicine. Psychiatric clinics concentrate all professional material capacity needed for psychiatric research and education in psychiatry, both pre- and postgraduate. They are usually joined with medical faculties.
  Charles University has 7 faculties (3 in Prague and 4 in large Bohemian and Moravian cities).
- Mental homes for children are expected to reduce the number of beds due to systematic development of outpatient and intermediary services. Mental homes for children are designed for children with poor academic and social performance who need long-term health and educational care. Typically, these would be CAP department patients where outpatient and intermediary care and treatment was not sufficient.

Currently, there are 5 mental homes for children, with 413 beds for psychiatric patients. The world standard would be 6-8 beds per 100,000 inhabitants, in the Czech Republic the ratio is 4 beds per 100,000 inhabitants.

Complementary services and rehabilitation

The Czech Republic lacks all complementary services helping children, but much more adolescents, to integrate back into real life. What we lack most are day and night care facilities, short-term boarding arrangements for youth, adolescent group homes, centers with specific programs designed not only for treated drug users, centers for under age delinquents, protected workshops and workplaces, rehabilitation facilities for children and adolescents with learning and developmental disorders, for psychotic patients in remission or chronic psychiatric patients (children and adolescents).

Foster homes and special foster homes for children with conduct disorders belong to the Department of Education. Pedopsychiatrists employed there are mere opinion givers.

In extreme cases there should be the possibility of sending 15–18 year-old adolescents to protected workshops with a production scheme designed for adults.

Personnel

The Czech department of psychiatry currently employs 1,539 fully qualified physicians. There are 130 CAP professionals (35 males, 95 females). Under the new concept the basic teams of professionals - pedopsychiatry is mainly a team type of work – should consist of the following:

- *CAP outpatient department:* 1 pedopsychiatrist, ideally 3–5 clinical psychologists, qualified psychotherapists, 1 nurse or social worker per 100,000–150,000 inhabitants, higher health personnel, bachelors.
- *Crisis center:* specialized physician or clinical psychologist, bachelors, qualified psychotherapist, nurse, social worker, rehabilitation professional, higher health personnel, lawyer, etc.
- *Daycare facility:* psychiatrist, nurse, other physicians, clinical psychologists, qualified psychotherapists, social worker, bachelors, rehabilitation professionals, ergotherapists, higher health personnel, specially trained teachers, speech therapists, and other paramedical personnel.
- *Bed care facility:* 1 pedopsychiatrist, ideally 3–5 clinical psychologists, qualified psychotherapists, 1 nurse or social worker per 100,000–150,000 inhabitants, higher health personnel, bachelors.

- *CAP departments under hospitals:* psychiatrists and other physicians, clinical psychologists, qualified psychotherapists, lower health personnel, higher health personnel, paramedical personnel, auxiliary health personnel, social workers, ergotherapists, physiotherapists, teachers, possibly specially trained teachers, speech therapists, other professionals with university education, and others.
- *CAP departments under mental homes:* 1 pedopsychiatrist, ideally 3–5 clinical psychologists, qualified psychotherapists, 1 nurse or social worker per 100,000–150,000 inhabitants, higher health personnel, bachelors.
- *Mental homes for children:* pedopsychiatrists and other physicians, clinical psychologists, qualified psychotherapists, lower health personnel, higher health personnel, paramedical personnel, auxiliary health personnel, social workers, ergotherapeutists, physiotherapists, teachers, possibly specially trained teachers, school masters, speech therapists, other professionals with university education, and others.

Funding of services

Health care in the Czech Republic is covered partly out of the state budget and partly by the insurance companies. The state budget provides for medical research, education of physicians, programs against drug abuse, the running of mental homes, etc.

Children and adolescents, university students, and the retired are insured by the state. All CAP bed and outpatient care, including rehabilitation is covered by insurance companies. Long-term care of under age patients is covered by the state. Once of age, these patients receive a disability pension from the Department of Labor and Social Affairs. Since the early 1990s, the cost of pharmaceuticals has risen sharply. As the West European investors entered the Czech market, the cost of pharmaceuticals rose by 500 % from 1990 to 1996. All pharmaceuticals administered in hospitals and institutions are covered by insurance companies. The same is true of the majority of prescribed pharmaceuticals. In the case of some foreign compounds, patients participate in the payment, with the exception of drugs with vital indication.

Evaluation

Admission to a hospital on the grounds of a mental disorder is still a social stigma in the Czech Republic. People are afraid of being "marked" and parents fear a psychiatric record will hinder the social achievements of the child. Charity organization and sponsorship is much more willing to allocate funds for the physically handicapped (e.g., leukemia, blindness) rather than the mentally retarded, let alone "madmen", i.e., mentally ill children. Whatever euphemism you use, what springs to people's mind is the image of some "crazy" individuals, generally feared and despised, and, what is worse, better to be eluded as if they did not exist. That is why many centers use "cover-up" names like Blue Key Center, Spiral, Green Court, etc. Many parents say at school that their child attends "psychological consulting".

In the Czech Republic there is not one global evaluation study of CAP care. There are several papers on the pedopsychiatric care in a defined administrative unit. What is available, though, is the Czech Health Statistics Yearbook, containing detailed demographic data concerning the state of health of the Czech population, network of health establishments, the manpower and the labor, and economic indicators. The international comparison includes basic demographic indicators and mortality rates by causes of death (infant mortality rate included). The psychiatry section contains dispensary services data, number of invalidity or partial invalidity benefits paid, number of psychiatric examinations, and the most frequent diagnostic categories. Very inaccurate and "tip-of-the-iceberg" kind of data are those concerning drug dependencies, but still are the only data available. On the other hand, very precise are the data concerning people placed into outpatient protected care (for forensic reasons).

In 1997, the following data stopped being collected and presented: dispensary services, number of psychiatric examinations of children and adolescents (with the exception of F 70–98 diagnoses), the number of drug dependencies. According to the 1997 yearbook (data collected through Dec. 31, 1996), there were 23,544 first examinations of patients with F 80–98 psychiatric diagnoses (i.e., developmental disorders in children and adolescents) and 16,270 examinations of patients with F 70–79 diagnoses (i.e., mental retardation). In the age group 18–19 years, 1,654 invalid benefits and 319 partial invalid benefits were paid.

4. Cooperation with medical and non-medical disciplines

Cooperation with pediatrics

The cooperation takes on the form of both consulting and double care (e.g., cooperation between a child neurologist and a child psychiatrist when treating a specific group of epileptic patients). The Czech Republic lacks special bed care units or outpatient departments for children with a combination of somatic and mental disorders. The psychiatric examination has a consulting nature: the child is hospitalized in a pediatric department and then is transferred to outpatient psychiatric care, always in cooperation with one or more child specialists of different medical branches.

Cooperation with psychiatry

CAP departments are often found under psychiatric clinics and mental homes. Family centers also nurture close cooperation of the basic branch professionals and specialized branch professionals. Research tries to answer questions like continuity or discontinuity of mental disorders, equal or different response to pharmaceuticals in different age groups, the possible prevention of future adult psychopathology through preventive care in childhood, etc.

Cooperation with doctors in private practice

The physicians who opened their own private practice usually remained at their original workplaces. The net of outpatient establishments is still sustained and the cooperation works well.

To perform a pedopsychiatric examination no pediatric note is required. Private physicians have signed agreements with insurance companies who cover the care these physicians perform. Children and adolescents are insured by the state who provides for them.

Cooperation with non-medical institutions and professionals

The closest form of cooperation is that with psychologists. Psychologists together with social workers constitute the basic pedopsychiatric team. Still before the 1989 "Velvet Revolution", school guidance counseling centers were set up, employing a psychologist and sometimes a social worker. Psychologists and psychiatrists today are separate and independent entities. Each works on his/her own, reporting to his/her insurance company, and the basic team is disintegrating. The cooperation, however, is still present, but its quality and frequency now mainly depends on interpersonal relationships.

One of the important parts of pedopsychiatric care is cooperating with the school facility that the patient attends. (This is particularly true of patients with hyperkinetic disorders, specific developmental and conduct disorders.) Cooperation with schools for the educationally subnormal (ESN schools), staffed by specialists who have studied the handicapped, is of vital importance. Schools for children with special needs are designed for handicapped children. Upon the completion of the compulsory school attendance, the pedopsychiatrist, together with a psychologist, helps the children choose their profession and a suitable workplace.

The Department of Care for Child and Family, under city councils and local government offices, fall under the jurisdiction of the Ministry of Labor and Social Affairs. These departments in cooperation with a child and adolescent psychiatrist address the problem of parental custody when a marriage breaks up, placement of children in foster families, children's homes, and foster homes with a special regime (when parents cannot handle the child). Typically, these would be socially disrupted families due to alcohol or other drug dependency, delinquency, prostitution, etc., in rare cases families where one of the parents suffers from a serious mental disorder. The handicapped and mentally retarded children and adolescents are also placed in institutes of social care.

Issues like juvenile delinquency prevention, child sexual abuse, mistreatment and neglect are addressed with the participation of the Ministry of Justice. In the last three years, juvenile delinquency has become a matter of serious concern in the Czech Republic. The number of aggressive criminal offences and racially motivated offences is rising (skinheads attacking gypsies). Moreover, the unemployment rate is increasing.

5. Graduate/postgraduate training and continuing medical education

Graduate training: The role of medical faculties

There are 7 medical faculties in the Czech Republic. Psychiatry (both general and special) is part of the syllabus in all of them. However, none of the faculties offers a CAP course. Some faculties offer courses in practical psychotherapy, e.g., communication skills, usually as an optional subject during the 7th or 8th term. The general and special psychiatry course in the fifth year of study has the form of a 3-week block of theoretical lectures and practical exercise, concluded by a final exam. CAP is made an integral part of general and special psychiatry. Also, a couple of questions in the tests, evaluated through computers, cover pedopsychiatry. On October 31, 1996, there were 6,355 students studying at the 7 aforementioned medical faculties.

Postgraduate training, a joint effort

Upon the completion of the 6-year study and passing the final exams, students of medicine graduate and receive an M.D. diploma. (There is an obligatory 1-year draft for men.) Further, there are two levels of specialized boards (residency boards and fellowship boards). After 2–3 years of professional practice in hospitals (practical experience in internal medicine, surgery, gynaecology and obstetrics of at least 3 months is required), the physicians choose where they wish to work. They register at the Ministry of Health and in the IPT. The IPT then sets the date when they can take the residency boards in one of the five basic branches of medicine – internal medicine, gynaecology and obstetrics, surgery, psychiatry, and pediatry. The exam consists of a test and a practical part, and the following day a theoretical part takes place before a committee of experts. Having passed the boards, they become officially experts in the given branch. The above mentioned boards are obligatory for all physicians.

If a physician wishes to specialize in CAP, having passed the residency boards in psychiatry or pediatry, he has to work for at least 3 years in the given branch. Six years after graduation he can enroll in the IPT to take the CAP fellowship boards. The special CAP postgraduate program embraces the following:

- 1 year of psychiatric practical experience (working with physicians who passed pediatric residency boards)
- 3 years of CAP practical experience (working with physicians who passed psychiatric or pediatric residency boards)

Three months of practical experience in neurology is recommended to all physicians and for those who passed psychiatric residency boards a 3-month practical experience in pediatrics is deemed fit. Both theoretical and practical preparation takes place at clinics, in mental homes, hospitals, outpatient departments of health centers, in surgery departments, and various other centers.

Physicians have to work under supervision and at least once a year attend an IPT course. Having enrolled to take their boards, they take a test evaluated by a computer. If they score less than 70 %, the date of the boards is postponed. Before taking the exam, physicians undergo a 6-week preparatory study at an IPT clinic.

The CAP fellowship boards breaks down into two parts: practical (case report with emphasis placed on differential diagnosis and all specific forms of treatment) and theoretical. During the theoretical part the trainee defends his scientific paper (minimum 20 pages) before a committee and answers 4 questions (one concerning legislation and health care system, 2 concerning general psychiatry, and 2 concerning particular issues connected to his/her specialization). The committee consists of a chairman, a CAP expert (member of the Medical Chamber), one specialist from the Ministry of Health, and one other professional. The committee assesses the trainee's knowledge and decrees whether he/she passed or failed. In the case of an excellent result, the grading is copied down into his/her record book and a note is sent to his/her boss. Physicians who passed their CAP fellowship boards receive a diploma and become CAP experts. With this diploma they are granted permission to open their own private practice.

Within the cooperation with the EU (both IACAPAP and ESCAP), IPT recommends the harmonization of CAP educational programs according to objectives set by the EU.

The new postgraduate training program has the following structure:

- 1 year of psychiatry
- 4 years of CAP (1-year practice in hospitals, mental homes, clinics or day care facilities, 2.5-year practice in outpatient establishments, centers, and surgeries, 3-month pediatric, and 3-month neurological practice)
  - theoretical training – 680 hours of professional training (including congresses, conferences, workshops, and interdepartmental commissions)
  - practical training – 170 hours of clinical supervision
  - psychotherapeutic training – 170 hours of theoretical workshops, 100 hours of individual or group self awareness training
  - research – 170 hours of supervised research

Continuing medical education in child and adolescent psychiatry and psychotherapy

The IPT organized 32 professional courses. In the 1960s and 70s the courses lasted 2 weeks. Later, each course was dedicated to one topic taking 1-2 days. To date, 92 CAP courses have been organized. Theoretical lectures are offered in the IPT and at the special psychotherapeutic faculty. Practical experience can be obtained through individual or group self-awareness training. In 1997, a sub-department of psychotherapy was set up in the IPT, under the department of psychiatry. Since the establishment of IPT, all physicians have their record books, where all theoretical training and practical experience is recorded. All activities and evaluation of their work is carried out by their boss (typically a senior consultant – head of clinic), who is in charge of the postgraduate training. Before passing the fellowship boards, IPT holds a 6-week study at the psychiatric clinic, seat of CAP sub-department.

Since 1961, the first Wednesday every month, the Medical Association of J. E. Purkyne holds a workshop, attended by psychiatrists coming from all over the Czech Republic. Through 1997, 360 workshops had taken place. Every 2 years, a "Youth Mental Health" workshop is held in Brno, the capital of Moravia. Through 1997, there were 18 of them. For more than a decade now, every other year a 2-day discussion meeting of pedopsychiatrists called "Oparanské dny" (Oparany days) is held. (Oparany is the seat of the oldest and largest child mental home in the Czech Republic.)

6. Research

Research fields and strategies

CAP research activities in the Czech Republic are rather scarce. Some studies (e.g., in schizophrenia, Tourett's disease, co-occurrence of diseases, hyperkinetic disorders, tics) are carried out at clinics and typically are part of dissertation or thesis projects. There is no global systemic research concept in CAP. Pedopsychiatrists sometimes participate in genetic, pediatric or psychiatric research teams studying, for example, fragile X syndrome, stomach ache in children or eating disorders. Under the Psychiatric Research Institute pedopsychiatric research is occasionally carried out, e.g., a longitudinal study of exposure to negative life events, drug dependencies, delinquency, deprived and sub-deprived children. Recently, thanks to grants, studies were carried out concerning aggressiveness, mental development of unwanted children and their adoption, sexual abuse, use of biofeedback in hyperkinetic children, etc.

Other types of studies recently launched are usually financed by pharmaceutic companies and are dedicated to standardization of dosages and use of new, atypical antipsychotic drugs in children and adolescents.

A study on new brain imaging methods used in tics and hyperkinetic disorders is still missing.

Research training

Under the new concept, research is made part of CAP postgraduate training. However, so far no CAP research educational programs (including practical training) have been carried out.

Funding

Funding of research is usually taken care of by grant agencies, sometimes pharmaceutic companies. Despite money being usually the very prerequisite of research, the financial question still has not been settled.

7. Future perspectives

Research

It is important to pick out educational centers fit for postgraduate training to become a place for research activities and education and training in scientific methods and approaches.

In cooperation with basic psychiatry researchers and foreign CAP research professionals, it is vital to train experts ready to become heads of CAP postgraduate training.

It is necessary to pick out basic research projects to be harmonized within the international cooperation framework.

New legislation addressing funding of research should be drafted and both state and non-governmental organizations should be solicited to get involved in the support of CAP research projects.

EU countries research centers should be contacted in order to learn to choose suitable projects and avoid repeating mistakes.

Training

It is important to pick out the best training centers, appoint trainers in research, theoretical training and clinical practical experience, including psychotherapeutic training.

The Czech Republic also aspires to become a member of EFTA (European Forum for All Psychiatric Trainees).

Improvement of services and care systems

It is necessary to

- streamline the system, network, and activity of health establishments
- gain support from the government and the parliament to launch the establishment of departments for adolescents, construction of daycare facilities and the so-called intermediary psychiatric services network, including rehabilitation and complementary services, under the new concept
- train experts and provide care for drug addicts younger than 15 (currently there is no care offered to these minors) and gradually also expand the care for adolescents (who, in the most severe cases, are handed over to adult psychiatrists and placed in detoxicant departments for adults, with little possibility of any after-treatment care).

Child and adolescent psychiatry in Denmark

P. H. Thomsen

1. Definition, historical development, and current situation

Definition

Child/adolescent psychiatry provides diagnoses and treatment for children and adolescents suffering from psychiatric disorders and conditions. The majority of these patients have normal cognitive abilities, while others suffer mental retardation. The core group of patients have psychotic disorders, affective disorders, personality disorders, and pervasive developmental disorders (i.e., conditions similar to that of autism). Other patient groups include those with conduct disorders, emotional disorders, and somatic disorders. Child/adolescent intervention is closely connected to the patient's family and surroundings. Community-based working methods are frequently required in the case of adolescents whose treatment methods include psycho-education, psychotherapy, pharmacotherapy, and environmental therapy.

Historical development

The first child-psychiatric outpatient unit was opened in Copenhagen in 1935. During the forties, two further units were opened, one in Copenhagen and the other in Aarhus. During the seventies and eighties, further units were established, covering the majority of Danish counties. Prior to 1953, child psychiatry was not considered an independent entity, but was established by way of a clinical and theoretical education. In 1994 the new independant entity of child/adolescent psychiatry was established. It was created on the basis of the 40 year old specialist child/adolescent-psychiatry, which was formerly placed within child/adult psychiatry. The new specialist core groups are children and adolescents between the ages 0 and 18 years suffering from psychiatric disorders. The upper age limit is, however, flexible.

Current situation

Denmark has an approximate population of 5 million inhabitants. The country is divided into 14 counties. Twelve of these counties have a child-psychiatric unit, while adolescent-psychiatric units are also found in nine counties. Emergency facilities are found to a limited degree, with several units offering emergency or sub-emergency admittance within a two to three day period. Development over the past 10 years has not led to any increase in the number of available beds within child-psychiatry. For example, in the county of Aarhus (which has a population of 650,000), 72 beds were available to 0–16 year olds in 1972. Today, only 26 beds are available, together with a further 30 day beds only. In accordance with the principle of district-psychiatry, there has, therefore, been a significant expansion in the outpatient facility. Personnel from the wards have subsequently been transferred to outpatient departments.

2. Classification systems, diagnostic and therapeutic methods

Classification systems

In Denmark, the ICD-10 classification system is used in all child/adolescent units. All relevant information regarding the diagnosis (main diagnosis, second diagnosis, somatic diagnosis, etc.), including sex, age at referral, and admission details are collected in the Nationwide Psychiatric Case Register, which covers the entire country. This register serves as the basis for all extensive research, partly in a diagnostic division on a national level, and partly in a description of the course. This register has provided the opportunity to conduct anonymous research, has made it possible to observe specific diagnoses, etc., as well as providing the opportunity to follow-up particular patients, with the approval of scientific-ethical committees. Use of the diagnostic system was changed in 1992, where a direct switch was made from ICD-8 to ICD-10. The register has formed the basis of numerous research projects (Nielsen & Mølbak 1998, Thomsen et al. 1992, Thomsen & Jensen 1994, Thomsen 1996, Lorenzen 1997).

Diagnostic methods

In all child/adolescent psychiatric wards, diagnoses are based on a thorough knowledge of symptomatology, environmental and genetic relations. As yet, no standardized interviews or rating scales have been used, although they are now being introduced as part of the routine evaluation in several areas. In many places, function-neurological and neuro-psychological examinations now serve as part of the evaluation in children and adolescents. In a few places, specific diagnostical interviews are utilized for younger patients, whereas family-diagnostical instruments are utilized in other areas.

Therapeutic methods

Most frequently, treatment methods are eclectic. Some wards still use a psychodynamic approach as a primary option, while others utilize a systematically orientated family approach. However, the cognitive principles of therapeutic behavior are becoming more widely accepted. At the same time, an increased utilization and fine-tuning of the psycho-educational principle has been experienced. Medication has traditionally been used rarely within the child/adolescent group. In later years, however, an increase has occurred, particularly in the field of anti-depressant medications. This is partly due to a decrease in side-effects, and partly due to the biological connection of causes being gradually introduced in the treatment of patients. In the adolescent psychiatric wards, antipsychotics are widely used, as well as antidepressants, anti-epilepsy, prophylactic medicine, lithium, etc. No specific reference program for the treatment of individual, mental illnesses in children and adolescents has yet been developed, although work in this area is commencing in separate wards, as well as in the Danish Psychiatric Society's organization.

3. Structure and organization of services

Guidelines for services for children and adolescents with psychiatric disorders

Child and adolescent psychiatry is a separate entity, covering the age group 0–18 years. Twelve of Denmark's 14 counties have a child-psychiatric unit; 8 counties offer full-admittance, as well as day and outpatient treatment. One county offers a dayfacility and an outpatient facility, while 4 counties have an outpatient facility only. The majority of child/adolescent psychiatric wards are attached to the hospital sector and are administrated from the county's hospital administrations. In some counties, child/adolescent psychiatry was separated from the hospital sector (during the late eighties/early nineties), being transferred to social administration, either with adult psychiatry, or as a separate unit.
In spring 1998, the study by the Danish Health Board "Targets for the quality of child/adolescent psychiatry" was released; the study illustrates the following objectives for out-patient treatment:

- All counties must provide access to a child/adolescent psychiatric facility.
- All authorities dealing with children and adolescents must be in a position to refer a child/adolescent for psychiatric evaluation as well as be able to provide treatment.
- In cases of emergency, specialist advice must be available by telephone 24 h a day. Instant admittance, or in sub-emergencies, outpatient treatment (followed by full treatment within a couple of days) should also be available.
- In the case of normal referrals, an evaluation should be offered within a few weeks, no more than two months, and this should be followed by treatment, if required, at the earliest possible convenience.
- Where possible, parents of children/adolescents below the age of 18 years should be included.
- The child/adolescent and the parents should be provided with the appropriate treatment options, psycho-therapeutic, as well as social-psychiatric and biological.

- ▶ Immediate access to child/adolescent psychiatric counseling should be available at all times.
- ▶ Continuity of personnel during examination and treatment should be given high priority.

Furthermore, the following criteria have been listed for admittance:

- ▶ The child/adolescent psychiatric consultation during admittance should be on a professional basis, ensuring a cross-professionally/cross-technically based overall view of the child's/adolescent's symptoms and resources. It must, also, ensure the child's/adolescent's and the parent's positive participation during the course of the admittance.
- ▶ The child/adolescent and the parents should be given the option of individual-, family-, and group-orientated psycho-therapeutic treatment by well-educated personnel, dependent on requirements.
- ▶ The biological treatment methods must be constantly updated and meet the accepted, clinical practice in order that a rational pharmacotherapy can be fulfilled.
- ▶ Work within this field should be based on environmental therapeutic principles.
- ▶ The law of psychiatry regarding coercive measures must be strictly adhered to, and the use of force must be reduced to a minimum.
- ▶ Admittance must be a possible option and, if necessary, steps must be taken to protect particularly anxious, uneasy, aggressive, and suicidal children/adolescents in psychiatric units.

Furthermore, the study states that the objective of child/adolescent psychiatric counseling is to ensure a high professional standard, as well as ensure the development of liason work towards pediatrics, in adult psychiatry, obstetrics, and other special units.

At the same time, the study also stresses that the county's dissimilar expansion of the child/adolescent psychiatric field, coupled with the desire for decentralization into smaller units, as well as the expansion of the child/adolescent psychiatric counseling function, constitutes a real danger of decreasing professional expertise. It is, therefore, of paramount importance that individual units are developed as specialist education and research centers in order to strengthen the professional network and increase the level of professionalism. The study has drawn-up objectives for treatment consultations provided to groups of patients with particular ways of presenting a specific problem. It recommends that special areas be developed in accordance with the university hospitals in Aarhus, Copenhagen, and Odense. These so-called leading functions apply to the following areas:

- Severely complicated eating disorder cases
- Particularly complicated procedures for neuro-psychiatric sufferers
- Complicated psychotic conditions in children and youths
- More severe atypical development disruptions

With regard to separate county units or, perhaps, cross-county units (where several counties participate), it is recommended that expertise be developed to deal with the following special groups:

- Infant psychiatry
- Children whose parents suffer from mental-illness
- Mentally handicapped
- Those with neuro-psychiatric disruptions
- Eating disorders
- Sexually abused children and adolescents
- Suicidal children and adolescents.

In Denmark, the number of child/adolescent psychiatrists with a private practice is extremely low. In the majority of counties, no private pratice is found at all.

Regarding the social area, treatment homes for children with varying categories of mental illness have been established throughout the entire country, and in all counties psychological-pedagogical counseling centers have been established, modeled after the American Child Guidance Clinics. Furthermore, during the 1980s, several so-called "family workshops" were established in a number of municipalities. Here, family therapy is undertaken normally by social workers and social educationalists.

Personnel

Child/adolescent psychiatry is characterized by cross-professional/cross-technical participation, as well as family involvement and the remaining network. Work in the individual ward is undertaken by a leading specialist in child/adolescent psychiatry and also involves child/adolescent psychiatrists, trainee doctors, psychologists, social workers, nurses, educationalists, teachers, caregivers, physio- and occupational-therapists, as well as speech therapists and secretaries.

Funding of services

As in the case of all alternative medical treatment, referral for child/adolescent psychiatric treatment is free in Denmark. As yet, no private insurance schemes exist and all hospital treatment is financed by the state. The hospitals, including child/adolescent psychiatric units, are administered by the counties (there are 14 counties in Denmark). As in all other specialist areas, free choice of hospital is provided, providing the family with the option of a child/adolescent psychiatric unit outside their home county. In these cases, the home county would be responsible for financing the treatment. Exceptions to free choice of hospital are, however, the three university hospitals situated in Aarhus, Copenhagen, and Odense. Referrals to these units require a guarantee from the home county (i.e., a written guarantee that the home county is willing to finance treatment undertaken by the university hospitals). Referral to a private practice child/adolescent psychiatrist is also provided free of charge, as well as the right to at least 12 consultations per year.

As previously mentioned, an expansion of child/adolescent psychiatry has been agreed in the majority of Danish counties. Due to the present general lack of doctors and, therefore, the lack of qualified specialists, it has, however, been difficult to fill the positions, particularly in counties some distance from the university hospitals. Nationwide, there is a long waiting list for both evaluation and treatment. At present, the waiting list is between six and nine months.

There has been a great deal of political debate regarding these unusually long waiting lists. From a professional point of view, possible consequences have also been a major cause of concern.

4. Cooperation with medical and non-medical disciplines

Cooperation with pediatrics

The majority of child/adolescent psychiatric wards are responsible for counseling and ensuring liaison with the pediatric wards. This cooperation often functions in the form of unscheduled inspections, as well as routine weekly conferences, where children with suspected mental illnesses (psychosomatic symptoms, etc.) can be presented by the pediatricians and their symptoms discussed. Furthermore, neuro-pediatricians participate in planned conferences, where children from neuro-psychiatric wards are frequently discussed. Within the country's only existing infant ward in Copenhagen, there is close cooperation with pediatrics as well as the gynaecological/obstetrical wards. This cooperation focuses particularly upon those children whose mothers suffer from mental illness and children in "risk groups".

Cooperation with psychiatry

Child/adolescent psychiatry in Denmark has a traditionally, close cooperation with adult psychiatry. In most areas, the wards are actually linked geographically as well as administratively to one another. A natural field of cooperation is adolescent psychiatry which is organized in such a way that both the evaluation and treatment of patients up to 20–21 years of age is accommodated within the same facility. The decision to place adolescent psychiatry with child/adolescent psychiatry has been made. At the same time, however, adolescent psychiatrists with an adult psychiatry education have been chosen in order that both professions can be represented. In the majority of places, there is also cooperation regarding children whose parents are mentally ill. In just a few areas, there is also a positive research-related cooperation with psychiatry.

Cooperation with non-medical institutions and professionals

Child/adolescent psychiatry receives many referrals from non-medical professionals. Infants and school-children are frequently referred from pedagogical-psychological advisors, as part of a school system, supervised by psychologists. These groups are normally the first people to identify that a child has difficulties either via a teacher or via parents. Cooperation between those who provide educational and psychological advice is close, both leading up to referral and following evaluation or treatment. In many cases, the child/adolescent psychiatrist will suggest special educational measures, which must be implemented by the persons offering educational and psychological advice. In addition, child/adolescent psychiatry has close cooperation with county counselors, who are responsible for referring people for treatment within the appropriate institutions – an often vital link in the after-care of children and adolescents. Furthermore, there is close cooperation between the social services in the individual municipalities, regarding the effectuation of familial support, support for the child and, naturally, in cases where the admittance of a child is a possible option.

5. Graduate/postgraduate training and continuing medical education

Graduate training: The role of medical faculties

Lectures on child/adolescent psychiatry are offered as a medical speciality by Denmark's three medical schools in Copenhagen, Aarhus, and Odense. At the present time, however, the country boasts only one professorship in child/adolescent psychiatry. This was instituted in 1998 and is based at the University of Aarhus with a direct connection to the Child and Adolescent Psychiatric Hospital in Aarhus, Denmark. Until 1992, the professorship in the former "child psychiatry", was based at the University of Copenhagen, being directly connected to the hospital's child psychiatric ward. Since that time, however, the Copenhagen professorship has existed only as an unfilled position. Within the universities of Odense and Copenhagen, there are a number of associate professors in child/adolescent psychiatry. These staff members are responsible for education in the field of child/adolescent psychiatry. Medical students receive a theoretical education on the subject and are provided with the opportunity of spending a shorter period in child/adolescent psychiatric wards. Particularly interested students are given the opportunity to spend a "free choice month" in a child/adolescent ward. Examinations in child/adolescent psychiatry are placed during the penultimate year of medical studies. It has also been merged with the psychiatric examination of all three universities. Within the universities of Copenhagen and Aarhus, the examination is written, whereas, at Odense University, the examination is oral and video-based. The degree in child/adolescent psychiatry represents one third of the total psychiatric grade.

Postgraduate training, a joint effort

Following a concluded medical university examination, together with the following compulsory post-graduate terms of hospital service (six months of medicine, six months surgery and six months practical experience), the child/adolescent psychiatric specialist education consists of a 5.5 year long clinical education, which is constructed as follows:

Practical clinical education (4.5 years in all), consisting of an introductory period of employment (12 months duration), a teaching position (18 months duration, including 9 months of child psychiatry and nine months of adolescent psychiatry), as well as a position of senior registrar (24 months), divided into 12 months of child psychiatry and 12 months of adolescent psychiatry. Furthermore, supplementary education (12 months duration) is required, including six months psychiatry and six months pediatrics.

In addition to the clinical education, a theoretical education must be undertaken, frequently preceded by a psychiatric introductory course (approximately 60 h). The theoretical course on child/adolescent psychiatry consists of an obligatory course of a number of subcourses, covering the most vital aspects of the field. Finally, a basic education in psychotherapy is also required. In recent years, the clinical education has become more stringent, including the introduction of check lists, evaluation interviews, the appointment of doctors in charge of the education, as well as a newly introduced inspector arrangement (inspectors appointed by the Danish Psychiatric Society, who make evaluation visits to units having an educational obligation).

Until recently, only four specialists per year obtained a degree. However, owing to recent development in the field, as well as expansion, the decision to educate eight specialists per year has been made.

Continuing medical education

Despite the fact that child/adolescent psychiatry is a separate medical entity, it is not part of its own scientific society. The specialty is part of the Danish Psychiatric Society, as an addition to adult psychiatry. There is a joint board, as well as having joint treatment and research groups; however, child/adolescent psychiatry organizes its own separate section meetings. These are of specific interest to child/adolescent psychiatrists. From the approximate 1000 members of the Danish Psychiatric Society, 150 are child/adolescent psychiatrists. The Danish Psychiatric Society arranges courses for inservice training, which is relevant to psychiatrists as well as child/adolescent psychiatrists. At present, there is no formal requirement for continuing medical education (CME) in Denmark. On a more superior level, covering all specialties, the possibility of a more formal (and in some cases perhaps, obligatory, continuous inservice training) is being considered.

6. Research

Research fields and strategies

Research and guaranteed quality are two important aspects of the daily work within the field of child/adolescent psychiatry. Research and guaranteed quality ensures that daily treatment in the field of child/adolescent psychiatry is based on the best possible foundation. In recent years, a positive development has occurred with increasing research activities within child/adolescent psychiatric wards in Denmark. Among other things, this has resulted in more completed theses and Ph.D dissertations. Previously, the tradition of research has been minimal on a nationwide scale. A lack of resources has resulted in child/adolescent psychiatrists being obliged to give the urgent, clinical assignments higher priority than research.

The decentralized structure of child/adolescent psychiatry, with smaller clinical units (which do not form a satisfactory basis for a prosperous research environment), has resulted in scarce development of research within this field. Organizationally, however, there have been improvements. To this end, a professorship in child/adolescent psychiatry with an attached clinical assistant position has been established. Furthermore, active research environments have been established at all three university wards in the country.

Child/adolescent psychiatric research has focused largely upon clinically descriptive, epidemiological projects and clinical follow-up studies (Tolstrup 1957, Dahl 1965, Brask 1959, Thomsen 1996b, Aarkrog 1994, Larsen et al. 1990, Mouridsen et al. 1998, Lier et al. 1995). In these cases, the main focus has been set around attention disturbances, obsessive compulsive disorder, and borderline conditions in adolescents. In addition, a number of research centers participate in nationwide, clinical and international multicenter investigations relating to eating disorders in children/adolescents, as well as obsessive compulsive disorder. Furthermore, research in treatment methods among other things, pharmacological treatment of depression in adolescents and pharmacological/psychotherapeutic treatment methods in children/adolescents with obsessive compulsive disorder. Throughout the country, high level research into infant psychiatry has also taken place. One particular research center has also specialized in the standardization and validation of diagnostic interviews and screening instruments.

7. Future perspectives

Significant future research themes will relate to clinical research with a view to diagnostic classification as well as follow-up studies, in order to illustrate the long-term follow-up. Treatment research attempting to illustrate both psycho-pharmacological and psycho-therapeutic treatment will also be given a high priority. Furthermore, genetic research is improving, as is neuro-psychiatric research, where among other things an updated technique of brain imaging, together with quality control projects have been developed, all with the aim of ensuring quality in the daily work regarding clinical evaluation and treatment.

Organizationally, it has been necessary to establish research units which are connected to the three university wards and which have direct association with the clinic. The Danish Psychiatric Society has emphasized the importance of all three universities establishing professorships in child/adolescent psychiatry.

Selected references

Aarkrog T (1994) Borderline adolescents – 20 years later. Thesis. Bispebjerg Hospital, Dept. of Adolescent Psychiatry, Copenhagen. ISBN 87-984982-0-7

Brask BH (1959) Borderline Schizophrenia in children. Acta Psych et Neurol Scand 34 (4): 265–283

Dahl V (1965) The course of mental disorders in childhood. Thesis (in Danish). Munksgaard, Copenhagen

Danish Health Board (1997) Målsætning for kvalitet i børne- og ungdomspsykiatrien (in Danish) Sundhedsstyrelsen, Copenhagen

Larsen FW, Dahl V, Hallum E (1990) A 30-year follow-up study of a child psychiatric clientele. Acta Psych Scand 81: 39–45

Lier L, Gammeltoft M, Knudsen IJ (1995) Early mother-child relationship. The Copenhagen model of early preventive intervention towards mother-infant relationship disturbances. Arctic Medical Research 54 (1): 15–23

Lorenzen C (1997) The course and mortality of psychosis in adolescence. A Danish register-based investigation 1970–93. Thesis (in Danish). Psychiatric Hospital for Children and Adolescents in Aarhus, Denmark and Institute of Basic Psychiatric Research Department of Psychiatric Demography, Psychiatric Hospital in Aarhus

Mouridsen SE, Rich B, Isager T (1998) Validity of childhood disintegrative psychosis – General findings of a long-term follow-up study. Br J Psychiatry 172: 263–267

Nielsen S, Mølbak G (1998) Eating disorder and type 1 diabetes: Overview and summing-up. European Eating Disorders Review 6 (1): 4–26

Thomsen PH (1996a) A 22- to 25-year follow-up study of former child psychiatric patients: A register-based investigation of the course of psychiatric disorder and mortality in 546 Danish child psychiatric patients. Acta Psych Scand 94: 397–403

Thomsen PH (1996b) Obsessive-compulsive disorder in children and adolescents. A clinical follow-up study. Thesis. Institute of Basic Psychiatric Research Department of Psychiatric Demography, Psychiatric Hospital in Aarhus and Psychiatric Hospital for Children and Adolescents in Aarhus, Denmark. ISBN 87-900017-07-2

Thomsen PH, Møller LL, Dehlholm B, Brask BH (1992) Manic-depressive psychosis in children younger than 15 years. A register based investigation of 39 cases in Denmark. Acta Psych Scand 85: 401–406

Thomsen PH, Jensen J (1994) Obsessive-compulsive disorder: Admission patterns and diagnostic stability. A case-register study. Acta Psych Scand 90: 19–24

Tolstrup K (1957) Anorexia nervosa in childhood and adolescence. Thesis (in Danish). Munksgaard, Copenhagen

Child and adolescent psychiatry in Estonia

J. Liivamägi

1. Definition, historical development, and current situation

Definition

The field of child and adolescent psychiatry in Estonia is guided by Estonian "Law of Psychiatric Care" (1997) including the prevention of mental disorders, their diagnosis, treatment, psychological and social rehabilitation. Child and adolescent psychiatry is not at this time an independent specialty in Estonia. Thus, there are no special child and adolescent psychiatric hospitals or policlinics, and for that reason almost all child psychiatrists are working at general psychiatric hospitals and policlinics. Although their main activities concern child psychiatry, they must take part in duty work of general psychiatric institutions as well.

Historical development

The Republic of Estonia is a small country, situated on the coast of the Baltic Sea. The distance from east to west is 350 km and from north to south 240 km. The population is 1,496 million (1995); 71.6 % of whom live in urban settlements (Põlluste 1998). Trends and traditions in Estonian psychiatry and particularly in child psychiatry have had close relations with the history of Estonia as a country through history. In the 13th century the Estonian area was conquered by Germans and Danes, in 16th century by Sweden. The period of Swedish rule was a relatively prosperous time in Estonian history. Swedish King Gustav II Adolf opened in 1632 a university at Tartu, which played a central role for Estonian life, culture, and education in the coming centuries. As the result of the Great Northern War (1700–1721), which was started by Russian Csar Peter the First to "open a window to Europe", Estonia was annexed to the Russian Empire. Nevertheless, the German aristocracy in Estonia preserved all their rights, privileges, orientation, and cultural connections with Germany. Professors at the University of Tartu were also mostly invited from Germany (Laur 1989).

In the beginning and middle of 19th century, cursory recordings of persons with mental disorders in Russia demonstrated that their number in the three gubernias (Estlandia, Livlandia, and Kurlandia) was considerably higher than in other parts of the Empire (Saarma et al. 1981). Thus, based on this, philanthropic groups started to establish maintenance and help for children and persons with disabilities. Following examples of other European countries, between 1845 and 1901 7 special institutions for children were opened in Estonia for teaching, education, and guardianship. The czarist government did not take part in the material or moral support of such institutions (Kõrgessaar et al. 1987). Thanks to the activity and tenacity of surgery professor Eduard-Georg von Wahl (1833–1890) and his congenial associates, a psychiatric hospital as a basis for training for students of the medical faculty was opened in 1877 at the University of Tartu. Then, in 1880 the department of psychiatry and neurology at the University of Tartu was officially opened. Hermann Emminghaus (1845–1904), an assistant professor from the University of Würzburg (Germany), was elected as the first professor of psychiatry and neurology at Tartu. There is indirect evidence that Professor Emminghaus was also occupied with problems of mental health disorders in children during his Tartu period (1880–1886). During this period, he wrote the chapters "Children and irresponsibles" and "Dementia and Oligophrenia" for a forensic medicine textbook. After returning to Freiburg, Germany (1886), H. Emminghaus wrote "Psychic disturbances in childhood" (1887), the first textbook of child psychiatry in the world. The next professor of psychiatry after H. Emminghaus at the University of Tartu was Emil Kraepelin (1856–1926), who worked in Tartu from 1886–1891. Although Professor Kraepelin's influence to further develope Estonian psychiatry was very high for decades, there are no data about his and his successors Vladimir Tsiž (1855–1922), A. Justsenko (1868-1936), and M. Bresovsky (1877–1945) activities in the field of child psychiatry.

As a result of economic and political deterioration of the Russian Empire, the defeat of Russia in the First World War, and the revolution in February 1917, the majority of institutions for care of disabled children were closed. After establishment of the independent Estonian Republic (1920) by the initiative of physicians, intellectuals, feminist organizations, and with support from the Estonian government, some institutions to help disabled children were opened again. In the first period of the Estonian Republic (1920–1940), 7 more schools or maintenance institutions were additionally opened. At this time 450 children were in special schools and institutions (Kõrgessaar et al. 1987) (about 1,000,000 inhabitants lived in Estonia at that time). Estonian psychiatry had mainly followed the practices of the German school. In this period, there were 4 psychiatric hospitals in Estonia. Children with psychiatric problems were consulted and even rarely treated at the Psychiatric Clinic of the University of Tartu, but there was no systematic work with child psychiatry in Estonia.

During the Second World War the Estonian territory was completely occupied by the Soviet Union (1944). Connections with the "bad capitalistic West" were severed (associations with colleagues, subscription of literature, participation in international congresses, training in European countries, etc.). All medical and particularly psychiatric aid for the population was reorganized according to the principles of the Soviet Union. In 1944, Elmar Karu (1903–1996) was assigned as a professor of psychiatry and chief of Estonian psychiatrists. Estonian psychiatrists could take part in courses of specialization or continuing studies in central institutes of psychiatry in Moscow, Leningrad (St. Petersburg), and other places in the Soviet Union. They were invited to congresses/conferences in the Soviet Union and good personal connections arose between specialists. Still the unvaried conditions, preference and dictation of one-sided ideas or views and depreciation of others, the impossibility of first source acquaintance with trends, methods, and practice of psychiatry in other countries of the world formed general trends in psychiatry of the Soviet Union and in Estonia as well.

In Estonian psychiatry traditions and views that stemmed from Professors Emminghaus, Kraepelin, Tsiž and Bresovsky were alive; therefore, Estonian psychiatry did not follow the extreme tendencies of Soviet psychiatry. Professor Karu was also interested in child psychiatry, and later (1975) he delivered lectures about mental retardation and psychopathology of childhood and wrote a textbook on mental retardation (1981). In 1952 he sent one of the assistants to Moscow to study child psychiatry and then to deliver the psychiatric help to the children of Estonia. In the following years (after 1960) some psychiatrists also repeatedly went to Moscow and/or Leningrad, where they received training in the field of child psychiatry and started to work as child psychiatrists in Tartu (1963) and in other towns of Estonia (in the capital city – in Tallinn – 1963). In 1967 in Tallinn, in 1970 near the town of Viljandi, and in 1983 at the Psychiatric Clinic of the University of Tartu, child psychiatry wards for children at general psychiatric hospitals were opened. At that time in Estonia, there were about 120 beds for psychiatric services for children (ages 3–15 years) and 60 "neuropsychiatric" beds for children 1–3 years old with neurological disorders and deviations in development. Assistant Professor Lembit Mehilane (head of the Psychiatric Clinic 1983–1992) also had training in Moscow in the field of child psychiatry. He managed and stimulated the development of Estonian child psychiatry, delivered lectures about psychopathology of childhood, and wrote short textbooks about psychopharmacology and psychopathology of childhood (in cooperation with J. Liivamägi).

In the Soviet Union, psychology was underestimated for many years. Therefore, psychologists started to work in psychiatric hospitals in Estonia only in 1971, the first child psychologist in 1983. Thanks to the support of colleagues mainly from Scandinavian countries, Estonian psychiatry (and particularly child psychiatry) and psychology started to pay increasing attention to psychotherapy and family therapy.

Recent advances

After the collapse of the Soviet regime and reindependence of Estonia (1991), the number of beds in all psychiatric hospitals (including child psychiatric wards) has decreased and duration of hospitalization shortened by almost half. At the same time the number of outpatient visits has increased. These data indicate that emphasis in psychiatric care has shifted from inpatient treatment to outpatient treatment.

Current situation

On January 1, 1997, 1,462,130 inhabitants lived in Estonia, among them 25.6% children between 0–18 years (Põlluste 1998). Child and adolescent psychiatry and psychotherapy is represented in 3 hospitals (1 in a university department), with altogether 60 beds. There are a total of 46 specialists for child and adolescent psychiatry and psychotherapy, among them 20 child psychiatrists (2 of them are men).

Estonia has 1 child psychiatrist per 69,962 inhabitants or per 17,890 children and adolescents between 0–18 years of age. The ratio of child psychiatrists who work only in private practice (5 persons is 1 per 292,546 inhabitants or 1 per 75,140. Estonian psychiatrists are generally members of the Estonian Society of Psychiatrists, which has a section of child and adolescent psychiatry. Officially we have 10 members, but other child psychiatrists or specialists and some general psychiatrists are also taking part, in our specialized meetings on various child psychiatric topics.

2. Classification systems, diagnostic and therapeutic methods

Classification systems

In 1993 on the initiative of the Department of Psychiatry, ICD-10 was translated into Estonian and is used for diagnostic and scientific purposes. In all departments a case report as a basic document for each patient is completed, which includes family history, psychological and social problems, symptoms of disease, data of clinical investigations and opinions of specialists, multiaxial ICD-10 diagnosis, and a short description of therapeutic recommendations.

Diagnostic methods

To unify data about developmental dynamics and to describe the mental status of patients, special lists and several diagnostic scales are used. In all 3 child psychiatric wards EEG-recordings and in 2 hospitals MRI investigations are possible. Thanks to the material and moral support of Swedish colleagues of the child psychiatric ward at university hospital, the lekotek (toy library) was opened in 1993. In the lekotek a special teacher uses the special methodology of psychologic-pedagogic assessment for preschool children. Thanks to the good cooperation with neighboring disciplines, neurologic, genetic, and somatic examinations and consultations are used in all 3 wards. In complicated cases, teamwork has been used since 1994.

Therapeutic methods

The spectrum of therapeutic methods in Estonian child psychiatry depends on the availability and training of specialists. The psychodynamic approach in Estonian psychiatry is quite narrow (many child psychiatrists have studied child psychoanalysis in a course, which was supervised by Scottish and Finnish lecturers). The majority of child psychiatrists have completed courses in family therapy (thanks to the support of Sweden), and in cooperation with psychologists they use different psychotherapeutic methods in treatment. If it is indicated, we also use medication in the complex therapeutic process.

3. Structure and organization of services

Guidelines for services for children and adolescents with psychiatric disorders

Guidelines for services of Estonian child psychiatry are

- Psychiatric aid for children and adolescent with mental disorders will be provided in the broarder sense by family doctors, pediatrics, and/or the counties general psychiatrists;
- Child psychiatric aid can be delivered only by psychiatric institutions, doctors, and other specialists, who have the corresponding license;
- Mentally disturbed children and adolescents have all rights to receive treatment and guardianship in the same way as children with other disorders;
- The aim of services is to go closer to patients. That is, we train many child psychiatrists for work in pediatric hospitals, policlinics, and special schools.

Types of services

In our opinion there are now enough inpatient beds in Estonia, but the wards are too large (20 beds) and patients in wards are poorly differentiated by age. We cannot be content with outpatient service: although the number of child psychiatrists working in private practice will slowly increase, patients from outlying districts have difficulties coming for consultation.

Table 1. Services for mentally disturbed children and adolescents in Estonia

I Outpatient services
• Child and adolescent psychiatrists in private practice. • Other child and adolescent non-medical specialists in private practice (speech therapists, child psychologists). • Outpatient departments at pediatric, at general psychiatric hospitals, many child psychiatrists at pediatric institutions. • Family counseling services.
II Daypatient services
• One daypatient ward (10 beds) in a child psychiaric inpatient ward at a general psychiatric hospital.
III Inpatient services
• Inpatient service at the child psychiatric ward of the university hospital. • Inpatient services at child psychiatric wards of general state psychiatric hospitals.
IV Complementary services
• Rehabilitation services for special groups of patients (for patients with severe mental retardation, with autism, etc.). • Safeguard homes.

Outpatient services

The majority of outpatient consultations are carried out by child psychiatrists in outpatient units at child psychiatric wards, the minority by child psychiatrists in private practice. As a rule child psychiatrists provide help for children aged 3 to 18 years. Outside the medical field, 181 speech therapists, psychologists and special teachers take part in outpatient consultation and treatment to a certain extent. Several preschool children with mental and/or neurologic disabilities can additionally be evaluated and expanded in the lekotek (toy library) at the University Clinic of Tartu.

Daypatient services

There is only 1 daypatient ward (10 beds) at the general psychiatric hospital in Tallinn. It is closely linked with the inpatient department.

Inpatient services

In Estonia, there are 3 child psychiatric wards with 60 beds at the general psychiatric hospitals, including 1 university department. For young children up to 3 years of age, there is a neurologic ward at the Child Clinic of the University of Tartu for early detection and intervention.

Complementary services and rehabilitation

In connection with the reorganization of Estonian economics, complementary services are developing slowly. There are some child support centers, family counseling and support centers in towns, and also "Child Voice Center" and Crisis Center of Estonia for all people (in Tallinn). There is one rehabilitation institution for the handicapped with severe mental retardation, with autism, and neurologic damages.

Personnel

The number of child psychiatrists in Estonia has been around 20 for many years. There are 31 child psychologists.

Funding of services

In Estonia all people must pay 13 % of their earnings as social insurance. All patients are insured via the sick-fund, which pays the costs for outpatient, daypatient, and inpatient treatment, for investigations in psychiatric institutions, etc. directly to these institutions, family doctors or specialists in private practice. The costs for treatment of chronically ill, for children and adolescents with severe conduct disorders or for handicapped psychiatric children and adolescents in special institutions (special schools, maintenance service) are paid by the state.

Evaluation

From 1997–1998 an epidemiologic investigation of children's and adolescents' mental health and mental disorders was underway. One task of an epidemiological investigations is to obtain data about psychiatric disorders in the child population and on this basis ascertain the adequate need for child psychiatrists, psychologists, special teachers, speech therapists, etc. in Estonia.

4. Cooperation with medical and non-medical disciplines

Cooperation with pediatrics

In Estonia, pediatric hospitals have no wards for psychosomatic disorders. In some pediatric institutions (policlinics, support centers, in the Child Clinic at University of Tartu), there are also child psychiatrists working. Children and adolescents with somatic disorders, who need psychiatric help, will always be consulted by a child psychiatrist. Annually the Department of Psychiatry in Tartu organizes advanced courses (mainly 3–4, à 30 hours) for pediatricians, family doctors, and other specialists on current topics of child psychiatry.

Cooperation with psychiatry

Child and adolescent psychiatry in Estonia is very closely linked with general psychiatry. There are 2 common contact points with general psychiatry. First, the majority of child psychiatrists work in child psychiatric wards of general psychiatry hospitals. They take part in duty-work of the general hospital, have common clinical conferences, etc. Second, in many cases general psychiatric services are needed if there are emergency conditions, because child psychiatric wards are not equipped with closed sections of the ward for such patients, and in one ward are children of all ages.

Cooperation with doctors in private practice

In Estonia, private practice is developing very quickly. The cooperation with specialists in private practice is generally very good. Many child psychiatrists and other specialists, who are working in state or county/town psychiatric hospitals, are also working in private practice.

Cooperation with non-medical institutions and professionals

There have been rapid changes in the development of the non-medical system for children and adolescent services. Estonian child psychiatrists have the closest collaboration with the education system. By our investigations (1998), around 20% of pupils in our schools have learning difficulties, behavior problems, and/or depression, and the use of alcohol and drugs is increasing at a high rate. In Estonia there are special schools for children and adolescents with mental retardation, separate schools for teenage boys (two) and girls (one) with conduct disorders, 1 school for criminal adolescents (ages 15–18), and 2 boarding schools for children with long-lasting neurotic disorders. There are many special schools for children with severe impairment of vision (1), hearing (1) or damage of motor functions (1). An important institution for the cooperation with child psychiatry are inspectors for children and adolescents within the police force. They deal with children of asocial or divorced families, with children in support centers, with users of alcohol and/or drugs, etc. In legal proceedings with children or teenagers under 18 years, an examination and a statement must be made by a child psychiatrist.

5. Graduate/postgraduate training and continuing medical education

Graduate training: The role of medical faculties

In Estonia only the University of Tartu is training medical doctors. Child psychiatry is not represented by a separate department or chair. Thus, in the Department of Psychiatry at the University of Tartu, 1 assistant professor is working, who is a consultant in the field of child psychiatry. He carries out courses/lectures about childhood psychopathology for students in the department of special teachers. For medical students, lectures and practical works about child psychiatry are integrated into general psychiatry.

Postgraduate training, a joint effort

After six years of studies, medical students should pass the final examinations and practical training, which ends with the granting of a certificate to practice medicine. In Estonia doctors, who desire to receive the qualification in the field of child psychiatry must first undergo the training in general psychiatry. After 4 years of theoretical education and practical work in basic psychiatric hospitals, all trainees of general psychiatry must take an exam given by the Certification Board by Social Ministry to become professionals in general psychiatry. General psychiatrists or trainees, who want to obtain the level of competency in child psychiatry, must additionally work 1 year in a child psychiatric ward of a basic psychiatric hospital under the supervision of experienced colleagues. Theoretical education in child and adolescent psychiatry consists of 120 h of lectures, seminars, and case discussions, 60 h is the individual work of trainees. The training ends with an oral board examination at the commission of child psychiatrists by the Society of Estonian Psychiatrists.

Continuing medical education in child and adolescent psychiatry and psychotherapy

In Estonia all psychiatrists (and child psychiatrists) must pass an assessment of the level of competence in psychiatry every 5 years by a Certification Board. There are elaborate methods for assessment of the work and level of competence of psychiatrists. Psychiatrists and other specialists should continue psychiatric/ psychological education in courses of supplementary teaching by the Department of Psychiatry in Tartu or abroad.

Training programs for other disciplines

Topics of child and adolescent psychiatry are included in teaching programs for family doctors, teachers, special teachers, psychologists, and nurses.

6. Research

Research fields and strategies

Research in the field of child psychiatry in Estonia is carried out mostly at the Department of Psychiatry, University of Tartu. During the period of Soviet power, complementary services in psychiatry were developed weakly, and the leading form of therapy was biological therapy. Therefore, research in general psychiatry was dedicated to clinical psychopharmacology and to investigation of neurophysiological mechanisms of neurotic and psychotic conditions. In child and adolescent psychiatry through the 1980s investigations were dispersed. After the 1980s we investigated nootropic drugs (nootropil, phenibut) for neurotic and conduct disorders (enuresis, fears, ADHD, etc.) in children and adolescents. Since 1990, Estonian child psychiatrists have been engaged with 3 topics of research: 1) the epidemiological investigation of the mental state of children and childhood disorders; 2) risk factors in Estonia for mental health disorders of children; 3) children's temperament and its influence on structure and duration of mental disorders.

In the Department of Education of Children with Special Needs at the University of Tartu and at the Institute of Education of Tallinn investigations of learning disabilities and school problems have been carried out as well.

Research training and career development

Our young scientists take part in courses/lectures at the University of Tartu, but also in training seminars abroad (in Sweden) to increase the quality of research. In Estonia, research training seminars take place at the University of Tartu but there are no postdoctoral training programs yet.

Funding

Research work in Estonian child psychiatry is covered at relatively modest level by several sources:

- the Estonian Scientific Fund (Eesti Teadusfond),
- a part of studies is covered by Estonian Social Ministry,
- research work, which is supported by the sick-fund, and
- support from pharmaceutical companies.

7. Future perspectives

Research

There are three main directions in Estonian child psychiatry for the next few years: 1) the epidemiological investigation of the mental health state of children and adolescents will be continued in other counties of Estonia; 2) symptomatology and biology of childhood depression; 3) risk factors for mental disorders in childhood.

Training

- In the areas of undergraduate and graduate training there is an urgent need to deepen and expand knowledge of medical and pedagogic students in the field of child psychiatry.
- The postgraduate training scheme to become a specialist in child and adolescent psychiatry and psychotherapy (5 years) will be changed to expand the time for training in child psychiatry.
- Continuing postgraduate training for child psychiatrists and other doctors will be carried out in the form of meetings or renewal courses on miscellaneous topics in child psychiatry.

Improvement of services and care systems

Although since reindependence (in 1991) of Estonia great changes have occurred in Estonian psychiatry, further progress is still needed:

- In the field of child psychiatry and psychotherapy, the main focus of service should be toward outpatient care and development of private praxis.
- Child psychiatry should be brought closer to patients, that is a child psychiatrist or general psychiatrist with deeper knowledge of common problems of child psychiatry should work in all large counties of Estonia.
- Different special schools with highly qualified personnel and available child psychiatric service should be opened for 3 groups of delinquent children and adolescents: with severe conduct disorder, with criminal activity, and for teenagers with delinquency and mental retardation.

Estonian child psychiatrists and other non-medical specialists hope that these necessary changes will be gradually realized.

Selected references

Emminghaus H (1887) Die psychischen Störungen des Kindesalters. Laupp, Tübingen
Kõrgessaar J, Veskiväli E (1987) Eripedagoogika Eestis (In Estonian). Tartu Riiklik Ülikool
Laur M (1989) Estonian History. In: Villems A (ed) Estonia and Tartu. Tartu University, pp 2–6 (in Estonian)
Mehilane L (1996) (ed) Mental Health Care Reforms in the Baltic States. University of Tartu. Geneva Initiative, 1996
Põlluste K (ed) Eesti Rahva Tervis. Tartu, 1998 (in Estonian)
Saarma JM, Karu EJ (1981)Razvitie psihiatrii v Tartuskom Universitete (in Russian).Tallinn, "Valgus"
Saarma J (1982) Psühhiaatria minevik ja tänapäev. Tallin (in Estonian)

Child and adolescent psychiatry in Finland*

J. Piha, F. Almqvist

Finland is one of the five Nordic countries with high living standards. The country was a part of royal Sweden for 600 years and after that for around one hundred years an autonomous grand duchy of czaristic Russia. Finland became an independent republic in 1917 and never belonged to the former Soviet Union. Since the beginning of 1995 Finland has been one of the EU countries. The present population of Finland is 5.1 million inhabitants. The proportion of children and adolescents is approximately 22 %. The geographical area of Finland is huge; it is a bit larger than Italy where the population is eleven times that of Finland.

1. Definition, historical development, and current situation

Definition and historical development

In Finland, child psychiatry was recognized as an independent medical specialty already in the beginning of 1950s, like in the other Nordic countries (subspecialty in 1951, main specialty in 1955, Piha 1991). Despite the name ("child"), the expertise of the specialty covered the whole age range of development from birth to the end of adolescence.

The roots of Finnish child psychiatry originate in the 1920s when the first child guidance clinics were founded and the first child psychiatric ward was opened. For decades, the main emphasis in the development of child psychiatry has been promoting the clinical services. The academic and scientific part of the discipline was not given high priority. The limited professional child psychiatric resources were constantly engaged in heavy clinical duties, often even outside the medical field. As a consequence, the scientific activities suffered, and child psychiatry has had difficulties in reaching the ordinary standards of academic medicine.

In Finland there are five universities with a medical faculty and each of them now has a full professorship in child psychiatry. The first chair was established in 1973 in Helsinki, at the same time as the establishment of a corresponding chair in London (Sommerschild & Groeholt 1989, Wardle 1991). The other universities

* This chapter is an updated modification of an article by Piha and Almqvist (1994).

received associate professorships (Turku 1973, Tampere 1974, Kuopio 1977, Oulu 1983) that were later transformed into full professorships (Kuopio 1985, Tampere 1986, Turku 1987, Oulu 1992). Since the beginning of June 1993, all the five professorships have been for the first time permanently occupied. It took twenty years to create this basic university structure. The slow development and the mediocre result can be regarded as a consequence of the adulto-centrism prevailing in the academic world and in society.

The Finnish Child Psychiatry Association was founded in 1956, and its predecessor, the Child Psychiatry Club, already in 1951 (Forsius 1986). The association has very actively offered opportunities for continuing medical education and emphasized the importance of international contacts. The association has continued the same traditions but, in addition, has concentrated on the promotion of the professional interests of child psychiatrists. In 1985 the association established the Finnish Child Psychiatry Research Foundation. The following year in connection with the 30-year anniversary of the association the first grants for child psychiatric research were awarded. The foundation has a great impact on the identity of child psychiatry in Finland.

Recent advances and current situation

In 1979 adolescent psychiatry was established as a subspecialty of child psychiatry and general/adult psychiatry. The roots of adolescent psychiatry in Finland were anchored in child psychiatry. In hospital settings, however, adolescent psychiatry was, since its administrative establishment, associated more with general/adult psychiatry than with child psychiatry. This was contrary to the situation in Europe and in the USA where child and adolescent psychiatry has traditionally meant one unified specialty.

Quite recently, the European Union of Medical Specialist acknowledged child and adolescent psychiatry/psychotherapy as its own medical specialty (European Union of Medical Specialists 1992). In Finland, however, the development took different lines. A new Decree on Medical Specialties in Finland defined, at the beginning of 1999, four distinct independent main specialties in the field of psychiatry: child psychiatry, adolescent psychiatry, adult psychiatry, and forensic psychiatry. As a consequence, Finland is the only country in the whole world, where child psychiatry and adolescent psychiatry are disunited specialties. At the moment, it is quite difficult to foresee how the academic and clinical fields for psychiatry of minors will develop. One problem is that there are no university posts for adolescent psychiatry. (See also: postgraduate training, p. 99.)

2. Classification systems, diagnostic and therapeutic methods

Classification systems and diagnostic methods

In Finland, the International Classification of Diseases is in use, currently, the ICD-10 version. A diagnostic manual for clinicians has been prepared. The manual combines the ICD-10 clinical ("blue book") and scientific ("green book") descriptions and diagnostic guidelines. In scientific research, the Fourth Edition of the Diagnostic and Statistical Manual of Mental Disorders (DSM-IV) is mainly used.

The diagnosis is based on clinical child and family psychiatric evaluations, child psychological testing, and on somatic and child neurological examinations, if necessary.

Therapeutic methods

Open care child psychiatry work has for decades been very individually oriented. The main treatment method has been supportive psychotherapy. The psychotherapy of the child has been accompanied by parental guidance. Since the beginning of the 1980s, the family therapy approach has become more prevalent. This shift is, of course, natural because the treatment of the child is difficult or impossible without the family. In addition, many family therapy training programs on the specialist level have been arranged at the same time in several localities throughout the country, and this has made it easy to obtain the necessary skills in family therapy. In the 1990s, different forms of professional network therapy have emerged in the child psychiatric field.

In inpatient treatment, the therapeutic approach is also mostly individually oriented. The two most frequently used treatment modes are a dyadic relationship with a personal nurse and parental guidance. Individual psychotherapy and family therapy are applied in about one third and medication in one fifth of the cases (Piha, Salmisaari & Koskinen 1990). Half of inpatients stay in the hospital less than 2 months. The length of stay is for 30 % between 2 and 6 months and for 20 % more than 6 months (Sourander, Korkeila & Turunen 1998). There are only a few beds for child psychiatric emergency treatment.

3. Structure and organization of services

The main resource of every branch of health care is the number of public offices and positions. In the fields of child psychiatry and child psychosocial work, those resources have been in Finland provided through three channels: the central hospital organization, the former adult mental hospital districts, and the network of child guidance clinics. There seems to be a lot of resources devoted to psychiatric and psychosocial work for children, but in practice nearly all of the different agencies, units, and centers within each sector are small and isolated, and they have had only limited cooperation on the level of service delivery planning. As a consequence, the infrastructure of the field is scattered and disconnected. There are only a few child psychiatric centers which are big enough to be able to maintain the high level of clinical and research expertise necessary for successful development of child psychiatry.

Guidelines for services for children and adolescents with psychiatric disorders

Finland is divided into 20 health care districts which carry the responsibility of specialized medicine. In each district, there is a main or central hospital and each has a child psychiatric outpatient unit, and most of them also have an inpatient unit. In some of the districts, there are a few child and adolescent psychiatry outpatient centers which previously were part of the former adult mental hospital districts. In addition, there are child guidance clinics in all districts but administratively they belong to the social sector. Adult psychiatrists did not show much interest in the development of child and adolescent psychiatric service delivery (during the time of adult mental health districts) because they have been satisfied with and relied on the services provided by the social sector (Lääkintöhallitus 1991).

Outpatient services

The first outpatient units within hospital settings were opened in Helsinki University Hospital in the late 1950s, and ten years later in Helsinki Children's Castle Hospital and in Turku University Hospital. According to instructions given by the National Board of Health, every central hospital had to establish a child psychiatric outpatient unit before 1982. These units represent the highest expertise in child psychiatric outpatient care in the health care districts. However, the resources provided for these units are very limited: in each unit there were in 1990 on average only 4.2 professionals involved in clinical work (Piha & Sourander 1991). Child psychiatry has not had high priority in the central hospital administration. There are around 30 small child and adolescent psychiatry outpatient centers outside the central hospitals.

Daypatient services

There are only 8 wards (with around 50 "beds") which offer child psychiatric daycare services. This is a serious shortcoming in the Finnish child psychiatry delivery system.

Inpatient services

The first beds for child psychiatric hospital treatment were reserved in 1924 in an adult mental hospital in Helsinki, and the first true child psychiatric ward was opened in 1927 in Tampere (Forsius 1991). This ward and the second ward, established in 1950 in Helsinki, were later changed to adolescent psychiatry units. In the late 1950s, new child psychiatric wards, which still operate, were established in Children's Castle and Aurora hospitals in Helsinki. Ten years later new inpatient units were opened in Oulu and Turku University Hospitals. Most of the child psychiatric inpatient treatment facilities in central hospitals were established at the beginning of 1980s in accordance with the instructions of National Health Board. Four central hospitals are still missing an inpatient unit.

At present, there are about 290 beds for child psychiatric inpatient treatment in 21 different hospitals (Piha & Aronen 1989, Piha & Korhonen 1991). Only two family wards exist. The number of professionals is on average 15 for 8 beds. Of those professionals, 1.1 are physicians (specialists and trainees), 1.5 clinical psychologists and social workers, and 9.9 belong to the nursing staff. There are considerable variations between different wards with regard to the number of professionals (Piha & Korhonen 1991).

There is a shortage of child and adolescent psychiatric inpatient facilities. This shortage is reflected in the institutions of the social sector: about half of the 2500 children and adolescents living in those institutions are in the need of psychiatric treatment (Kaivosoja 1992).

At the beginning of the 1990s, only 6 % of the child psychiatric hospital patients were under 7 years old, 37 % were between 7 and 11 years, and 58 % were older than 11 years (Sourander & Turunen 1999).

Complementary services

Complementary services are provided for children and adolescents who will need very long-lasting psycho-social rehabilitation. Out-of-home placement is considered as a last measure when open care services have proved to be inadequate and the child's psychosocial development is seriously endangered. These services include foster homes, group homes, and children's homes. Residential care in Finland is a social work responsibility and is run under social legislation.

Funding of services

In Finland, all child psychiatric inpatient services, and almost all outpatient services, are provided by the public sector, which is funded by the state and communities. There are no private child psychiatric hospitals, and the private outpatient service centers are small and are located only in the main cities in the southern part of the country. Visits to private practitioners are reimbursed by the National Health Insurance.

4. Cooperation with medical and non-medical disciplines

Cooperation with pediatrics and psychiatry

The relations between child psychiatry and pediatrics, and child psychiatry and general/adult psychiatry have been ambiguous and enigmatic (Wardle 1991). In the pioneering years of child psychiatry, both pediatricians and psychiatrists were active in facilitating the new field. After these early years, it was more in the interest of pediatrics than of general/adult psychiatry to develop child psychiatry. As a consequence, academic and clinical child psychiatry has in Finland been close to pediatrics and distant to general/adult psychiatry.

At present, however, the main issue seems to be that it is hard for pediatrics and general/adult psychiatry to recognize and acknowledge the proper qualities of child psychiatry. The creation of relations based on equality and mutuality has proved to be complex (Solnit 1988, Steinhauer, Bradley & von Gauthier 1992). Thus, at present in Finland it seems to be that the pediatricians understand psychiatry better than the adult psychiatrists understand the child.

Cooperation with doctors in private practice

There are only a few child psychiatrists in private practice (around 25), and the private sector does not play any significant role from the perspective of the whole country (Kaivosoja & Säntti 1991). Most of them are involved with long-term individual psychotherapies. Specialist level 3-year training programs in child psychotherapy have been carried out since the late 1970s but only in Helsinki (Arajärvi 1990). This is the reason why the number of child psychiatrists working in the private sector has increased only in the southern part of Finland.

Cooperation with non-medical institutions and professionals

The first child guidance clinics in Finland were opened in the middle of the 1920s, only a couple of years after the foundation of the famous guidance clinic in Boston (Forsius 1991). Unfortunately, the activities of these clinics had to be stopped a few years later. Five still operating clinics were founded between 1938 and 1949 in Helsinki, Turku, and Tampere, and this meant the real beginning of the child guidance clinic movement in Finland. Since 1950, the child guidance clinics have received financial support from the state, thus, stimulating the establishment of new clinics. Before the Act on Child Guidance Clinics in 1972, there were 37 different units. In the ten years after the Act, the number more than doubled to 89 clinics. Currently about 120 child guidance clinics are operating, and the network covers the whole child and adolescent population. In fact, this network forms the basis of child and adolescent psychosocial open care services.

The staff of child guidance clinics consists principally of clinical psychologists and social workers. Many units have suffered from the absence of a child and adolescent psychiatrist.

5. Graduate/postgraduate training and continuing medical education

Graduate training: The role of medical faculties

Child psychiatry has since the 1960s been included in the training of all medical students. The teaching volume in the curriculum is minimal, varying between 20 and 40 hours at the different universities. The child psychiatric courses are mostly running parallel to the courses in pediatrics, obstetrics, and gynecology.

Postgraduate training, a joint effort

In Finland a major change in the specialist training took place in 1986 when the responsibility of organizing, co-ordinating and controlling the training was transfered from the National Board of Health to the universities (Arajärvi 1986). The child psychiatry university departments now have the responsibility for and the university professors act as the heads of the training programs.

The structure and content of the specialist training program has gone through many transformations during past years. Those changes reflect the growing sense of the clearer identity of child psychiatry (Almqvist 1987, Piha 1989, Moilanen 1997). The total length of the training is 6 years. The current training program, from the beginning of 1999 is the same in every university and can be summarized as follows:

- Training in basic medical care (health care center) (6 months) is the same for all specialties.
- Common trunk training (18 months) includes 6 months in acute adult psychiatry and 12 months in child psychiatry, adolescent psychiatry, adult psychiatry, and/or forensic psychiatry.
- Specialty training (48 months) consists of 36–48 months training in child psychiatry and of 0–12 months training in adolescent psychiatry. There must be at least 18 months training in outpatient care and at least 18 months training in inpatient care. Six months of the training can be replaced with full day clinical research work.

In addition, the training in basic medical care or specialty training must include 6 months training in the fields related to birth, somatic development, health, and diseases of child (e.g., pediatrics, child neurology, obstetrics, maternal, or well baby care).

It is required to have at least 2 years of the above mentioned child psychiatric specialty training in university hospitals. During the training, the trainee needs to have 80 hours of theoretical seminars (of which 20 hours on health administration, management and economics), in addition to the daily and weekly clinical and theoretical training and supervision provided by the training department.

In the beginning of the 1990s, there were 11.9 child psychiatry specialists for 100,000 inhabitans under 20 years in Finland; at that time the figure was one of the highest among EU countries (Piha 1997). The number of child psychiatrists has increased during recent years by 8–10 new specialists a year. At the beginning of 1998, the number of working-aged specialists was 176 (total number being 196; the respective figures in 1993 were 144 and 158) (Finnish Medical Association 1993, 1998).

In spite of these high numbers, there were at the beginning of 1998 more than 40 child psychiatry specialist vacancies (over 30 % of all vacancies) open or without a qualified professional. There is an urgent need to increase the specialist training capacity.

At present, no formal psychotherapy training is included in the curriculum, but in practice every trainee will become acquainted with psychodynamic individual psychotherapy and systemic family therapy through seminars, supervision, and clinical work. In addition, most trainees attend psychotherapy training for at least three years (specialist level training). An inquiry from 1990 showed that only one fourth of child psychiatrists had no formal training, 41 % were trained in individual psychotherapy, and 26 % in family therapy.

In 1993 the Finnish Medical Association launched a system of special competencies which allows confirmation of further education in focused fields inside medical specialties. Child psychotherapy has since 1996 been such a special competency in child psychiatry. This competency can be acquired in psychoanalytic and cognitive individual psychotherapy, group psychotherapy, and family psychotherapy. Under consideration are the special competencies of infant psychiatry and child and adolescent forensic psychotherapy.

Continuing medical education in child and adolescent psychiatry and psychotherapy

Currently there are no official regulations concerning continuing medical education (CME) in either child psychiatry or in other medical specialties. The Finnish Medical Association has given recommendations on CME stating it desirable but not compulsory. The Finnish Child Psychiatry Association and several other associations, institutions, and organizations provide CME for child psychiatry specialists.

6. Research

Research fields and strategies

There were some research interests in child psychiatric issues before the Second World War, in essence, before the time of the specialty. The first child psychiatric dissertation was published in 1936. However, this dissertation remained as the only genuine child psychiatric thesis for 30 years. The other researchers in the field were mostly pediatricians interested in social psychiatry. After the war in the 1950s many articles were published but the themes emphasized more somatic than psychiatric topics (Taipale 1986).

During the 1960s and 1970s, only six child psychiatric dissertations were published. The dissertations were still done outside the child psychiatry university and university hospital departments due to the lack of child psychiatric resources. The departments of social medicine and public health provided possibilities for research work, especially in epidemiologically oriented child psychiatry.

An increase in the number of dissertations took place during the 1980s and especially during the 1990s. In the 1980s eight dissertations and in the 1990s (until 1998) twelve dissertations have been published. During the on-going decade, the child psychiatry university departments have been able to provide younger researchers the needed support.

The major on-going research projects are focused on child and adolescent psychiatric epidemiology, development of twins, infant psychiatry and early mother-infant interaction, and child psychiatric inpatient treatment. Most of these projects have international contacts or are based on international cooperation. These research activities have been recognized during recent years at international congresses with many Finnish participants and presentations.

There still are some minor research projects which are too small and too isolated, and as a consequence some beginners in research still have to encounter alone the difficulties of research work. There is an urgent need to use the available resources more efficiently and to concentrate on larger study programs.

Research training and career development

During the early years of child psychiatry, the scientific training took place on an irregular and vague basis and was mostly connected with pediatrics. In the 1960s and 1970s, child psychiatrists interested in research still had to train themselves without the support of any research community and research tradition.

An important turning point in this regard took place at the beginning of the 1980s when the first Nordic Child Psychiatry Research Meeting was organized in Finland in 1982 and when the planning of a systematic scientific training program in child and adolescent psychiatry began in 1984. The training program was realized from 1985–87 by the combined efforts of the five child psychiatry university departments with the main financial support from the Ministry of Education (Almqvist 1986). This program was, in fact, the first nation-wide research training program within medical sciences in Finland.

After the training program, research seminars have been arranged on regular basis in the child psychiatry university departments. In addition, a tradition of an Annual Postgraduate Research Meeting in Child Psychiatry was created. These research meetings are arranged by each university department in turn. Internationally well-known researchers have been invited to give lectures and to supervise on-going research projects. Owing to the long-standing cooperation between the five university departments, a collaborative Finnish child psychiatry center has been developed.

7. Future perspectives

The main problem of the child and adolescent psychiatric service delivery system is the dispersed and scattered infrastructure. The service delivery units are too small and, as a consequence, ineffective and vulnerable. The current economic pressure on the whole medical service delivery system will affect child and adolescent psychiatric services, too. It is hoped that this pressure will lead to the unification of distinct units to produce a more functional infrastructure.

There are at least two different sub-fields of child and adolescent psychiatry which in the future will expand both in research and in clinical activities: infant psychiatry and child and adolescent forensic psychiatry. The progress in infant psychiatry has already considerably changed our understanding of the early infant development and mother-infant interaction. Clinical intervention techniques in this area are evolving. In the modern society, there are several circumstances where difficult child and adolescent psychiatric problems relate with social and legal issues. Problems linked, e.g., with custody, child sexual and physical abuse, and involuntary psychiatric care of minors, seem to be increasing in western European countries. Special child and adolescent psychiatric expertise will be needed to deal with these complex clinical problems.

The proper core of child and adolescent psychiatry is the developmental approach. In the future, this approach will be accentuated in research, training, and treatment. Close collaboration between medical specialties (e.g., pediatrics, child neurology, child surgery, child and adolescent psychiatry) sharing the developmental view is necessary. Only in this manner will a real integration of psyche and soma be achieved.

Selected references

Almqvist F (1986) Lastenpsykiatrisen tieteellisen tutkimuksen kehittäminen – Suomen lastenpsykiatrien yhteinen tieteellinen jatkokoulutusohjelma. In: Kaivosoja M (ed) Lapsen etu. 30 vuotta lastenpsykiatrista työtä ja tutkimusta Suomessa. Lastenpsykiatrian tutkimussäätiön julkaisu 1. Jyväskylä: Gummerus, pp 117–22

Almqvist F (1987) Lastenpsykiatria tieteiden joukossa. Sos.lääk Aikakl 24: 327–30

Arajärvi T (1986) Suomalaisten lastenpsykiatrien koulutuksen vaiheita. In: Kaivosoja M (ed) Lapsen etu. 30 vuotta lastenpsykiatrista työtä ja tutkimusta Suomessa. Lastenpsykiatrian tutkimussäätiön julkaisu 1. Jyväskylä: Gummerus, pp 99–103

Arajärvi T (1990) Child psychiatry in Finland in the past and now. Psychiatria Fennica 21: 69–75

European Union of Medical Specialists (1992) Compendium of Medical Specialist Training in the E.C. Brussels

Finnish Medical Association: Register on physicians, 1993 & 1998

Forsius H (1986) Suomen Lastenpsykiatrisen Yhdistyksen historia. In: Kaivosoja M (ed) Lapsen etu. 30 vuotta lastenpsykiatrista työtä ja tutkimusta Suomessa. Lastenpsykiatrian tutkimussäätiön julkaisu 1. Jyväskylä: Gummerus, pp 91–97

Forsius F (1991) Lastenpsykiatrian historia. In: Arajärvi T, Varilo E (eds) Lastenpsykiatria tänään. 3rd edition. Tampere: Weilin+Göös, pp 21–36

Kaivosoja M (1992) Lasten psykiatrinen sairaalahoito: kohtaavatko tarve ja tarjonta? Suom Lääkäril 47: 2082–5

Kaivosoja M, Säntti R (1991) Ongelmanuoret ja palveluiden ongelmat. Kehittämisosaston selvityksiä 1991:1. Helsinki: Sosiaali- ja terveysministeriö

Lääkintöhallitus (1991) Psykiatrisen erikoissairaanhoidon ja mielenterveystyön kehitysnäkymät 1990-luvulla. Lääkintöhallituksen julkaisuja 172. Helsinki

Moilanen I (1997) Child and adolescent psychiatry in Finland. Eur Child Adol Psychiatry 6: 241–243
Piha J (1989) Lastenpsykiatria yliopistollisena ja kliinisenä erikoisalana. Suom Lääkäril 44: 2495–7
Piha J (1991) Lastenpsykiatria ja psykiatria. Suom Lääkäril 46: 1142
Piha J (1997) The status of child and adolescent psychiatry in EU- and EFTA countries. Eur Child Adol Psychiatry 6: 116–118
Piha J, Almqvist F (1994) Child psychiatry as an academic and clinical discipline in Finland. Nord J Psychiatry 48: 3–8
Piha J, Aronen E (1989) Lastenpsykiatrian sairaansijojen alueellinen jakautuminen. Suom Lääkäril 44: 3187–92
Piha J, Korhonen A-K (1991) Lastenpsykiatrisen osastohoidon henkilöstöresurssit. Suom Lääkäril 46: 3162–7
Piha J, Salmisaari T, Koskinen M (1990) Characteristics of recent child psychiatric in-patient treatment in Finland. Psychiatria Fennica 21: 77–86
Piha J, Sourander A (1991) Keskussairaaloiden lastenpsykiatrian poliklinikoiden henkilöstöresurssit. Suom Lääkäril 46: 1173–5
Solnit AJ (1988) Child and adolescent psychiatry should stand separate from general psychiatry. J Am Acad Child Adol Psychiatry 27: 658–69
Sommerschild H, Groeholt B (1989) Laerebok i barnepsykiatri. Oslo: TANO
Sourander A, Korkeila J, Turunen M-M (1998) Factors related to length of psychiatric hospital stay of children and adolescents: A nationwide register study. Nord J Psychiatry 5: 373–378
Sourander A, Turunen M-M (1999) Psychiatric hospital care among children and adolescents in Finland: a nationwide register study. Soc Psychiatry Psychiatr Epidemiol 34: 105–110
Steinhauer PD, Bradley SJ, von Gauthier Y (1992) Child and adult psychiatry: Comparison and contrast. Can J Psychiatry 37: 440–449
Taipale V (1986) Lastenpsykiatrisen tutkimuksen juurista. In: Kaivosoja M (ed) Lapsen etu. 30 vuotta lastenpsykiatrista työtä ja tutkimusta Suomessa. Lastenpsykiatrian tutkimussäätiön julkaisu 1. Jyväskylä: Gummerus, pp 87–90
Wardle CJ (1991) Twentieth-century influences on the development in Britain of services for child and adolescent psychiatry. Br J Psychiatry 159: 53–68

Child and adolescent psychiatry in France

P. Jeammet

1. Definition, historical development, and current situation

Definition

In France, psychiatry was separated from neurology after the events of May 1968. Prior to this, both fields belonged to "neuropsychiatry". There is only one specialty: psychiatry. Child psychiatry represents an additional option of general psychiatry.

Generally, it is therefore impossible to practice child and adolescent psychiatry unless one has acquired the qualification to be a psychiatrist. Yet, recently it has become possible for pediatricians to obtain a degree in child psychiatry (which does not involve becoming a child psychiatrist), if they have completed certain courses and internship requirements during their residency. The age of the patients relevant to the competence of child psychiatry is not strictly defined and can range up to 16 to 18 with a tendency to develop services for adolescents and young adults until 20 and sometimes 25 years old.

Because child psychiatry is not in itself considered as a specialty, theoretically, any medical doctor specialized in psychiatry can practice child and adolescent psychiatry. Actually, in most high-ranking positions offered in child and adolescent psychiatry, it is generally required that candidates have completed the additional option for the title of child psychiatrist. Yet the majority of French psychiatrists support more versatility in psychiatric practice to avoid a split between general and child psychiatry.

The postgraduate training schedule to become a psychiatrist requires four years of study in medical or psychiatric services as a resident ("interne") after a competition and very selective examination at the end of the medical curriculum. No more than the first year can be spent in a medical department. The three other years have to be spent in a psychiatric unit, and two of them in child and adolescent psychiatry if qualification in child and adolescent psychiatry is desired. You also have to have had a stage in pediatrics during your medical studies. The training curriculum is completed at the end by a "memoire", which means a research and clinical work argued in front of a jury.

Historical development

In the field of psychiatry, adult psychiatry reigned as master in France as in most countries for almost 150 years. The model referred to was mental illness in its most complete clinical expression as found among adults. Little interest was given to children, except in cases of infirmity or hereditary defects (degenerates) and later, little by little, in research concerning an adult-like form of psychiatric pathology (the infantile schizophrenia of Sancte de Sanctis).

Two events were to create the groundwork for an interest in childhood and the troubles that could have an effect on it: Freud's description of infantile neurosis, and the weight of childhood experiences in the emergence of psychopathology; mandatory education and learning difficulties which it revealed (the invention of the I.Q. by Binet). Later in Germanic countries, social behavior difficulties that created an interest in adolescence and psychopathologies were described by K. Schneider. Attempts were made to understand the psychology of delinquent youth and to engage therapeutic approaches (Aichhorn). But child psychiatry had to become an entity of its own before the two extremes, adolescent psychiatry and infantile psychiatry, could be fully taken into account.

The individualization of child psychiatry took place immediately after the Second World War in the late 1940s. It came about as the result of the evolution of psychiatry itself both in Europe, especially in France, and in the U.S. This evolution was due to the joint influence of psychoanalysis, the development of institutional therapy, and the discovery of psychotropic medicine. The conjugation of these three factors had the effect of "dealienation" psychiatry, of opening new therapeutic perspectives, and of re-centering psychiatry on the individual. Psychoanalysis in particular considered an individual's past history and childhood to be an important, if not primordial factor. In 1950, the first international congress of psychiatry was held in Paris.

It was at this time that a chair of childhood psychiatry was created at La Salpetrière under Professor Heuyer. Later, emanating from this unit came psychiatrists with a psychoanalytic orientation, such as S. Lebovici and R. Diatkine, who were decisive in extending work on childhood psychology, notably with the creation of the Alfred Binet Center in the XIII arrondissement of Paris in 1961. This center, along with the adult unit to which it was attached, was to become a renowned center for childhood psychology and training, consecrated by the creation of the review "La Psychiatrie de l'Enfant", which was created under Professor Ajuriaguerra.

Concomitantly, under the guidance of another psychoanalyst, Professor R. Mises, the Fondation Vallée located in Gentilly near Paris was transformed from a boarding house for so-called mentally deficient children into a care-giving unit which was to become a model of long-term hospitalization in the treatment of mentally deficient and psychotic children. Professor Mises contributed immensely to differentiating deficiencies from severe developmental difficulties. He created the term "dysharmonie d'évolution" to describe developmental difficulties which were not accompanied by outright symbiotic, schizophrenic or autistic psychosis but which consisted of diverse interpersonal troubles and praxic or gnosic learning difficulties. He brought to light the importance of early affective deprivation and of distortions in the interaction between the infant or the children and their parents in the development of these troubles.

Adolescent psychiatry also began to emerge with the consultations of yet another psychoanalyst, Dr. Pierre Male at Ste. Anne's Hospital. Contact with the judiciary system gave rise to a specific approach toward adolescents with psychosocial difficulties.

In the 1970s and 1980s, under the leadership of Professor S. Lebovici, both infant and adolescent psychiatry greatly expanded in France.

Official organizations

The Société Française de Psychiatrie de l'Enfant et de l'Adolescent et des Professions Associées publishes a journal, Neuropsychiatrie de l'Enfance et de l'Adolescence. The society was first created in 1937. It disappeared during the Second World War but was reestablished under the same name at the war's end. There are also other publications concerning child psychiatry, such as Psychiatrie de l'Enfant, Journal de la Psychanalyse de l'Enfant, and the Revue Adolescence. A new pluridisciplinary review has just come out: Enfance et Psy.

Recent advances

In France, the treatment of psychiatrically disturbed children and adolescents is funded by the social security system. In the public services the children and their families do not pay anything. In private practice, they are generally reimbursed by social security; sometimes with a certain category of medical doctor, they have to pay a part. In private practice, the psychologists fees are not reimbursed.

Certain categories of services, mainly residential services, for children and adolescents with a large part of education do not depend on the social security system but on the welfare system payed by the general council of each territorial department.

Current situation

In 1997, the population of France was 58,500,000, among them 11,245,000 children and adolescents between 0 and 15 years and 3,9000,000 adolescents and young adults between 15–19 years. At the time being (1998), child and adolescent psychiatry is represented in about 150 child psychiatric hospitals and departments, among them 33 university departments. Out of the 2000 specialists for child and adolescent psychiatry (half of them are also adult psychiatrists), 1200 are participating in some way in private practice, covered by insurance. In relation to the general population, there is one child and adolescent psychiatrist per 30,000 inhabitants or per 8000 children and adolescents between birth and 19 years of age. The French Society for Child and Adolescent Psychiatry has now about 550 members.

2. Classification systems, diagnostic and therapeutic methods

Classification systems

The classification used to fill out the diagnostic forms is the Classification Française des Troubles Mentaux de l'Enfant et de l'Adolescent (French classification system). However, the WHO ICD-10 classification and sometimes the DSM (Diagnostic and Statistical Manual) are also used for international publications.

French practitioners on the whole remain quite attached to the first classification. They reproach the two other systems for being too concerned with behavior and outward manifestations. On the other hand, catamnestic studies pinpoint the need to decipher symptoms in order to evaluate the nature of the disorder, to find adapted therapy, and to make short- and long-term prognoses.

There is an equivalency between the ICD and the French classification which now includes a classification of child and adolescent mental handicaps based on the work of Ph. W. Wood.

Diagnostic methods

The whole spectrum of diagnostic procedures is used.

Therapeutic methods

Also in the field of therapy, a broad spectrum of methods is used. However, the orientation of the different departments varies. Psychodynamic approaches (from psychoanalytic theories) continue to have a large influence on the majority of child and adolescent psychiatrists. Hence, this influence can be found on the psychological approach, remediation, institutional work, individual or group therapy, or work with the family, all of which are favored in child therapy. Pharmacological treatments have only a limited use. For example, the use of Ritalin today remains rare.

The majority of the inpatient and outpatient departments use an eclectic approach with the integration of different methods including family counseling and family therapy, and also, if indicated, medication.

3. Structure and organization of services

Guidelines for services for children and adolescents with psychiatric disorders

A number of practitioners work in both the public and private domains. Some of them practice in only one domain. Public sector care in child psychiatry is well developed in France. In 1972, the government created child and adolescent psychiatry sectors. There is one child and adolescent sector for three adult sectors. The population of each catchment area for child and adolescent is about 210,000 inhabitants.

In 1995, there were 315 child psychiatry sectors. They received 330,000 children and adolescents (15% more than in 1993). It was the first contact for half of them, 17 % had been seen only once in the year, and most of them were between 5 and 14 years old. The children before 5 years represent 14% and the adolescents more than 15 years 15 %. Among these 330,000 children, only 10 % had a part-time treatment and 3 % a full-time treatment. For the latter, the mean duration of the hospitalization was 69 days. For the ambulatory treatment the mean frequency of the consultations was 12 times a year.

The main goal of the child psychiatry sectors was to carry out, in their geographical areas, the entirety of the preventive and treatment activities concerning child and adolescent mental health. Thus, the child and adolescent psychiatry sector is in charge of:

- a complete psychiatric examination of the child, if necessary, psychological, speech, and psychomotor evaluations, and even a school assessment. This examination includes a thorough interview with the parents.
- the treatment of the child, if necessary. Theoretically, every type of therapeutic action can be carried out within each sector: therapeutic consultations, family guidance consultation, or more frequent and more regular therapy (psychotherapy, speech therapy, psychomotor or educational therapy) individually or in groups.

All the therapies proposed within the sector are free and are performed as close as possible to the families' homes.

Types of services

Sectors may have at their disposal five types of facilities for performing treatments. However, not every sector has all the existing facilities available. The five types of facilities are listed below.

- *Medical Psychological Centers* (Centres Médico-Psychologiques). Outpatient consultation and treatment centers, which are the operational bases of the coordinated activities.
- *Daycare hospitals.* Institutions in charge of children with serious mental disorders during the day, providing intensive treatments as well as the necessary educational programs (the latter are carried out by special education teachers from the public education system).
- *Part-time therapeutic centers.* Institutions in charge of therapeutic treatments for a number of hours each day, while allowing the child to stay in the regular school system; this facility is for less serious cases.
- *Full-time residential treatment centers.* For long-lasting psychotic pathologies, residential treatment is justified by the seriousness of the illness or by family

disorganization. For more acute pathologies, particularly with adolescents (depression, suicide attempt, anorexia nervosa), shorter confinements are possible, allowing the implementation of a therapy that can be continued after leaving the hospital.

- *Therapeutic family placement.* The patient is placed in a family setting for children with psychiatric disorders through assistance paid for by the hospital and supervised by a sector's specialized team.

Of the sectors 90 % have a part-time therapeutic center and/or a day-hospital. Half of them have a full-time residential center.

Some public or semipublic healthcare units working in the field of child psychiatry are nevertheless independent from child psychiatry administrative structures. These are mainly:

- *The medical-psychological-educational centers* (CMPP: Centres Médico-Psycho-Pédagogiques). These are managed by nonprofit, private associations. The CMPP have done pioneering work in ambulatory treatment of children with psychological disorders and difficulties in school. They function within the same framework as the child psychiatry structures and represent an important part of the child psychiatry care system.
- *The early intervention medical-social centers* (CAMSP: Centres d'Action Médico-Sociale Précoce). They take care, very early on, of the special education and treatment of preschool children with somatic disorders, and motor, sensory or mental handicaps. The CAMSP can be multipurpose or specialized in treating a specific handicap. They propose the treatment and remediation required by the child's condition/state which can be performed in groups or individually at the center or at home.
- *The medical-educational institutions* (Instituts Médico-Educatifs or Médico-Pédagogiques). Managed by nonprofit private associations, they provide, under medical supervision, educational and pedagogical activities with children who generally have a mental deficiency, sometimes associated with psychotic disorders or a physical handicap.

4. Cooperation with medical and non-medical disciplines

Psychiatry sectors are in close contact with the other agencies dealing with childhood: mother and child protection agencies, public healthcare centers, daycare centers, schools, child social workers, family court, and childcare services in hospitals. Concurrently, the psychiatry sector is developing a series of training, teaching, and research programs that will contribute to setting up primary prevention. The team in charge of these preventive actions is multidisciplinary. The multidisciplinarity is based on significant work done during clinical and administrative meetings.

5. Graduate/postgraduate training and continuing medical education

Graduate training: The role of medical faculties

As is the case within other medical fields, psychiatry is taught by professors of psychiatry in different university hospitals, called CHU. The professors are seconded by assistant clinical head doctors "chefs de clinique" in French, named after their internship for a renewable two year period. They are chosen by professors for their personal qualities as well as the work they have accomplished. Professors are designated for life, and the clinical head doctors are designated on a temporary basis. All of the above are recruited and paid by the university. Professors are government employees. Both professors and clinical head doctors also receive payment from the CHU to which they are necessarily attached. Clinical activity takes up at least 50 % of their time (in reality, practically always more). Government employees are not allowed to have two salaries. For this reason, the pay received from the CHU is considered as an indemnity even though it is more consequential than the university pay. However, the CHU indemnity is not taken into account for retirement pensions, which are calculated only on the lesser university salary.

Professors are allowed to have a private practice within the hospital (not more than two half-days of consultations) and a possibility 10 % of the unit's beds. Few psychiatrists take advantage of this opportunity.

There are presently 33 professors of child and adolescent psychiatry in France within 49 CHU, 11 of which are in Paris. This is barely just more than half of what exists for adults (52). Certain CHU have several child psychiatry professors (some 2, and in one case 3) but 20 university hospitals have no child psychiatry professor.

The number of medical students has drastically diminished over the past ten years because of the numerus clausus of medical students. A competitive examination is held at the end of the first year, and the minister offers only a limited number of places for those who wish to continue. A student can take this exam two times. After the exam, from 60 to 120 students are allowed to continue. This varies from one CHU to another. About 50 % of these students will become specialists after an internship exam. Every year the health ministry decides on the number of specialists that can be accepted as interns for each specialty. In psychiatry this number is about 180 for the whole CHU a year which means that there will be a significant decline in the number of psychiatrists in the years to come.

There is a mandatory course in psychiatry of about 30 hours for all medical students. There is also a course in medical psychology which varies from 30 to 60 hours depending on the CHU. This course is usually given by psychiatrists and consists of information on childhood and adolescent development, personality formation, and doctor/patient relationships.

Postgraduate training, a joint effort

Recruitment of psychiatrists as child psychiatrists in France is carried out through a competitive examination (considered as both democratic and very selective), common for all the specialities. When you succeed, you have to choose between four kinds of specialities: medicine, surgery, psychiatry, biology, public health. This examination evaluates candidates more for their abilities to learn and to memorize a great amount of information than for their clinical abilities, their creativity, or their motivation to become involved in the field of psychiatry.

Thus, the internship begins with a competitive examination at the end of the medical curriculum. The exam can be taken only twice. It gives access for 4 years to positions of responsibility in specialized services in which the intern can acquire the qualification of psychiatrist. The child psychiatry option can be granted to interns who have the qualification in psychiatry if they have also spent four semesters of their internship in services qualifying for child psychiatry and regularly attended a certain number of seminars which fulfill the child psychiatry requirements.

For a period of time, long ago, there was a specialized internship in psychiatry that one could enter if one had an inclination toward psychiatry. This is not the case today, and it can happen that candidates choose psychiatry based on their rank for the internship, regardless of personal interest in psychiatry.

During the internship there is a mandatory curriculum organized for specialized interns on a regional basis: the DES (diploma of higher studies) which groups psychiatric interns from all the university hospitals in the region. During the four years of specialized study, this curriculum consists of several yearly seminars, some of which are mandatory. Others are optional. At the end of the four years there is a short thesis, in addition to the final medical thesis. However, most of the curriculum is followed within the units to which the students are assigned. Students change units every six months, with the possibility of extending to one year. The interns go to different units in their region, alternating between university hospitals and non-university psychiatric units (specialized hospital centers) directed by psychiatrists without the title of professor. The last year of the internship can be done in a psychiatric unit in a different region from the one where the student had been and which he had chosen according to his rank at the outcome of his examination.

The most delicate problem of this curriculum is the place reserved for training in the different types of psychotherapy. This question has not yet been resolved. This training is essentially done in private institutions outside the university and the students have to pay for it. This is so for psychoanalysis, cognitive-behavioral therapy, and family therapies.

The aim of the majority of the teachers is not to establish a program with a content and a method and a specific number of hours as is done in certain countries. In France, there are obstacles due to regulation: courses for specialists must allow for a wide margin of individual initiative. Added to this is the fact that training in psychotherapy depends on personal engagement and motivation and cannot be the same for all psychiatrists. On the whole, teachers feel that there should be a basic university curriculum, completed by a more specific and probing curriculum based on personal options. Later, personal training can be followed outside the university. Teaching psychoanalysis is the perfect example of this.

This type of training puts affective dynamics and mechanisms of identification (or counter-identification) into play. These could be influenced in a system involving hierarchy. Possible conflicts and fears concerning grades could be disturbing for personal development. Inversely, phenomena of fascination could induce positions of transfer with regard to the trainers, leading to psychological weakening.

The basic curriculum should aim at helping the student to acquire a personal aptitude for a psychiatric relationships. This should be followed by training in therapeutic methods. All the DES curricula should include information about the different types of therapies. In general the programs of all universities do include seminars on the four main trends: psychoanalysis, behaviorism, and cognitive and systemic therapy. Sometimes hypnosis and relaxation training are also included.

The main problem addressed is what exactly is transmitted in this way: is it information, that is to say the transmission of theoretical knowledge in a given field, leaving aside practical training, or rather training with reviews and discussions concerning therapeutic follow-ups. Opinions vary on this subject: certain teachers feel that the DES curriculum should be limited to dispensing knowledge and that it is not qualified to insure training. Others feel that seminars led by an experienced teacher can create good conditions for practical training enabling the student to take charge of patients within the framework of the therapy studied.

There is a satisfactory method which is widely used: seminars concerning the handling of specific pathologies such as reactions to trauma, personality disorders, eating disorders or particular situations: including family pathology, liaison psychiatry, and outpatient care.

It is essential that beyond information the student be able to have hands-on training in therapy, as well as supervision. There is a certain amount of supervision that can be done in the university framework. The methods used are case discussions, groups called "inter-control" groups in which each participant relates his personal experience followed by group discussions of the problems encountered. This allows for an awareness of preconscious and even unconscious phenomena. In order to go further, it is necessary to call in supervisors who are not part of the university hierarchy and to enlarge those models which work well: using trainers from the outside who do not give their opinion of the interns, having cross-university training with discontinuous interventions, and calling in consultants who do not hold a position of power.

How can this training be validated? From the moment it is decided that the teachers do not grade the students, an absolute validation is not possible. However, attendance can be controlled in the seminars and the group discussions. The choice of a subject of dissertation or thesis is indirectly linked to this question. There is a whole area of psychiatry which is objective, and excellent theses have been written that do not allow for subjectivity as to subject matter or methodology. One can wonder whether it is not necessary for a psychiatrist to have done at least one study on psychopathology demanding personal involvement. Rules allow students to use their thesis as a dissertation subject in psychiatry. Some teachers have a rule which could be generalized: if the thesis is purely objective, the dissertation must be different and it must concern psychopathology.

Personal involvement appears indispensable. The model is that of didactic psychoanalysis and the path followed in psychoanalytic training. There are other orientations: psychoanalytic psychodrama, family therapy (systemic or psychoanalytic), behavior therapies, and hypnosis. These trainings are more in-depth than those which can be given in a curriculum shared by all psychiatrists. Often they correspond to a hyper-specialization. The job of the university is not to give such training, and it is not the best qualified place to do so.

What is desirable, on the other hand, is that the universities not be estranged from different schools of thought. It is important that the university hire professors who are capable psychoanalysts, cognitive therapists, or systemic therapists. Even though the university's job is not to insure training in these areas it must remain open minded to all areas of human science. Students may also obtain a "university diploma" (DU) by enrolling in courses that give complementary training on specific subjects. These are part of the university but not part of the DES nor of the DESC in psycho-pediatrics.

Continuing medical education in child and adolescent psychiatry and psychotherapy

At the time being, the government is trying to organize formal requirements for continuing medical education.

Training programs for other disciplines

Besides private practice, work in child psychiatry is the result of a multidisciplinary team. Associated with psychiatrists, we find psychologists, speech therapists, diverse educators, psychomotor specialists, social workers, and nurses.

All these professionals, except psychologists, are trained outside the universities in specialized schools into which candidates can enter after their high school degree. Currently, these short training periods tend to be 1 or 2 years longer than before, for a total of 3–4 years of schooling. The training acquired in these schools is most often multipurpose. It occurs mainly through daily work in child and adolescent psychiatry departments so that these professionals become competent in child psychiatric disorders.

Psychologists are trained in universities for 5 years. During their final year, they can specialize in child or adolescent psychology. Only a psychology degree with training in clinical and abnormal psychology theoretically allows one to work in child and adolescent units. In France, these allied professions have a lower economic status than in other European countries (United Kingdom, Scandinavia, etc.) or in the United States.

6. Research

Research fields and strategies

French organizations for medical research are now helping research networks which group together several teams, especially foreign ones, on a common project.

This grouping allows the members to have a common protocol, larger cohorts, and more efficient methods, notably for statistical purposes. It also means that a certain number of teams can add on to these common projects more specific projects related to their special interests. There are networks concerned with autism, bulimia, adolescent mood disorders, personality traits common to addictive disorders, the effect of early maternal depression on childhood development, etc. Projects with follow-ups on cohorts in the area of risk factors and resilience to drug abuse are under study.

French practitioners remain concerned with maintaining research in the area of the specificity of child and adolescent development and the importance of interpersonal interactions. This is even more necessary at a time when the impact of psycho-social changes on the mental health and the behavior of children are manifest. This concern should not hinder the expansion of research in other timely areas such as the genetics of mental illness, the evaluation of therapies, the impact of mental illness on public health, and the field of cognitive approaches. These studies, which started later in France than in other countries, are developing rapidly. Unfortunately, they are curbed by lack of funding.

Research training and career development

There is a diploma called the DEA (diploma of advanced studies) organized by the university and considered as a requirement for doing research. The curriculum lasts one year and involves full-time enrollment and an interruption in the internship. Students can obtain scholarships but these are largely insufficient in number. A doctoral thesis may be obtained after about three years of preparation. In order to obtain a university appointment, candidates have to have previously obtained an accreditation to supervise research, delivered by a jury upon the recommendation of an interdisciplinary university council. To obtain this recommendation, a DEA and a doctoral thesis are becoming increasingly necessary along with the publication of numerous articles in peer-reviewed, international journals.

Funding

The sector's budget does not mention research funding. Funding has to be obtained from other sources, such as the Institut National de la Santé et de la Recherche Médicale (INSERM), the Centre National de la Recherche Scientifique (CNRS), or organizations that can support research or conduct research networks in child psychiatry.

An important research funding organization is the Ministry of Health which announces at regular intervals special programs in the field of health care, etiology of disorders, health services, etc. A large number of foundations are also important for research funding such as the Foundation for Research or Foundation de France. Child psychiatric departments are participating at a modest level in the programs of all research funding organizations.

7. Future perspectives

In France, as in other countries, the behavioral and psychological difficulties of children and adolescents have brought to light the fact that psychiatry must develop ways to understand and treat specific pathologies of this age. These difficulties point out the necessity for psychiatrists to network with partners working with children in other fields: education, justice, and sociology. Information must circulate from one field to another. Specialists should be able to join forces without jeopardizing their specificities.

These actions are not easy to accomplish for financial reasons. This is why partnerships are essential. There is a risk that social action be favored over medical action, because the latter is more expensive. Social actions are of course useful but they may lead to an underestimation of the importance of psychopathology and, thus, delay specific treatments. The ongoing treatment of psychopathology at an early stage is a factor of success especially in childhood and adolescence where prevention and treatment are tightly interwoven. These are the stakes, but unfortunately those who make the decisions are often guided by short-term goals related to forthcoming elections.

Selected references

Braconnier A (1998) Psychologie dynamique et psychanalyse. Paris, Masson, p. 173

Delay J, Pichot P (1992) Abrégé de Psychologie. Paris, Masson

Jeammet Ph, Raynaud M, Consoli S (1996) Abrégé de Psychologie médicale. Paris, Masson

Lebovici S, Diatkine R, Soule M (1995) Nouveau traité de psychiatrie de l'enfant et de l'adolescent. P U F, 2ème édition, 4 vol

Marcelli D, Braconnier A (1996) Adolescence et Psychopathologie. Paris, Masson

Mazet Ph, Stoleru S (1995) Abrégé de Psychopathologie du nourrisson et du jeune enfant. Paris, Masson

Widlocher D (1994) Traité de psychopathologie, P U F

Child and adolescent psychiatry in Germany

H. Remschmidt

1. Definition, historical development, and current situation

Definition

The field of "child and adolescent psychiatry and psychotherapy" in Germany is defined as follows: "Child and adolescent psychiatry and psychotherapy comprises the diagnosis, non-operative treatment, prevention, and rehabilitation of psychiatric, psychosomatic, developmental and neurological diseases or disorders as well as psychological and social behavior disturbances during childhood and adolescence" (German Medical Association 1994). This definition has been modified several times since being first inaugurated in 1968, when child and adolescent psychiatry became an independent specialty. At that time, the specialty was called "child and adolescent psychiatry". Psychotherapy was added to the title in 1993, taking into account the importance of psychotherapeutic treatment methods. The post-graduate training schedule to become a child and adolescent psychiatrist and psychotherapist requires five years of training out of which one year can be completed either in pediatrics or in general psychiatry. The training curriculum for child and adolescent psychiatrists and psychotherapists can be completed in all 16 states of the Federal Republic of Germany and ends with an oral board examination at the Office of the Medical Association (Landesärztekammer) of each state.

Historical development

German child and adolescent psychiatry is very closely connected to European and international developments. Its roots go back to several other disciplines, especially pediatrics and psychiatry, but also clinical psychology, pedagogy (therapeutic education), and with regard to many regulations, also to social sciences and law. These influences, however, did not lead to a type of child and adolescent psychiatry as a kind of mixture of other heterogeneous disciplines, but as an independent specialty that has integrated all these influences in order to give psychiatrically ill and disturbed children and adolescents and their families the best possible support.

An important milestone in the history of German child and adolescent psychiatry was the textbook by Hermann Emminghaus (1887) entitled "Psychic disturbances in childhood" which was called the "hour of birth" of child psychiatry (Harms 1960). In 1899, the term "child psychiatry" was first used by the French psychiatrist M. Manheimer who called his book "Les troubles mentaux de l'enfance", subtitled "Précis de psychiatrie infantile" (Stutte 1974).

Further development was characterized by the books by Wilhelm Strohmayer (1910) "Psychopathology of childhood", Theodor Ziehen (1915) "Mental disorders in childhood", August Homburger (1926) "Lectures on childhood psychopathology", and Moritz Tramer (1942) "Textbook of general child psychiatry". After the second world war, the handbook article by Hermann Stutte (1960), the textbook by Jakob Lutz (1961), and the "Textbook of special child and adolescent psychiatry" by Harbauer, Lempp, Nissen, and Strunk (1971) were influential. These textbooks were followed by several others and by the three volume handbook "Child psychiatry in clinic and practice" edited by Helmut Remschmidt and Martin Schmidt (1985, 1988).

As far as the journals are concerned, three developments were important:

- In 1898, the journal "Children's Faults" (Die Kinderfehler) was founded which was continued as "Journal for Child Research" (Kinderforschung) and ceased to appear with its 50th volume during the second world war in 1944. After the war, this journal was continued as "Yearbook for Youth Psychiatry" (founded in 1956) and has been running since 1973 under the title "Journal of Child and Adolescent Psychiatry" (Zeitschrift für Kinder- und Jugendpsychiatrie). According to the change in the name of the specialty, this title was changed to "Journal of Child and Adolescent Psychiatry and Psychotherapy" in 1996.
- In 1934, Moritz Tramer founded the "Journal of Child Psychiatry" (Zeitschrift für Kinderpsychiatrie) which continued from 1984 as "Acta Paedopsychiatrica" and ceased to appear in 1994.
- As a third journal with a more psychoanalytic and, later, more interdisciplinary orientation, "Practice of Child Psychology and Psychiatry" was founded in 1951 by Annemarie Dührssen and Werner Schwidder, still exists, and has a large readership.

The establishment of a new discipline, however, is only possible by the foundation of scientific and professional organizations that push forward the further development of the discipline. The official foundation of a German association for child and adolescent psychiatry took place on September 5, 1940, in Vienna as "German Society for Child Psychiatry and Therapeutic Education". Its first president was Paul Schröder, head of the department of psychiatry at the University of Leipzig. During the second world war, under the Nazi regime, German child psychiatry was also involved in the euthanasia program, and thousands of mentally handicapped and psychiatrically ill children were murdered, with its cooperation.

In 1950, the "German Association for Youth Psychiatry" was refounded as a medical association, but with intensive cooperation with other disciplines such as therapeutic education, law, clinical psychology, psychiatry, and pediatrics.
German child and adolescent psychiatry has developed from four traditions:

- The neuropsychiatric tradition goes back to roots in neurology and psychiatry from which child psychiatry evolved at several places. This tradition was pronounced in the former German Democratic Republic where the specialty was called "child and adolescent neuropsychiatry". It is continued nowadays by neuropsychological approaches in several fields of child psychiatry.

- A tradition in therapeutic education developed mainly in pediatrics, which can be considered as a precursor of the departments of psychosomatics in pediatric hospitals.
- The psychodynamic-psychoanalytic tradition, based on psychoanalytic theories, which goes far back to the beginning of psychoanalysis and was also responsible for the inclusion of psychodynamic psychotherapy into the curriculum for child and adolescent psychiatrists as well as for the establishment of "psychagogues", who have changed their name to "psychoanalytic child and adolescent psychiatrists".
- The empirical-epidemiological tradition. This orientation was established in the sixties and seventies and was influenced to a great extent by empirical research from England and the United States.

After the German reunification, a "Society for Neuropsychiatry of Childhood and Adolescence" was founded in February 1990 in East Germany which was later integrated into the "German Society for Child and Adolescent Psychiatry". This society, whose name was changed to "Society for Child and Adolescent Psychiatry and Psychotherapy" in 1994, organizes its official meetings once every two years in different locations in Germany. The last (25th) congress took place in Dresden in May 1997. There exist two other organizations of child and adolescent psychiatry in Germany: the professional organization (Berufsverband) which was founded in 1978 and now has (1997) 623 members. This organization represents the group of child and adolescent psychiatrists and psychotherapists in private practice. The second organization is the Conference of Directors of Child and Adolescent Psychiatric Hospitals in Germany, which was founded in 1990 and has 112 members.

These three organizations have established a close cooperation and have joint working groups for quality assurance, training, and research.

Recent advances

In Germany, the treatment of psychiatrically disturbed children and adolescents is funded by the insurance for acute disorders, by the youth welfare organization, and by the social security system after the acute phase for rehabilitation and reintegration. The social security system is responsible only for physically handicapped and severely mentally handicapped children and adolescents, whereas the youth welfare organization is responsible for psychiatrically handicapped children and adolescents up to the age of 18.

With regard to the progress of child and adolescent psychiatry in Germany in general, four developments during the last twenty years have been decisive:

- The Psychiatry Enquête of the Federal Government of Germany (report 1975),
- the Model Program Psychiatry of the Federal Government of Germany (1980 – 1985),
- the Psychiatry Personnel Equipment Act (stepwise introduction between 1991 and 1995), and

- the inclusion of psychotherapy in the training curriculum and as a specialty which is since 1992 “child and adolescent psychiatry and psychotherapy”.

These four developments have influenced current child and adolescent psychiatry and psychotherapy in a remarkable way. The Psychiatry Enquête inaugurated by two members of the parliament opened the possibility for a broad inquiry about the situation of psychiatry and child and adolescent psychiatry throughout West Germany. After the report of the commission (1975), the Model Program Psychiatry was created which was carried out in 14 regions of the Federal Republic of Germany and evaluated different types of services and created new ones. One region (Marburg) was devoted exclusively to the evaluation and establishment of child and adolescent psychiatric services. Many newly created services could be continued. The Psychiatry Personnel Equipment Act was responsible for more satisfactory staffing of psychiatric hospitals and services which led to a remarkable improvement of every day work. The inclusion of psychotherapy into the curriculum for child psychiatrists and for general psychiatrists was not only important for the individual professional training of each child and adolescent psychiatrist, but also improved the status of child and adolescent psychiatry.

Current situation

On December 31, 1994, the population of Germany was 81,538,600, among them 15.9 million children and adolescents between 0 and 18 years, which is about 19.5% of the total population. At the present (1997), child and adolescent psychiatry and psychotherapy is represented in 114 child psychiatric hospitals and departments, among them 25 university departments. Out of the 781 specialists for child and adolescent psychiatry and psychotherapy (half of them are women), 311 are participating in some way in private practice, which is covered by insurance. In relation to the general population, there is one child and adolescent psychiatrist per 104,402 inhabitants or per 20,358 children and adolescents between birth and 18 years of age. If we calculate the same proportions for child and adolescent psychiatrists in private practice, the relations are 1:262,182 or 1:51,125.

The German Society for Child and Adolescent Psychiatry and Psychotherapy has now 650 members; in 1975, there were only 200 specialists for child and adolescent psychiatry, among them 34 women. This is a remarkable development.

But there are still several needs: Though the Federal Government of Germany has accepted the proposal of the Expert Commission for the Model Program Psychiatry to establish a department of child and adolescent psychiatry at every university, ten out of 35 faculties are still lacking our discipline. There are not enough child and adolescent psychiatrists in private practice, and there is an enormous need for research in many fields in order to improve our knowledge on the etiology of disorders and to provide adequate and effective treatment programs.

2. Classification systems, diagnostic and therapeutic methods

Classification systems

In Germany, the ICD-10 classification system is widely used, in nearly all departments in a multiaxial framework (Remschmidt and Schmidt 1994). Some departments also use DSM-IV, especially for scientific purposes. Nearly all academic departments and many other departments use a basic documentation for all cases, including the most important data from the history, a symptom list, a multiaxial ICD-10 diagnosis, and a short description of the therapeutic measures carried out or recommended.

Diagnostic methods

The whole spectrum of diagnostic procedures is used. In most departments, neurological examinations and EEG recordings are also possible. With regard to laboratory methods and special imaging techniques, the cooperation with neighboring disciplines is fairly good. Special diagnostic methods have been developed in Germany in the field of neuropsychology, with regard to mother-child interactions, family diagnosis, and in the field of diagnosis and therapy of developmental disorders as well as in the field of evaluation.

Therapeutic methods

In the field of therapy, a broad spectrum of methods is also used. However, the orientation of the different departments varies. Some departments still follow a more psychodynamic approach and consequently use more psychodynamic methods; the majoritiy of the inpatient and outpatient departments use a more eclectic approach with the integration of different methods dominated by behavior therapeutic techniques, including family counseling and family therapy, and also, if indicated, medication.

3. Structure and organization of services

Guidelines for services for children and adolescents with psychiatric disorders

The Expert Commission of the Federal Government of Germany proposed guidelines for services based on the following general principles (Report of the Expert Commission, Expertenkommission der Bundesregierung, 1988, pp. 383-385):

- Services for psychiatrically disturbed children and adolescents should be equated with services for children with other disorders or diseases. Ideally, children with psychological disturbances and their parents should pass through the same door as children suffering from an infectious disease, a broken leg or in need of an operation.

- This equation requires an integration of the relevant services into the field of medicine, though there is a broad overlapping with other non-medical services.
- The services should be community-based, avoiding too long distances and too high thresholds for consultation. It was proposed to define a region of approximately 250,000 inhabitants for outpatient services and a region between 500,000 and 750,000 inhabitants for inpatient and complementary services. It should be the aim of service planning to treat most of the children and adolescents within their home region. However, there are some disorders or diseases that need special services and are not frequent enough to provide a center for them in every region. These groups are (1) children with chronic epilepsy and severe psychiatric problems, (2) children and adolescents with severe head injury, (3) psychiatrically disturbed delinquent children and adolescents who cannot be made responsible for the delinquent acts for psychiatric reasons, and (4) severely mentally handicapped children and adolescents with a high load of psychopathological disorders.
- The services should be qualified and respect age and developmental stage, the peculiarities of each child and his family as well as risk factors and protective factors in the patient and his environment.

Table 1. Services for psychiatrically disturbed children and adolescents in Germany

I.	**OUTPATIENT SERVICES**
1.	Child and adolescent psychiatrists in private practice
2.	Analytical child and adolescent psychotherapists in private practice
3.	Outpatient departments at hospitals
4.	Child psychiatric services at public health agencies
5.	Child guidance clinics and family counseling services
6.	Early intervention centers, social pediatric services
II.	**DAYPATIENT SERVICES**
1.	Daypatient clinics Two types: Integrated into inpatient settings or independent
2.	Night clinic treatment possibilities
III.	**INPATIENT SERVICES**
1.	Inpatient services at university hospitals
2.	Inpatient services at psychiatric state hospitals
3.	Inpatient services at general community hospitals or pediatric hospitals
IV.	**COMPLEMENTARY SERVICES**
1.	Rehabilitation services for special groups of patients (e.g., children with severe head injuries, epilepsy)
2.	Different types of homes
3.	Residential groups for adolescents

Types of services

Table 1 gives an overview of the different types of child and adolescent psychiatric services in Germany. On the whole, there are enough inpatient places, but they are not well distributed over the whole country. There are not enough outpatient services. This applies to outpatient services associated with hospitals as well as to private practice. Child psychiatry is one of the few medical disciplines in Germany in which private practice is still offering good prospects and is not restricted.

There is also a shortage of daypatient facilities and a paucity of complementary services (rehabilitation programs, programs for chronic patients and for special groups such as drug-dependent children and adolescents, delinquent adolescents).

Outpatient services

The majority of outpatient consultations are carried out by child psychiatrists in private practice (n = 311), by outpatient units of child psychiatric state hospitals, and university departments (n = 25). Outside the medical field, more than 1,000 child guidance clinics and also more than 1,000 analytic child and adolescent psychotherapists (most of them in private practice) participate in outpatient consultation and treatment. In 1988, the Expert Commission for the Model Program Psychiatry of the Federal Government of Germany proposed a relation of one child psychiatrist per 200,000 inhabitants. But from the current point of view, this is an underestimation of the actual needs. With regard to child guidance clinics, WHO proposed a relation of one child guidance clinic per 50,000 inhabitants. This figure has not yet been reached in any of the 16 states in Germany. For young children in the first three years of their lives, there are centers for early detection and intervention. There is an obligation for the counties of every state to provide those services that have mainly a pedagogic orientation, but not all of them have a physician as a consultant.

Daypatient services

Daypatient services are important and, if well organized, effective and efficient services for the treatment of psychiatrically disturbed children and adolescents. There are three types of daypatient services: associated ones working in close relationship with inpatient departments, integrated ones carrying out their daypatient work in inpatient wards, together with inpatients, and independent daypatient services without any connection to an inpatient unit, most of them being associated with an outpatient department. The Expert Commission did not support the model of an independent and more or less isolated day hospital, because of a lack of flexibility between inpatient and daypatient treatment modalities. Instead, the Expert Commission proposed a triadic service system consisting of outpatient, daypatient, and inpatient services responsible for a circumscribed region. No proposal was made with regard to a certain relationship of one day hospital per a certain number of inhabitants.

Inpatient services

At the present time, there exist 114 inpatient services, including 25 university departments. On the whole, there are enough inpatient treatment places. However, these are distributed inadequately throughout the country. Thus, the Expert Commission proposed to provide a better distribution of services in the future, to provide more community-based inpatient services, to care for adequate buildings and personnel equipment, to provide the possibility that mothers be admitted to hospital together with young children needing inpatient treatment (rooming-in), and to respect a minimum size of an inpatient department (not less than 30 beds) in order to take care of different groups of patients who have to be separated in different wards.

In 1988, the Expert Commission proposed seven beds per 100,000 inhabitants in rural areas and up to 11 per 100,000 for an inner-city population. The current recommendation is 5–7 beds per 100,000 inhabitants, depending on the kind of the population to be served.

Complementary services and rehabilitation

The task of complementary and rehabilitative services is to provide care for children and adolescents with long-lasting and chronic psychiatric disorders. There is a great need for these types of services, especially for those patients who cannot be reintegrated into normal life and their former environment after inpatient treatment. There are special laws regulating the financial support of these services (Bundessozialhilfegesetz). Different types of services are summarized under the headline of complementary services:

- "Transitional homes" (Übergangswohnheime) that provide educational and vocational help after inpatient treatment for those patients who are not able to return to their former environment (family, school, occupation). There should be approximately 15 places per 500,000 – 750,000 inhabitants.
- Group homes for adolescents preparing them for their next step into independence while providing a certain guidance and counseling through adult professionals. The proposal is to have two group homes with 6 – 8 places per 500,000 – 750.000 inhabitants.
- Youth centers: In contrast to the two institutions above, the adolescents are quite independent in these centers; only the meals and some leisure activities are provided. These institutions provide support for those adolescents who cannot return to their families and who are preparing themselves for their professional work or are already continuously working.
- Foster homes/family nursing: This is an effective alternative to youth centers, especially for children and adolescents with a chronic psychiatric illness or handicapped children and adolescents. The advantage is that this type of institution provides a kind of family framework for the patient that can take into account his special needs and/or peculiarities.
- Rehabilitation services concentrate their activities on three fields: medical rehabilitation, scholastic and vocational rehabilitation, and social rehabilitation.

There exist special workshops for adolescents with chronic psychiatric disorders that provide also professional training, education, and continuous work under flexible conditions that take into account the abilities and handicaps of the patients.

Personnel

Great progress for all psychiatric services and particularly for child and adolescent psychiatric services was made with the Psychiatry Personnel Equipment Act which was stepwise realized between 1991 and 1995. The main advantage of this new personnel act is that the personnel needed for a certain ward or institution is no longer calculated in relation to the number but to the specific needs and requirements of the patients. Therefore, the patients are subdivided into several groups according to the amount of care, support, supervision, and treatment they need. The time required for every activitiy of the personnel with regard to different patients' groups is registered, and on this basis the adequate number of staff members (doctors, psychologists, nurses, etc.) is calculated.

Funding of services

In Germany, inpatient, outpatient, and daypatient facilities are paid in one form or the other by the state. Germany has a compulsory insurance system. All patients and families are insured and the insurances usually pay the costs for outpatient, daypatient, or inpatient treatment directly to the hospitals. This applies to all acute treatment necessities. The responsibility for chronically ill psychiatric children and adolescents is taken over by the youth welfare system and the social security system, depending on the kind and severity of the disorder. For example, for multiple handicapped children and adolescents in the sense of a combination of somatic and psychiatric disorders, the social security system is usually responsible. For children and adolescents suffering from chronic psychiatric disorders, however, the "youth welfare system" is responsible since 1991. This change in responsibility has imposed a heavy burden on the youth agencies who were not prepared to handle these problems.

As far as the complementary services are concerned, the same funding agencies are responsible (youth welfare system and social security system). Several of these purposes are in the hands of non-governmental welfare organizations and charities who obtain their financial support from different sources, mainly the youth welfare system and the social security system.

Rehabilitation services are paid partly by the insurances, and partly by the social security system.

Evaluation

There are not many studies in Germany that have so far evaluated psychiatric services for children and adolescents. In the region of Marburg which was the only region for the evaluation of child and adolescent psychiatric services within the Model Program Psychiatry of the Federal Government, we had the unique opportunity to do a comprehensive evaluation study of all services of three counties within a certain time-span (Remschmidt & Walter 1989; Remschmidt, et al. 1990; Walter, et al. 1988).

Within this program, psychiatric services for children and adolescents in three rural counties comprising 575,000 inhabitants were evaluated. During a one-year period, the referred population was almost completely recorded (n = 5,307). According to these data, the utilization of outpatient services was influenced by the local supply of outpatient care. In well-equipped areas, the referral rates reached a comparatively high level; however, they did not exceed 3.8 % of the unreferred peer group. Markedly higher rates had been found in community surveys, where the prevalence estimates amounted to 7 % at least. The attendance of child and adolescent psychiatric hospitals depended on the availability of community-based outpatient care as well as the distance between living place and the place of residential care. With growing distance, admission rates decreased, whereas the duration of hospital stays increased. The provision of specialized outpatient services was correlated to a high percentage of hospital referrals from that area; on the other hand, the duration of hospital stays was reduced. Inpatients from counties not appropriately served by outpatient facilities had significantly longer inhospital stays. During an interval of 42 months, hospital admissions (referred to the number of inhabitants) shrank in those counties where outpatient services for children and adolescents had been improved (Walter, et al. 1988).

4. Cooperation with medical and non-medical disciplines

Cooperation with pediatrics

Several, but not all, academic departments of pediatrics have a ward for psychosomatic disorders, usually headed by a child psychiatrist or a pediatrician with some training in child and adolescent psychiatry. In most departments of pediatrics, there also exist liaison or consulting services carried out by the neighboring departments of child and adolescent psychiatry and psychotherapy. Other fields for the cooperation with pediatrics are chronic somatic disorder, neonatology, and intensive care. Cooperations with regard to these fields have been developed in many university departments of pediatrics, but also in community pediatric hospitals.

Finally, there is a need to cooperate with neuropediatrics, not only in the field of epilepsy, but also with regard to brain damage, metabolic disorders, disorders of the central nervous system, and especially in the field of prevention and early intervention.

Cooperation with psychiatry

The departments of child and adolescent psychiatry in Germany mainly belong to a center of psychiatry; they are rarely associated with pediatric hospitals with the exception of psychosomatic departments. Child and adolescent psychiatry shares a diagnostic approach with general psychiatry, but deals with the same age group as pediatrics. So, associations with both are possible, but from a historical point of view, child and adolescent psychiatry is more often associated in institutions with general psychiatry. With regard to every day practice, there are three common fields with general psychiatry: (1) Adolescent psychiatry, which is in the hands of child and adolescent psychiatry up to the age of 18 – 21. In adolescent psychiatry, general psychiatric services are needed if there are emergency cases, because the departments of child and adolescent psychiatry and psychotherapy are not always equipped with a closed ward. (2) Family psychiatry: A common task in this field is the treatment of children of psychiatrically ill parents, where cooperation is necessary with regard to treatment of parents, and (3) the longitudinal perspective concerning psychiatric disorders in children and adolescents who have reached adulthood. This longitudinal developmental approach has not yet been developed in many places in Germany, but is a very important field for the future.

Cooperation with doctors in private practice

Cooperation with specialists from different fields who are working in private practice is generally very good. The German medical system gives priority to private practice, and the doctors in private practice are expected to cope with the needs of outpatient treatment and refer only those patients to hospitals who definitely need inpatient treatment or special medical investigations that cannot be carried out in private practice. The use of private practice does not mean that patients have to make their own insurance arrangements. A compulsary insurance system requires that every person be insured by law. Only those who earn above a certain level of income, are allowed to choose a private insurance which guarantees on average the best available service. This system means that nearly all patients first have to see their doctor in private practice who is either a general practitioner, a pediatrician, or a specialist in any other field and whose service is covered by the insurance.

Cooperation with non-medical institutions and professionals

Child and adolescent psychiatrists and psychotherapists have to cooperate with several other non-medical institutions. In the first place, the child guidance clinics have to be mentioned. There are more than 1050 in Germany with approximately 3600 full-time staff members, mainly psychologists and social workers. The average relation is one child guidance clinic to 79,000 inhabitants in the states of the former West Germany (1993) and one to 66,000 inhabitants in the states of the former East Germany (1995). The majority of child guidance clinics are headed by clinical psychologists and only a few by child and adolescent psychiatrists and psychotherapists. Close cooperation between child psychiatric services and child guidance clinics is necessary, although it is not as good as it should be everywhere.

The most important non-medical institutions for the cooperation with child and adolescent psychiatry are the local youth agencies. There are several common fields of activity: adoption, child protection, children of divorced families, children in homes and other institutions, child guidance services, etc. Through the new German child and adolescents' support law (Kinder- und Jugendhilfegesetz, in force since 1991), the youth agencies are responsible for the extrafamiliar placement of psychiatrically handicapped children and adolescents. Thus, they play an important role in the cooperation with child and adolescent psychiatry.

Other cooperating institutions include the school psychological services and the different types of special schools (special schools for children with learning disabilities, with speech and language disorders, with behavioral disturbances and conduct disorders, and for mentally handicapped children).

In the field of psychotherapy, the group of the analytic child and adolescent psychotherapists (formerly called psychagogues; there are more than 1,000 in Germany) has to be mentioned. Most of them are working in private practice along the lines of the psychoanalytic model, their patients being delegated to them by physicians.

Finally, consulting services are delivered by child and adolescent psychiatry and psychotherapy to different types of children's homes and in some places to the public health agencies.

5. Graduate/postgraduate training and continuing medical education

Graduate training: The role of medical faculties

In 1997, child psychiatry was represented by a separate department or chair in 25 out of 35 medical faculties in Germany. This means that in 10 medical faculties, there is no formal teaching program in child and adolescent psychiatry and psychotherapy for medical students. This is compensated in some faculties by lecturers from other universities, but there is still an urgent need to establish a department of child and adolescent psychiatry in every medical faculty. This was also stated by the Federal Government of Germany in its statement on the report about the Model Program Psychiatry. In 1997, two new chairs of child psychiatry were established, one at the medical faculty in Aachen and the other at the medical faculty in Mainz. At the moment (1997), the following medical faculties do not have child and adolescent psychiatric departments: Bonn, Düsseldorf, Gießen, Greifswald, Halle, Hannover, Homburg, Regensburg, Ulm, and one of the two faculties in Munich.

At those medical faculties with a department of child and adolescent psychiatry, the curriculum of child and adolescent psychiatry for medical students is integrated into general psychiatry and pediatrics, and there are also separate teaching

Table 2. Training curriculum for specialists in child and adolescent psychiatry and psychotherapy

Candidates must prove extensive knowledge, experience, and proficiency in the following subjects:	
1.	General and special psychopathology, including biographical aspects of anamnesis, behavior observation techniques, and exploration techniques
2.	Clarification and consideration of original causes of psychiatric disorders in children and adolescents, including preparation of a therapy plan
3.	Developmental psychology, psychosomatics, and neurotic disorders
4.	Methodology of psychological testing and rating of psychological findings
5.	Specific neurological methods of investigation
6.	Nosology and differential diagnosis of psychosomatic, psychiatric, and neurological disorders and diseases
7.	Indication for and techniques of psychotherapy, including different psychotherapeutic methods, participation in a Balint-group, self-experience, and psychodynamic treatment under supervision
8.	Indication for and techniques of functional therapies as well as indirect child and adolescent psychiatric treatment via behavior modification of parents or parent substitutes
9.	Somato- and pharmacotherapeutic methods and their indications in different psychiatric and neurological disorders
10.	Rating of laboratory values
11.	Indication for and methods of neuroradiological and electrophysiological techniques of investigation
12.	Documentation of findings, medical reports, including specific regulations of social legislation as well as legal norms of patient-doctor relationships
13.	Quality assurance in medical practice
14.	Expert opinion
Knowledge has to be imparted in the following subjects:	
1.	Development, anatomy, physiology, and pathology of the nervous system, biology and pathology of maturation, of human genetics, and metabolic disorders as well as of the endocrine system,
2.	Techniques of specific puncture methods
3.	Techniques of neuroradiological and electrophysiological methods of investigation
4.	Basic knowledge of principles of mental hygiene specific to different developmental stages
5.	Prevention and rehabilitation, including health counseling and health education

courses with special lectures in child and adolescent psychiatry and psychotherapy. Child psychiatry is also included in bedside-teaching. As far as the questions for the multiple choice examinations are concerned, approximately 25 % of the questions in psychiatry and 15–20 % in pediatrics belong to the field of child and adolescent psychiatry.

Postgraduate training, a joint effort

To become a specialist in child and adolescent psychiatry, after the final medical examination and the practical phase of training which ends with the so-called "approbation" (certificate to practice medicine independently), a candidate has to spend four years in child and adolescent psychiatry and psychotherapy and one year either in general psychiatry or in pediatrics. It is also possible to spend half a year in neurology. Of the four years of training in the field of child and adolescent psychiatry and psychotherapy, two years of training in inpatient services are obligatory. Two years can also be completed in a specialist private practice.

The different components of the training curriculum are listed in Table 2.

As the table demonstrates, a substantial part of the training curriculum is concentrated on psychotherapy (since 1993).

After having completed all the requirements for the specialist training, an oral examination has to be passed at the office of the medical society of the state (Bundesland) where the training has taken place.

For the documentation of the different parts of specialist training, there exists a log-book produced by the German Society for Child and Adolescent Psychiatry and Psychotherapy.

Continuing medical education in child and adolescent psychiatry and psychotherapy

At the time being, there are no formal requirements for continuing medical education (CME) in Germany, but the regulations for all medical specialists in Germany make it clear that continuing medical education is desirable, but is not obligatory.

Training programs for other disciplines

Child and adolescent psychiatrists and psychotherapists are included in several training programs for other medical and non-medical specialists. The main programs are carried out in the field of psychotherapy (especially with pediatricians and general practitioners), psychologists, teachers, nurses, pedagogues, and social pedagogues.

6. Research

Research fields and strategies

Broad and high-quality research has been carried out in German child and adolescent psychiatry and psychotherapy during the past two decades in four areas: (1) interaction and communication research within families, especially mother-child interaction, (2) neuropsychological and neurophysiological aspects of developmental disorders, (3) classification of child psychiatric disorders and behavioral disturbances, and (4) epidemiology, therapy evaluation, and quality control.

These issues are in line with a worldwide trend (Remschmidt 1996) that can be characterized by three tendencies:

- By an increased consideration of the biological basis of psychiatric disorders at all ages. The main topics here are molecular biology, genetics, and new imaging techniques.
- By a greater consideration of the principles of development. Main topics are developmental psychopathology, developmental psychology, developmental neurology, and developmental biochemistry.
- By the introduction of rational, effective, and efficient diagnostic and therapeutic measures. Main topics are standardized diagnosis, development of guidelines, quality assurance, and evaluation.

With regard to therapy, it is now quite clear that there is no single theory and no single therapeutic approach appropriate for the majority of psychiatric disorders in children and adolescents. It is necessary to develop treatment methods that are specific for a particular disorder which allow sufficient flexibility to provide for the individual characteristics of every case.

With regard to the further development of research in child and adolescent psychiatry and psychotherapy, a working group supported by the German Society for Child and Adolescent Psychiatry and Psychotherapy (Schmidt and Remschmidt 1989) developed a number of proposals as follows:

- Research in the etiology of psychiatric disorders in children and adolescents: In this field, research programs have already been carried out with the aim of detecting genetic mechanisms in several disorders such as dyslexia, autism, Gilles de la Tourette-syndrome, eating disorders, and obesity. New imaging techniques have also been used in these and other conditions, recently applying a functional-experimental approach.
- Multi-level research on stability and change in psychiatric disorders in children and adolescents.
- Research on externalizing disorders which are – due to their high stability – still an enormous problem for families, school, and society. The absence of effective treatment methods is a severe problem all over the world.
- Research on developmental disorders which are an important risk factor for the development of secondary psychiatric disorders and dissocial behavior.
- Research in the field of intervention, evaluation, and quality assurance: It is of great importance to evaluate therapeutic methods as well as services and to include quality assurance systems into a wide field of activities in diagnosis and psychotherapy.

The German Society for Child and Adolescent Psychiatry and Psychotherapy has set up a commission for the development of guidelines for diagnosis and therapy for the most important psychiatric disorders in children and adolescents in order to establish effective and efficient disorder-specific therapeutic programs that can be administered in different settings.

Research training and career development

There is no doubt that an appropriate and up-to-date research training is the most important precondition for high-quality research in the future (Remschmidt 1996). A good research training is, of course, also important for a future scientific career. For twenty years, the departments for child and adolescent psychiatry and psychotherapy at the universities of Heidelberg (located in Mannheim) and Marburg have been carrying out research training courses for young scientists, and these have been very successful. Meanwhile, several former participants of the seminars have qualified as professors of child and adolescent psychiatry. What we need, however, are regular research training seminars and postdoctoral training programs, and these have not yet really been developed in Germany. This will be an important task for the future.

Funding

Research in the field of psychiatric disorders in children and adolescents in Germany is carried out mostly at the universities and at special research institutes such as the Max Planck Institutes. At the time being, there is no special institution outside the universities devoted to research in child and adolescent psychiatry. Some research in psychopathological disorders in children and adolescents is also carried out at university institutes of psychology, but most of these are working mainly in the field of psychopathological disorders in adulthood within the departments for clinical psychology.

As far as funding is concerned, the German Research Association (Deutsche Forschungsgemeinschaft) plays the most important role allocating 656.3 million DM per year (1996) to all research fields of biology and medicine. Child and adolescent psychiatry and psychotherapy benefits in all four domains of funding, but only at a relatively modest level: single project funding, clinical research groups, point-of-main-effort programs, and special research areas (Sonderforschungsbereiche).

Other important research funding organizations are the ministries of the Federal Government, especially the Ministry for Health and the Ministry for Research and Technology which announce at regular intervals special programs in the field of health care, etiology of disorders, health services, etc.

Thirdly, a large number of foundations are important for research funding, most prominently the Volkswagen-Stiftung.

Child psychiatric departments are participating at a modest level in the programs of all research funding organizations described above.

7. Future perspectives

The future perspectives of child and adolescent psychiatry and psychotherapy cannot be seen independently from the development and the influences of society in general. It is difficult to predict how the framework for child psychiatry in Germany will be in the future. Nevertheless, the following perspectives seem to be reasonable.

Research

The situation in research can be looked upon in terms of two contrasting views: on the one hand, many mental and behavioral disorders in children and adolescents are not yet understood. On the other hand, the available findings are often not generally known and, therefore, not used in diagnosis, treatment, and prevention. Thus, three consequences have to be drawn from this situation:

- to stimulate basic and clinical research at all frontiers of scientific inquiry,
- to spread the available knowledge to all persons and institutions in the health care system, and

- to advocate child and adolescent mental health research among decision makers in politics and in the public.

In all three directions, initiatives have been taken by the German Association for Child and Adolescent Psychiatry and Psychotherapy as well as both other child psychiatric organizations in a joint effort by putting forward research projects, developing new research instruments, by facilitating the training of young researchers, by disseminating new results to mental health workers and to the public by special publications and newsletters, and by putting major emphasis on all issues of quality assurance and clinical evaluation research. At the moment, clinical guidelines are also being developed that include major disorders and their diagnostic and therapeutic implications.

As far as the advocacy for child mental health is concerned, negotiations with politicians, with members of the German Medical Association (GMA) and the National Association of Statutory Health Insurance Physicians (NASHIP) have been initiated. In addition, the third edition of the "Memorandum of the German Association for Child and Adolescent Psychiatry and Psychotherapy" is being revised. This document describes the current situation of child and adolescent psychiatry, including detailed proposals for the future development.

Training

Undergraduate, graduate, and postgraduate training has to be facilitated. As far as undergraduate training is concerned, there is an urgent need to establish departments of child and adolescent psychiatry at all medical faculties in Germany. At the moment, 10 faculties are still lacking a chair of child and adolescent psychiatry. With regard to postgraduate training, new regulations came out in 1994, and the German training scheme to become a specialist in child and adolescent psychiatry and psychotherapy is very much in line with the new European curriculum being discussed in all countries of the European Union and the EFTA countries. Continuing medical education (CME) has not yet been formally introduced, but initiatives have been taken in that direction.

Improvement of services and care systems

In spite of much progress supported by the Model Program Psychiatry of the Federal Government (1980–1985) and the Psychiatry Personnel Equipment Act (1991–1995), a lot of further progress is still needed. From the analysis of the current mental health system, the following conclusions can be drawn and should be realized:

- ▶ The main focus of services delivery is not any longer on inpatient care, but on outpatient services, daypatient facilities, and complementary services based on a community level.

- Specialized services are needed with highly qualified personnel and pragmatic, effective, and efficient treatment programs that have to be evaluated. The top priority of these services should be the treatment and care for children and adolescents with severe and persistent mental health problems.
- There are not enough child and adolescent psychiatrists in private practice. The conditions for this group of doctors have to be improved. It can, however, be expected that the situation will get better during the next few years, because private practice in child psychiatry is not restricted and still offers good prospects.
- The coordination of the different services has to be improved. The Expert Commission of the Model Program Psychiatry of the Federal Government has made proposals for coordination which have not yet been realized in many places.

There is hope that in all three fields (research, training, and service systems) the necessary developments will be initiated and stepwise realized. If this is the case, child and adolescent psychiatry in Germany will have a good future.

Selected References

Deutsche Gesellschaft für Kinder- und Jugendpsychiatrie (1990) Denkschrift zur Lage der Kinder- und Jugendpsychiatrie in der Bundesrepublik Deutschland, 2. Auflage, Marburg
Emminghaus H (1887) Die psychischen Störungen des Kindesalters. Laupp, Tübingen
Expertenkommission der Bundesregierung: Empfehlungen zur Reform der Versorgung im psychiatrischen und psychotherapeutisch/psychosomatischen Bereich. Auf der Grundlage des Modellprogramm Psychiatrie der Bundesregierung. BMJFFG, Bonn (1988)
Harbauer H, Lempp R, Nissen G, Strunk P (1971) Lehrbuch der speziellen Kinder- und Jugendpsychiatrie. Springer, Berlin
Harms E (1960) At the cradle of child psychiatry. Am J Orthopsychiatry 30: 186–190
Homburger A (1926) Vorlesungen über Psychopathologie des Kindesalters. Springer, Berlin
Kanner L (1957) Child psychiatry. 3. edn. Blackwell, Oxford
Lutz J (1961) Kinderpsychiatrie. Rotapfel Verlag, Zürich
Manheimer M (1899) Les troubles mentaux de l'enfance: Précis de psychiatrie infantile avec les applications pédagogiques et médico-légales. Sociétè d' éditions scientifiques, Paris
Remschmidt H (1996) Changing views: New perspectives in child psychiatric research. European Child and Adolescent Psychiatry 5: 2–10
Remschmidt H, Schmidt MH; Kinder- und Jugendpsychiatrie in Klinik und Praxis. Bd. I (1988), Bd. II und III (1985). Thieme, Stuttgart
Remschmidt H, Walter R (1989) Evaluation kinder- und jugendpsychiatrischer Versorgung. Analysen und Erhebungen in drei hessischen Landkreisen. Enke Stuttgart
Remschmidt H, Schmidt MH (eds) (1994) Multiaxiales Klassifikationsschema für psychische Störungen des Kindes- und Jugendalters nach ICD-10 der WHO. 3. Aufl. Huber, Bern
Remschmidt H, Walter R, Kampert K, Hennighausen K (1990) Evaluation der Versorgung psychisch auffälliger und kranker Kinder und Jugendlicher in drei Landkreisen. Nervenarzt 61: 34–45
Schmidt MH, Remschmidt H (1989) Forschung in der Kinder- und Jugendpsychiatrie: Perspektiven, Strategien, Schwerpunkte. Kinder- und Jugendpsychiatrische Klinik am Zentralinstitut für Seelische Gesundheit, Mannheim und Klinik für Kinder- und Jugendpsychiatrie der Philipps-Universität, Marburg (in Abstimmung mit der Deutschen Gesellschaft für Kinder- und Jugendpsychiatrie für den Bundesminister für Forschung und Technologie erstellt)
Stutte H (1960) Kinderpsychiatrie und Jugendpsychiatrie. In: Gruhle HW, Jung R, Mayer-Gross W, Müller M (eds) Psychiatrie der Gegenwart Bd II (Klinische Psychiatrie) (pp 952–1087) Springer: Berlin
Stutte H (1974) Zur Geschichte des Terminus "Kinderpsychiatrie". Acta Paedopsychiatrica 41: 209–215

Strohmayer W (1910) Vorlesungen über die Psychopathologie des Kindesalters. Laupp, Tübingen
Tramer M (1942) Lehrbuch der allgemeinen Kinderpsychiatrie, einschließlich der allgemeinen Psychiatrie der Pubertät und Adoleszenz. 3. Aufl., Schwabe, Basel
Virchow R (1869) Über gewisse die Gesundheit benachteiligende Einflüsse der Schulen. Zentralblatt für die gesamte preußische Unterrichtsverwaltung. pp 343–362
Walter R, Kampert K, Remschmidt H (1988) Evaluation der kinder- und jugendpsychiatrischen Versorgung in drei hessischen Landkreisen. Praxis der Kinderpsychologie und Kinderpsychiatrie 37: 2–11
Ziehen Th (1915) Die Geisteskrankheiten einschließlich des Schwachsinns und die psychopathischen Konstitutionen im Kindesalter. Reuther und Reichard, Berlin

Child and adolescent psychiatry in Greece

J. Tsiantis, S. Beratis, E. Tsanira, G. Karantanos

1. Definition, historical development, and current situation

Definition

The field of child psychiatry in Greece has been repeatedly redefined in recent years and has been accepted as covering "the diagnosis, therapeutic management and rehabilitation of psychopathological and developmental disturbances of childhood and adolescence, together with the promotion of mental health more generally among children, adolescents, and their families". In Greece, the term that has come to be used for the discipline is "child psychiatry" (one word in Greek), but it is taken for granted that this also covers adolescence. "Psychotherapy" is not included in the title. The age range is defined as 0–18 years. In practice, it is accepted that in the 16–18 year age group there may be an overlap with adult psychiatry.

Historical development

Child psychiatry is a relatively new discipline in Greece. The first efforts to set it up as an independent discipline began to take shape during the 1950s. The origins of child psychiatry were connected chiefly with the neuropsychiatric and psychiatric tradition. Until 1981, neurology and psychiatry were taught as a single postgraduate qualification, and the doctors who later decided to work on the mental disorders of childhood and adolescence had this background of training. Links with pediatrics and child-neurology have begun to develop in recent years. Psychoanalytic and psychodynamic theory and practice also account for a significant part of the psychiatric tradition in Greece. These orientations have contributed much to shaping child psychiatry in Greece. Other theoretical and therapeutic orientations have also been assimilated gradually. In Greece, a spirit of cooperation with the other professions involved in the mental health of children was promoted from the start and remains strong today. The professions of special teaching, psychology, and social work also began to develop during the 1950s. It is, of course, interesting that the first state special school, run by special teachers, opened in Athens (Kesariani) as early as 1937. These teachers defined special teaching even then as "therapeutic education" (Kalantzis, Vakareli-Kalantzis 1973). Where juvenile delinquency was concerned, the Associations for the Protection of Minors were set up (by Emergency Law 2724/40) and supplemented with the institution of probation officers (Law 2793/1954) in the larger cities.

In practice, the first important steps were those described below:

- The setting up of the country's first child psychiatry inpatient department in 1954. However, this department functioned on the premises of the Athens Neuropsychiatric Hospital, Greece's largest psychiatric hospital, to which it belonged.
- One early and very positive step was the founding of a semi-independent and non-profit organization entitled Kentro Psychikis Yginis (Mental Health Center). However, this organization received public funding, and its board of management was appointed by the Ministry of Health and Welfare. From the start it provided for children's outpatient services with an orientation towards the community, and this was of great importance given the spirit of the times. As a result, the first child guidance center was founded in Athens in 1956. This mental health center developed other services for children and expanded to cover 2–3 cities in Greece. It still provides useful services today, functioning in parallel and as a supplement to the National Health Service.
- The Hellenic Society for Mental Hygiene and Child Neuropsychiatry whose charter determined that care for the mental health of children and the promotion of related activities were its primary aims was founded in 1957. This association became a member of the International Association for Child Psychiatry and Allied Professions (1976), which expressly added adolescents to its chapter (Kaloutsis 1993).

Shortly afterwards (in 1963–1964), the State Neuropsychiatric Hospital for Children was opened near Athens. It remains the only hospital of its type in Greece. Its capacity has reached 180 beds, initially divided into two sections. It should be borne in mind that the approach prevailing at the time was that of "inpatient care and treatment", with an emphasis on the more serious and long-term disorders including mental retardation of various degrees. From the start, the two sections were obliged to admit children of this kind from all over Greece and also to engage in educational work with them. The accumulation of cases, the prolonged hospitalization of the children far from their families, and institutionalization were, as could have been expected, the consequences. Even today, individuals with physical and mental handicaps aged over 18 years are still treated in this institution.

Recent advances – psychiatric reform

In the early 1980s, child psychiatry in Greece entered a period of more active development. The most important points in this transition were as follows:

- The establishment in 1978 of a Department of Child Psychiatry in the Aghia Sophia Children's Hospital in Athens, the country's largest general pediatric hospital, with 650 beds. This was a new departure of the greatest significance. Within the Department of Child Psychiatry, there was an outpatient clinic from the start and liaison/consultation child psychiatry was practised, while by the mid-1980s an inpatient unit and a community child psychiatry unit was added.

- Recognition of child psychiatry as a separate discipline in 1981. This development took place at the same time as the separation of neurology and psychiatry, which became independent disciplines. Both developments were stimulated by Greece's accession to the (then) EEC.
- The formation by the Ministry of Health and Welfare in 1982 of a working party to study child psychiatric care in Greece and propose short-term and medium-term measures (Ministry of Health and Welfare 1982).
- The campaign for psychiatric reform which followed, in conjunction with promotion of the National Health System, then newly-founded. Efforts to reform the state system of psychiatric care in Greece had begun in the late 1970s. A significant role in the intensification of these efforts was played by the unsatisfactory conditions in the Greek psychiatric state hospitals, which became more widely known to Greek (and international) public opinion and particularly to the European press in the early 1980s. A report commissioned by the Greek government from the European Commission commented in harsh terms on the appalling conditions in which patients received care, with particular emphasis on the asylums of Leros. The report referred, inter alia, to the disgraceful state of the Leros PIKPA unit for children. The Greek initiative to reform the state psychiatric care system led to the approval of regulation 815/84 of the (then) EEC, and Greece received, by way of exception, considerable financial support in order to foster the initiatives being taken on the national level. The regulation was promoted on the basis of the proposals compiled by a team of experts (Commission of the European Community 1985).
- Within the framework of the National Health Service, provision was made for the formation of departments of psychiatry in general hospitals and for the establishment of mental health centers in the community, both including child psychiatry departments. This has facilitated the development of departments of child psychiatry in the children's hospitals (two fully-developed and two partly-developed departments) and of sections in child psychiatry in the mental health centers of various Greek cities. Changes have also been made to the one child psychiatric state hospital, with internal and external adjustments being made to its departments and services. The first child psychiatric department, with custodial cases, in the large psychiatric state hospital in Athens closed in 1986, as part of the efforts to bring about psychiatric reform in Greece. The psychiatric reform campaign has also included deinstitutionalization programs, the most important of which (in the field of child psychiatry) has been the Leros PIKPA program, which involved systematic intervention to transform and improve care and to set up a community home for children, adolescents, and young adults with mental and physical handicaps and associated psychosocial problems (Tsiantis 1995).
- The formation, within the Ministry of Health and Welfare, of the Central Health Council. The framework of the council includes a Mental Health Committee with a Child Psychiatry Sub-Committee. This authority is entitled to submit its expert opinions directly to the Minister of Health and the departments of the ministry.
- The formation of the Hellenic Society of Child Psychiatry in 1983 and the establishment – within the Hellenic Association of Psychiatrists – of a Child

Psychiatry Division (1987). These two bodies cooperate closely, especially on matters of postgraduate and continuous education, harmonization with the Union of European Medical Specialists (UEMS), etc.

- Publication of the first textbook: Contemporary Issues in Child Psychiatry by J. Tsiantis and S. Manolopoulos, in three volumes (Tsiantis, Manolopoulos 1987).

Current situation

The total population of Greece is approximately 10,000,000 (census of 1991); it is unequally distributed with almost 30 % of the population living in the Greater Athens area, 15 % in the northern city of Thessaloniki, and the remainder spread over smaller towns, villages, and numerous islands.

In the early 1980s, the number of child psychiatrists in Greece was very small. The incentives granted and the development that has taken place have now brought the number up to 150. Some of the frameworks in which they are active have links with university departments. Child psychiatry is also practised on a private basis, although in this respect, too, the Greek provinces are poorly supplied with services. There can be no doubt that throughout Greece, as a whole, the distribution of services and child psychiatrists lags far behind the specifications of the WHO. Among the positive developments in the field of child and family mental health is the establishment, in recent years, of autonomous and independent departments of psychology in a number of Greek universities. Postgraduate studies are now available in clinical and educational psychology.

2. Classification systems, diagnostic and therapeutic methods

Classification systems

Most of the child psychiatry departments in Greece seem to use the ICD-10 system for the diagnostic classification of their cases. Use of this system was encouraged by its official translation into Greek shortly after its publication (Stefanis et al. 1993). Some departments also use the DSM-IV system, and the need for familiarity with this system, too, is recognized, especially so that the literature can be followed with greater ease and for research purposes.

Diagnostic methods

Clinical child psychiatry assessments are often supplemented with psychological testing or examination by other professionals, depending on the case. It is established practice, both in public and private care, for there to be extensive collaboration among the professionals who make up the child psychiatry team. Depending on circumstances, cases are referred for paraclinical and laboratory investigations; EEG testing, imaging, genetic and metabolic testing, etc., are all widely used where indicated.

Therapeutic methods

The entire spectrum of therapeutic approaches is available, although, of course, fundamental orientations differ from department to department. In many departments, the psychodynamic approach and family therapy are stressed. It is also worth noting that the early 1990s saw the establishment of associations providing training in individual psychoanalytic psychotherapy for children and adolescents in collaboration with the European Federation for Psychoanalytic Psychotherapy. There are also programs providing training in family therapy.

3. Structure and organization of services

Guidelines for services, sectorisation of services

The instructions for the development of child psychiatry services include the proposals for their sectorization submitted by the Central Health Council subcommittee on child psychiatric care (Central Health Council 1995). These proposals were elaborated in collaboration between, on the one hand, the Hellenic Society of Child Psychiatrists and the Child Psychiatry section of the Hellenic Association of Psychiatrists and, on the other, almost all of the child psychiatrists working in Greece. The basic points of the proposals were as follows: sectorization of services, development of mobile units for mountain and island regions, provision of adequate staffing levels, development of intermediate child care structures (hostels, etc.) as well as the development of mental health services within the framework of primary care.

Types of services

Prior to 1981, there were seven child psychiatry services in Greece, mostly in the form of child guidance centers, which were concentrated in Athens and Thessaloniki. By 1990, the number of the different types of services had risen to 22 and by 1996 to 36. It is encouraging that the process of development of services in other Greek cities has begun, but in general child psychiatry services tend to be more highly developed and concentrated in Athens, Thessaloniki, and a small number of large cities, while extensive areas of Greece (especially in the mountains and on the islands) are not covered at all by the public care service. As a rule, these areas lack even child psychiatrists in private practice (Tsiantis 1997).

Outpatient services

Most of the cases referred are examined in child guidance centers (where the director is a child psychiatrist), in the child psychiatry departments of the general pediatrics hospitals, in community child psychiatry units or at the counseling centers for children and families operated by local government or non-profit making Non-Governmental Organizations (NGO). Such examinations are also carried out by child psychiatrists in private practice. Work of a largely clinical and diagnostic and counseling nature is also done in the private sector by psychologists, most of them trained in clinical or educational psychology. The number of these professionals working in the private sector is not known. There appear still to be questions of a statutory nature connected with the unimpeded exercise of psychology as a profession, and although there is a state mechanism granting licences to practise psychology (issued by the Central Health Council of the Ministry of Health), it applies only to those who intend to work in the public sector.

Daypatient services

Day services, if properly organized, can play an important part in diagnosis and therapy. In Greece, however, they are very little developed and meet only a small part of existing needs. In effect, there is only one day center for adolescents in a general hospital for adults (in Athens), another in a non-profit unit for children with psychotic and other developmental disorders (the Perivolaki, in Athens), and a third unit for children of latent and adolescent age groups with pervasive developmental disorders within the framework of a semi-governmental organization (the Kentro Psychikis Ygiinis, in Athens). Some day services are also available in the private sector. These services are addressed primarily to school-age children (5–14 years) with serious developmental disorders. They tend to be staffed by special teachers and psychologists and on rare occasions have a child psychiatrist as a consultant. The social security system meets part of the cost of the use of these services. The problem where they are concerned is the lack of supervision over the way in which they operate.

Inpatient services

There are two inpatient care units in general hospitals (10 beds in the Aghia Sophia Children's Hospital, Athens, and 15 beds in the Ippokrateio Pediatric Department, Thessaloniki), together with a short-stay unit (20 beds) in the Child Psychiatry Hospital of Attiki. Needless to say, there are needs which are not being met, especially in the adolescent age group and in rural areas. On the basis of the standards proposed, it has been calculated that there should be 6–8 beds for each million of the population and that figure should be doubled in order to cater to the needs of adolescence. This means that there is scope for the provision of more beds, correctly distributed in spatial terms. However, this has to be seen against the background of the tendency for the establishment of daycare centers rather than inpatient care units.

Complementary services and rehabilitation

Hostels for children and adolescents

Units of this kind, especially for adolescents with mental disorders or behavior disorders, are very limited in number: there are only three in the Greater Athens area. The shortage of such units creates an acute problem in connection with the post-hospital care which is sometimes necessary for children and adolescents from families with multiple psychosocial problems.

Pre-vocational training centers

In recent years, a number of pre-vocational training units for adolescents with mental disorders (with or without learning difficulties) have been set up. They are subsidized by the EU but there are usually problems with the continuation of their financing, which has a seriously harmful effect on their continued operation and on the continued provision of care.

Personnel

To date, there are no specific instructions covering all the types of child psychiatry services and laying down staffing levels. In the particular case of child guidance centers, it has been proposed that there should be an interdisciplinary team consisting of a child psychiatrist as director, 1–2 trained child psychiatrists, 1–2 psychologists, 1–2 social workers, 1 special teacher and 1 speech therapist. Theoretically, such a team could meet the needs of the families referred, who, it has been proposed, should be drawn from a population of between 100,000 and 300,000 people. The personnel of the other care structures (inpatient units, day centers, hostels, etc.) are developed on the basis of needs as they arise and of proposals submitted to the Ministry of Health – which are not always accepted.

Funding of services

The state child psychiatry care system in Greece meets the cost of the services provided by the state child psychiatry services, including those available from general hospitals (inpatient and outpatient care, liaison psychiatry, community programs) and at the child guidance centres.

All Greeks pay mandatory social security contributions, but the amount of social security funds is very large and the sums they are prepared to pay out are usually far below the cost of the services provided. When the services are provided by the public sector, the balance is met by the state, but when insured persons are compelled to turn to the private sector (especially for diagnostic or psychotherapeutic work) they themselves have to pay sums many times those which the social security funds can disburse. Cases of children and adolescents with serious motor or mental handicaps in combination with psychosocial problems are covered with the granting of allowances through the social welfare system, and rehabilitation and general care services are provided by the state.

Evaluation

No studies evaluating child psychiatry services have been published to date. The Directorate of Mental Health of the Ministry of Health and Welfare recently inaugurated a program under which all the psychiatric services of Greece will be monitored. A draft law "concerning the development and modernization of mental health services" is currently in the final stages of preparation, and it is hoped that provisions covering the appropriate development and organization of child psychiatry services will be contained in it. At present, there is a professor of child psychiatry at the University of Patra, another in Athens, and an assistant professor in Thessaloniki. The Ministry of Education recently issued a Presidential Decree establishing the first university department of child psychiatry, in the Athens Medical School, which has endorsed the decree. Step by step, similar departments will have to be established in the country's other medical faculties.

4. Cooperation with medical and non-medical disciplines

Cooperation with pediatrics

Several university and non-university hospitals have a collaboration between the departments of pediatrics and child and adolescent psychiatry. Primarily, this collaboration is based on the existence of a pediatric liaison service which administratively is a unit under the auspices of the child and adolescents department. The services offered by pediatric liaison attempt to cover all units of pediatrics such as inpatient general and special wards, various clinics and units (neonatology, endocrinology, thalassemic, etc.).

Special wards for psychosomatic disorders do not exist but such cases are being taken care of on an inpatient or outpatient basis, by the departments of pediatrics and child and adolescent psychiatry. The choice of hospitalization of the one or the other department depends on the nature of the case and the severity of the somatic condition.

There is a clear need for an increase in the number of child psychiatrists working in liaison services in order to improve the conditions of cooperation in the care of patients, and in teaching pediatricians psychosocial aspects of pediatrics.

Cooperation with psychiatry

In Greece certain departments of child and adolescent psychiatry are connected administratively to departments of general psychiatry, while others are completely independent. The ones connected with general psychiatry exist mostly in general hospitals or in psychiatric hospitals, while the independent ones are in general pediatric hospitals. Near Athens there is a large psychiatric institution exclusively for children and adolescents. Certain child and adolescent psychiatry departments cover individuals up to the age of 19–20 while others stop at the age of 14–15 years. There are also certain adult psychiatrists who see older adolescents above 16 years of age. There are not enough inpatient services for older adolescents and their hospitalization becomes often problematic. When adult and child psychiatry services belong to the same department, there is often collaboration in the care of child and adolescent patients and their parents.

Another area of collaboration involves the rotation of adult psychiatry residents in child and adolescent psychiatry services up to three months. However, not all adult psychiatry residency programs include this requirement.

Cooperation with doctors in private practice

There is no formal system of cooperation with doctors in private practice. Child and adolescent psychiatry patients and their families can see private doctors or attend the outpatient hospital clinic, as they wish. Private doctors may refer patients to the hospital for special medical investigations.

Cooperation with non-medical institutions and professionals

Child psychiatry in the public sector is usually practised within multidisciplinary teams in Greece. Therefore, there is a close cooperation between child psychiatrists and other non-medical mental health professionals. There is also a cooperation in the field of training in several child psychiatry services between undergraduate and postgraduate students in psychology or social work.

There is also a cooperation between child and adolescent psychiatrists and non-medical institutions but this cooperation is rather loose and not equally developed in the various parts of the country. There are various types of special schools, public or private, but not all of them necessarily have a consultant child psychiatrist. When they do not have their own consultant, they refer the children to child psychiatry clinics or to private practitioners. The same applies to other non-medical institutions such as adoption agencies, foster placement agencies, etc.

5. Graduate/postgraduate training and continuing medical education

Postgraduate training, a joint effort

The duration and content of postgraduate training are determined by decisions of the Minister of Health published in the Government Gazette. The appropriate scientific bodies submit their proposals in this respect, on their own initiative or when invited to do so. These proposals may be taken into consideration, but are not binding to the ministry.

At present (under arrangements introduced in 1994), training lasts 4 1/2 years, of which 2 1/2 years are in child psychiatry, 1 1/2 years in adult psychiatry, and six months in neurology. A recent joint proposal prepared by the standing committee of the Hellenic Society of Child Psychiatry and the Child Psychiatry division of the Hellenic Association of Psychiatrists suggested that the length of training should be extended to five years and that psychotherapy should be included in the training experience, thus harmonizing it with the UEMS guidelines. More specifically, it has been proposed that training should consist of one year in adult psychiatry, six months in neurology, and 3 1/2 years in child psychiatry. The proposals also deal in detail with the following:

- The objectives of the training and the criteria for recognition of training centers. The criteria to assure quality of training (Central Health Council 1998, see Table 1).

Four departments of child psychiatry in Athens and one in Thessaloniki have already been recognized as capable of providing complete training in child psychiatry. Certain other departments are in a position to provide part of the training. Postgraduate qualifications are awarded after written and viva voce examinations conducted in Athens and Thessaloniki before a committee of three child psychiatrists who are university professors or have served as directors of child psychiatry departments in the public sector. This committee serves for one year or two years and is appointed by decision of the Ministry of Health.

Continuing medical education in child and adolescent psychiatry and psychotherapy

At present, there are no formal requirements for continuing medical education (CME) in Greece, but it is encouraged. The joint standing committee of the Hellenic Society of Child Psychiatrists and the Child Psychiatry division of the Hellenic

Table 1. The training curriculum for child and adolescent psychiatrists

After training, trainees should possess sufficient knowledge, experience, and proficiency in the following subjects:

- Psychopathology (general and special)
- Nosology and differential diagnosis of psychiatric, psychosomatic, and neurological disorders
- Aspects of psychiatric intervention techniques and of techniques of observing children. Methodology of psychological testing and rating of psychological findings
- Training in neurological examination and knowledge of neurological methods of investigation
- Indications and techniques of the commonly-used methods of psychiatric treatment, including psychopharmacological treatments and psychotherapeutic techniques (individual and family psychotherapy). Quality assurance in the practice of child psychiatry
- Documentation of findings, medical reports and reports for the courts. Ethical issues in the practice of child psychiatry

Knowledge should be imparted on the following subjects:

- The psychological repercussions of physical illness (acute and chronic) and emergencies in pediatric practice. Intervention in psychosocial crises
- Effects of divorce, death, and loss on normal psychosocial development. Effects of physical, emotional, and sexual abuse
- Collaboration with the primary health care services. Management and intervention techniques for children and families suffering from malignant disorders
- The rehabilitation and social integration of children and adolescents with special needs
- Consultation services for education services (schools, daycare centers, etc.), social services, and community agencies. Basic knowledge of the principles of mental hygiene specific to the different developmental stages.

Society of Psychiatrists organizes various scientific activities in the field of continuous medical education, but these are not obligatory. Certificates are granted to participants, and activities have been made to harmonize the activities with the principles of the UEMS.

Training programs for other disciplines

Child and adolescent psychiatrists may be involved in training professionals from other disciplines. Such activities may occur (a) in child and adolescent psychiatry departments and services, (b) in training psychotherapy programs, and (c) through the supervision of psychotherapy cases on a private basis. Some departments have issued log-books to facilitate the documentation of the different components of specialist training, and efforts are being made to extend this procedure to all the child and adolescent training services. The log-book is based on the recommendations of the joint standing committee, and efforts have been made to follow the UEMS guidelines.

6. Research

Research into child psychiatry in Greece is not highly developed. There are a number of reasons for this, including the fact that until a few years ago there were no child psychiatrists on the staff of the medical schools and the very low level of funds allocated to research in Greece. The funds for child psychiatry research are almost non-existent. In recent years, however, some attempts to improve the situation have been made, with funding being sought outside Greece and from the European Union in particular. Proposals for research in Greece cover the following areas:

- Basic epidemiological research into the extent and incidence of childhood and adolescent mental disorders.
- Research into the various factors and methods by which the Greek family today can influence the normal (or otherwise) psychosocial development of children.

Needless to say, any future developments in the field of research will need to take into consideration the trends in child psychiatry world wide. These include among others:

- Considerations connected with the development of children and adolescents (the themes in developmental psychopathology and developmental psychology).
- The development of adequate and effective diagnostic and therapeutic tools, including standardized diagnosis, outcome studies, and quality assurance.
- Research into the various fields of preventive intervention (especially intervention in early life) and into the effectiveness of psychotherapeutic intervention.
- Longitudinal studies on stability and change in psychiatric disorders among children and adolescents.

It is among the intentions of the joint standing committee of the Hellenic Society of Child Psychiatrists and the Child Psychiatry division of the Hellenic Society of Psychiatrists to propose a strategy for the development of research. In this direction, a number of initiatives have been taken:

- The holding of training courses for young child psychiatrists.
- Encouragement of young child psychiatrists to take courses of a similar kind outside Greece when opportunities present themselves.
- Encouragement of child psychiatrists to publish in Greek and foreign-language journals.
- The assembly and translation into Greek of the various tools which have been used, and the publication of them in a booklet. Where expedient, such tools will be standardized for Greece. It is essential that high-quality research be developed in Greece, since through such a process child psychiatry will develop further and, by extension, the level of the child psychiatry services provided will rise.

7. Future perspectives

It is very hard to project what course child psychiatry will take, given the number of social, economic, political, and other factors on which developments will depend. However, despite these constraints, the following guidelines are proposed:

- Statutorily defined sectorization of the child psychiatry services provided throughout the country to ensure provision of care at a satisfactory level without social, economic, and geographical barriers. These services should be staffed by well-trained personnel
- Elimination of institutional/custodial care and replacement by community care. Upgrading of the undergraduate and postgraduate training of child mental health professionals. Establishment of departments of child psychiatry in all university hospitals. Development of primary health care services and the establishment of links with child mental health services. The state should invest more extensively in the mental health of children and their families, and lastly, it is important that Greek professionals in the fields of child health and mental health should be activated and should participate in upgrading the mental health services and in promoting research and training.

These proposals, if implemented, could serve as a foundation for hoping that the future of child psychiatry will be a satisfactory one.

Selected references

Central Health Council (1995) Report of the Subcommittee on Child Psychiatric Services (in Greek), Athens

Central Health Council (1998) Report of the Standing Committee of the Hellenic Association of Child Psychiatrists and the Child Psychiatry Division of the Hellenic Society of Psychiatrists (in Greek), Athens

Commission of the European Community (1984) Report of a Study of Mental Health Care in Greece. I. Brown, L. Liaropoulos, D. Lorenzen, P. Sakellaropoulos, J. Tsiantis, G. Katzourakis, Reform of Public Mental Health Care in Greece

WHO (1992) The ICD-10 Classification of Mental and Behaviour Disorders: Clinical Description and Diagnostic Guidelines. K Stefanis, K Soldatos, V Mavreas (eds) University Mental Health Institute Collaborating Center, Beta Publications, Athens 1993 (Greek translation)

Kalantzis C, Vakarelis-Kalantzis X (1973) Issues in Therapy, Education and Child Mental Health (in Greek), Karavias, Athens

Kaloutsis A (1993) The Hellenic Society for Mental Hygiene and Child Neuropsychiatry: Thirty Five Years of an Interdisciplinary Contribution to Child and Adolescent Mental Health (in Greek), Ellinika Grammata, Athens

Ministry of Health and Welfare (1982) Child Psychiatric Services in Greece. Report of a Working Party (J Andriakopoulos, S Giouroukos, G Karantanos, E Papathomopoulos, E Tsanira, J Tsiantis) (in Greek)

Tsiantis J (1987) Organisation of child psychiatric and preventive services in Greece. In: Tsiantis J, Manolopoulos S (eds) Contemporary Issues in Child Psychiatry, vol. 1, pp 404–443 (in Greek). Kastaniotis, Athens,

Tsiantis J (1995) The children of Leros PIKPA, British Journal of Psychiatry, vol. 167, supplement 28: 1–79

Tsiantis J (1997) Psychiatric services in Greece for the child. In: Child Mental Health Services (in Greek), Tetradia Psychiatrikis 57: 72–76, Athens

Child and adolescent psychiatry in Hungary

Á. Vetró

1. Definition, historical development, and current situation

Definition

Child and adolescent psychiatry in Hungary comprises the maintenance and development of the mental health of the 0–18 year old age group, the diagnosis and therapy of developed psychological disturbances, and the post-therapeutic rehabilitation of the patients in need.

This definition may sound a little general, as it does not specify the diversity of the various biological, psycho- or sociotherapeutic modes of treatment, but it does reflect the complex attitude to disease and therapy, which has recently been characteristic in Hungary.

Undoubtedly, however, it also reflects the disadvantage of the impossibility of isolating this profession a little more clearly from other medical and non-medical disciplines, making it more difficult for child psychiatry to develop its own identity.

Historical development

At the beginning of his career, the pioneer of Hungarian child psychiatry, Pál Ranschburg (1870–1945), dealt with general psychopathological questions. In his first prize-winning publication, a book entitled "Data on the psychology of the elderly", based on physiological factors, he wrote about the second pole of human life.

His work was of extreme importance for the establishment of experimental psychological methods in the field of psychopathology. While carrying out research into memory, he completed his research on children from elementary schools and from schools for defective children. In 1902 he relocated his laboratory to the National Institute for Defective Children, and the Psychological Laboratory for Defective Children was established.

Numerous of his scientific publications remain relevant today, e.g., "Schoolchildren with low intelligence", and "Imbecile schoolchildren" (1903), "The development and functioning of a child's psyche" (1905), "Monitoring plans for children exposed to moral deprivation" (1907).

Ranschburg's name became known internationally as a consequence of his doctrine "homogenous inhibition", though he also wrote many publications in foreign languages on child psychology. In Hungary, many of his students later became the "first generation" of therapeutic-educational professionals and researchers. The best representatives of the Ranschburg school are Mátyás Éltes, who elaborated the Binet-Simon test for Hungarian conditions, Margit Révész, László Focher, Lipót Szondi, Irén Kaufman, and János Schnell.

János Schnell (1893–1973) started his career as a school teacher, and later obtained a medical diploma as a teacher for children with mental disorders. Following Ranschburg's resignation in 1926, he became director of the research laboratory. As all of his interests were devoted toward the problems of psychological development in childhood, in 1935 he reorganized the institute, which continued its work as the Psychological Institute for Children. Although conditions in the institute at that time were poor, he worked with enthusiastic, caring fellow-workers, but an adjustment of salary scales and an appropriate number of civil servants was, nevertheless, out of the question.

The institution was able to survive only by charity or personal funding, rather than on the basis of a planned and organized national budget. The institute was merged into the Hungarian Academy of Sciences in 1951. In 1965, its profile was changed and it has since been functioning as the Institute of Psychology of the Hungarian Academy of Sciences.

Through Schnell's inexhaustible organizational capacity, his inextinguishable love for children, and the acknowledged needs in the capital, he organized the Central Child Neurological Institute, later the Metropolitan Mental Health Center for Children. The role of Schnell and the professionals who organized the metropolitan child mental health service was an essential one. There is a child neurology institute in every Hungarian county today, but their development and improvement of the quality of work in them still requires further well-planned efforts.

More and more eminent pediatricians were becoming interested in the problems of childhood neuropsychiatry in the 1930s. Under the direction of Édervári, for example, at the First Pediatric Clinic in Semmelweis Medical University, a separate outpatient department was established for the examination of children with hormone disturbances and psychopathic problems. In later years in the same department, outpatient care for children was organized by Pál Gegesi Kiss, a pediatrician, and Lucy Liebermann, a psychologist. Their observations were published in their book "Personality disorders in childhood".

In Hungary, the first child psychiatry department was established at the National Institute of Neurology and Psychiatry in 1950 by Blanka Lóránt, the then leading figure of child and adolescent neuropsychiatry.

In the "larger" psychiatry field, in cooperation with Angyal, she had learned the most modern neuropsychiatric views of the Viennese Poetzl School. During her active years, she was the first to deal with the symptomatology of "psychic focal symptoms", such as aphasia and anosognosia, and thereby with the physiology and pathology of speech development.

She performed important research in the field of "elective mutism" with catamnestic examination, accurately following the process of subacute progressive panencephalitis, and making symptomatic differences in childhood schizophrenia. She participated actively in the training of the new generation of child psychiatrists.

In the field of child development after Ranschburg, "asocial or disturbed" behavior was studied in Hungary by Júlia György, who directed the foundation of the Institute of Psychology in 1968. Her book "The antisocial personality" was published in 1967 and she received her Ph.D. degree in forensic psychology.

The work loads and organizational problems of national psychiatry did not allow child psychiatry to develop dramatically within neuropsychiatry. A children's department (with 14 beds) was established only in 1960 in Szeged at the Clinic of Neuropsychiatry of the Medical University, with Miklós Vargha as director.

This dramatically improved the training of the personnel and lessened the problems in research. In the 1980s, children's and adolescents' departments were established in many counties, but in recent years have been shut down. At present there are 7 inpatient departments.

Child psychiatry became an independent discipline in Hungary in 1965. Qualification as a child and adolescent psychiatrist and psychotherapist involves a specialization examination. More and more pediatricians have become interested in this discipline and it was predictable that, with better organization, Hungarian child psychiatry would gradually reach the necessary level of service as in other, more experienced countries. Unfortunately, in 1982 a new law relating to specialization examinations categorized child psychiatry among those fields where not a basic specialization examination but a more complex one was required, and repeated petitions to change the situation back to basic specialization examination have been in vain. Therefore, currently specialization in child and adolescent psychiatry can be achieved only secondarily, after specialization in pediatrics, psychiatry or neurology.

Until 1976, Hungarian child psychiatrists and neurologists were spread over sections of three separate scientific societies: Child Psychiatry and Child Neurology Section of the Society of Hungarian Pediatricians, the Child Section of the Hungarian Society of Neuropsychiatrists, and the Child Section of the Hungarian Neurosurgical Society. It was then decided that mutual scientific congresses would be held; the first was organized in Szeged in 1976 under the direction of Professor Miklós Vargha.

This was followed by annual events until 1989, when new scientific societies were founded: the Hungarian Association for Child Neurology-Neurosurgery and Child and Adolescent Psychiatry, which has been functioning since in two sections: the Child Neurological and Neurosurgical Section and the Child and Adolescent Psychiatry Section, and scientific meetings are now organized within these two sections.

Recent advances

The treatment of psychiatrically disturbed children in Hungary is funded by the Social Security System. Acute disorders are treated both on an inpatient and an outpatient basis. There are only a few beds for the rehabilitation of chronic cases in Child and Adolescent Psychiatry Departments. The treatment of permanent outpatients and chronic patients who need permanent hospitalization (physically handicapped and severely mentally retarded children) must be financed by each county from its social welfare budget.

Current situation

Hungary with an area 100,000 km^2 has a population of 10,354,000, of whom 52 % are females and 48 % males. Approximately 70 % of the population lives in cities, with 2 million in the capital, Budapest, and 30 % in villages or rural areas. The health coverage is provided by 34,255 doctors, who include 1,480 neuropsychiatrists. The total number of hospital beds available for the population is 105,097.

There are 17,225 hospital beds for neuropsychiatric patients (17 % of the total number of hospital beds), and there are 132 outpatient psychiatric institutes for this purpose.

Twenty-eight percent of the population (2.8 million) is under the age of 18 years, with a slight majority of boys. The organic patient care for the age group 0–18 years is carried out by 2,704 neonatal and pediatric specialists. For child patients there are 9,014 hospital beds; separate from the family doctor service, a successful preventive pediatric network has been established. Within the frame of the new health reform, through a union with the family doctor service, and as a consequence of declining child population, the number of non-utilized hospital beds is being reduced.

In 1998 child and adolescent psychiatry care is provided in 7 Child and Adolescent Psychiatry Departments. Concerning the general population, there are 172,833 inhabitants and 46,666 children and adolescents aged 0–18 years per child psychiatrist.

Of the 126 specialist child psychiatrists, only 50–60 work actively in their strict field; the others are retired, or work in their primary discipline (pediatrics, psychiatry or neurology). Private offices, which are funded by the Social Security System, function only part-time, and the numbers are low.

The number of members of the Hungarian Association of Child Neurology and Child and Adolescent Psychiatry is dynamically changing. At the end of 1997, there were 265 members, of whom 163 were Child and Adolescent Psychiatry section members or the members of the joint Child Neurology and Child and Adolescent Psychiatry section. There are only 17 male members.

Deficiencies remain. In the five Hungarian Medical Universities, Child and Adolescent Psychiatry exists independently only in Szeged, and only since January 1, 1998. None of the other universities have patient care units, even in the Departments of Pediatrics or Psychiatry.

Owing to the poor financial budget, in every county there is a deficiency of personnel in the child psychiatry care network, and the private centers face bankruptcy. Scientific research is also at a low level, as there are neither qualified teams nor financial support.

2. Classification systems, diagnostic and therapeutic methods

Classification systems

In Hungary, the compulsory classification system used by all patient care units is the ICD-10. For scientific research, DSM-IV is preferred.

Nationally, there is no integrated patient documentation, and each institute uses different methods to record patient data. Computer programs are increasingly being used.

Diagnostic methods

According to the traditions of neuropsychiatry, every patient undergoes internal and neurological examination as part of the diagnosic phase. Instrumental examinations (EEG, CT, MR, and laboratory tests) can be performed in most departments and outpatient units, with the cooperation of neighboring disciplines.

For psychiatric diagnosis, numerous questionnaires and symptom-estimating lists are widely used; the validity and standardization of these is a task for the future. The strong psychodynamic traditions mean that different projective tests are still widely used to establish the diagnosis and the type of therapy.

Therapeutic methods

In the majority of institutions, various methods are used in therapy, but emphasis is naturally placed on the dominant therapy of the given institutes.

In the departments, the psychodynamic approach is slowly moving into the background, and therapeutic behavior techniques are gradually taking precedence.

As concerns outpatient care, the majority of departments favor analytical therapy. Family counseling is widely practised, but classical family therapy is used by few professionals.

Between 20 and 25 % of outpatients receive pharmacotherapy; owing to the serious nature of the condition, the proportion of inpatients receiving such treatment is higher.

3. Structure and organization of services

Guidelines for services for children and adolescents with psychiatric disorders

The current Hungarian law laying down the guidelines for the operation of the health-care system, specifies neither the hospital norms nor the outpatient norms for child and adolescent psychiatry. In contrast with other disciplines, it does not specify the number of hospital beds, nor the activities of the health-care personnel in the pediatrics or psychiatry fields.

Therefore, after the law came into force, the county authorities had no way of either defining the number of hospital beds necessary for the psychiatric care of the population under 18 or specifying the working-hours of the specialist doctors. As far as we are aware, the current outpatient and inpatient care in some counties is regarded as partly involving pediatric and partly adult psychiatry without mentioning the hours and only taking into consideration the local conditions. Neither the maintainers nor the National Social Security Fund are obliged to provide the appropriate health-care on a population-proportional basis.

Since January 1, 1997 this has led to serious consequences. The 199 hospital beds available nationally in 1995 has been reduced to under 160, and the number of health personnel and treatments are being continually decreased.

Types of services

From the detailed information provided below, it will become clear that, except for the rehabilitation possibilities, child and adolescent psychiatric care is practiced in many forms, but the numbers of professionals, the infrastructure, and the size of the region covered differ widely. Unfortunately, the requirements proposed by the WHO are not met anywhere. The new financial system has led to the disease groups being changed, and family doctors are striving to treat more and more child psychiatric patients. Unfortunately, this generally consists only in including psychopharmaca in the prescriptions. As the family doctors lack the proper training, there is no possibility for a psychotherapeutic approach, let alone its application.

Outpatient services

Private practice in child and adolescent psychiatry

Private practice in child and adolescent psychiatry, although recognized by law, is almost unknown as a permanent occupation in Hungary. Some doctors are willing to work as child psychiatrists part time, but the numbers are fairly low.

One reason for this may be that the Social Security System does not appropriately reward the time spent with this time-demanding activity, and it is, therefore, not a viable financial option to run such a practice.

Child and adolescent psychiatric outpatient network

Child and adolescent psychiatric outpatient care is provided by child and adolescent psychiatrists. All 19 counties have one outpatient institute each, while in the capital there are 7. In these at present there are 40 child psychiatric specialists. The levels of both infrastructure and staffing differ widely within the country. In some places, such health care is provided by only one specialist; in other places, several multidisciplinary teams are available. The children and adolescents are referred to these centers by pediatricians, family doctors, and teachers.

Specialized outpatient units of hospitals

These do not generally provide preventive care or rehabilitation, but greatly help in the outpatient examination of ill children and in the post-treatment of hospitalized patients.

Specialized outpatient centers

These operate in different organizational forms (Training College for Teachers of Handicapped Children, hospital units, private practices funded by foundations, etc.), usually specializing in one certain particular disease (autism, hyperkinetic diseases, PTSD, etc.) or the whole field of child and adolescent psychiatry.

Network of child guidance clinics

This is usually run by a teacher or psychologist. Occasionally, a child psychiatrist is also employed, so that the psychiatric diagnoses should be adequate and the therapeutic work acknowledged. Children with behavioral disturbances or learning disorders are usually referred by the schools. The children's learning abilities are examined by committees, which can direct the children to special schools or classes.

Network of family help centers

These are organized by each county; every county has one or more institutes, funded by the social department of the regional local government office. The heads of such institutes are psychologists or social workers. Their major role is to establish a protective social network, but at times they deal with child psychiatric tasks as well.

Early developmental centers

Besides the perinatal intensive care centers, early developmental centers have also been established in many regions of the country. These were founded to screen out mental disorders and to provide the rehabilitation of physically handicapped and disturbed children between the ages of 0 and 3 years. These centers usually function in collaboration with hospital pediatric units.

Drug centers

In order to deal with the growing problems of drug abuse, regional drug centers have been established to monitor drug-addicted patients. In such centers, teenagers and young adults are treated on an outpatient basis.

Daypatient services

Despite repeated requests, the Social Security System has so far not acknowledged the existence of daypatient services. Patients treated in this way, therefore, occupy beds at the given hospital. Patients living nearby are admitted to the department, sent home in the afternoon, and readmitted next morning. This is the only way to provide them with full treatment in the department.

Inpatient services

In Hungary, 9 inpatient units were established over the past 45 years, only one of which is a university unit. In the last 4 years, however, owing to the drastic reduction of hospital beds in the health system, 2 have already been shut down and another one is in the process of being closed. There are 6 departments with 158 beds at present. These are divided unequally: in Transdanubia, for example, there is not a single inpatient department.

There is a rooming-in possibility for mothers in every department, although the Social Security System pays only a minimal fee for this to the institutions, and the majority of the institutions can, therefore, not take advantage of this. Child and adolescent therapy is generally performed separately in these departments. Other differentiated therapeutic care is usually not possible. There are no institutes for differentiated professional care (autists, forensic medical cases,etc.). Acute drug detoxification is performed at the adult psychiatry units; child psychiatric units do not undertake such therapy.

Complementary services and rehabilitation

Complementary services and rehabilitation therapy in Hungary are rare. The rehabilitation of drug patients has been proceeding for 3 years in the frame of model experiments and these drug centers continue to operate. Rehabilitation institutes that can accept 15–20 patients have been established for drug-dependent adolescents and young adults. There are also drug centers run by the churches. During the elaboration of the new law relating to child protection, the need arose for institutes where adolescents, who were not able to adapt to their original environment, could be treated. In such institutes, they may receive longer courses of therapy. Such a home was first established in Budapest in 1997.

The present child and adolescent psychiatry rehabilitation work is primarily carried out in educational institutions on a day-student or boarding school basis. Depending on the intellectual status of the children, there are two types of special schools for children with various grades of mental disorders. Special kindergartens and school groups have only recently been founded. These are for children with pervasive developmental disorders, mostly autistic patients. The therapy of children with conduct disorders or hyperkinetic (ADDH) children has not yet been solved. There are similar problems in schools in the case of anancastic or depressed children. Children unsuited to education live in foster homes. These are organizationally integrated with pediatric care and are typified more by an organic attitude than by rehabilitation or rehabilitation care.

Personnel

The number of health care personnel is determined by the number of hospital beds and not by the patients' individual needs. The minimum standards laid down in 1997 define the numbers of doctors and therapists needed in a certain department and the total number of personnel. These numbers are extremely low, but in the majority of workplaces not even these numbers are available. The staff of the departments are extremely overloaded, and only a moderate extent of differentiated therapy or health care is possible.

Funding of services

In Hungary, there is a compulsory insurance system. The National Social Security System pays the hospitals directly for all insured families (all children under the age of 14) for which inpatient or outpatient treatment is provided. The inpatient departments have introduced the American DRG financing system where the turnover of patients is very high, and therapeutic work is, therefore, more difficult. Switching to DRG has also meant that child psychiatric illnesses have become of low priority.

The average numbers of days of therapy were calculated according to tests run in general pediatric units. Therefore, because it falls in the 3–10 day therapy category, autism, for example, received a weighting factor of 0.7 as compared to the American factor of 3.5. The period of care is usually sufficient only to clarify the organic background of illnesses; psychotherapeutic intervention in child psychiatry, therefore, cannot be completed.

Since the new financial system was introduced, the general duration of care has been reduced from 3-4 weeks to 2–3 weeks; otherwise, the departments will go bankrupt and will be closed down. One chronic and one rehabilitation institute and department are financed by the Social Security System. The funding of the therapy of chronically ill or multiply handicapped children is a task of the social system.

Evaluation

In Hungary, no studies have been performed to evaluate the psychiatric services and their benefits for children and adolescents. The outpatient and inpatient institutions are overloaded and, without an increase of the number of personnel, it would be impossible to treat more patients. The Social Security System forces the hospitals to reduce the duration of treatment and the low average time that can be devoted to outpatients makes the effectivity of this kind of therapy questionable.

4. Cooperation with medical and non-medical services

Cooperation with pediatrics

The Pediatric Clinic at the Medical University in Pécs includes a child neuropsychiatry department where patients with neurological or psychosomatic complaints are treated with the cooperation of a specialized child psychiatrist. The Child and Adolescent Psychiatry Department at Albert Szent-Gyorgyi Medical University in Szeged collaborates with the Pediatric Clinic.

However, at present there has been no real breakthrough or really close cooperation in the above field. Pediatricians show great interest in the psychiatric diseases of children, but find the phrase "psychiatry" and its negative connotations, somewhat undesirable.

Cooperation with psychiatry

Some child and adolescent psychiatry units work together with adult psychiatry; the outpatient network, on the other hand, functions in cooperation with child neurology. Patients are directed here by pediatricians, but the diagnostic and therapeutic tools employed are similar to those of a psychiatrist.

The treatment of adolescents often demands the help of adults, as the units are not always prepared to treat aggressive psychotic patients.

Cooperation with doctors in private practice

At present there is no real possibility to consult family doctors. If they refer a patient, it simply means taking over the patient's treatment, and it certainly does not mean consultation about the child's problems. Although every patient has a family doctor, Hungarian law enables people to turn directly to a specialist if there is a psychiatric problem, without first consulting to the family doctor. The majority of patients are, therefore, brought in either by the parents or by the school, without the recommendation of a family doctor.

Cooperation with non-medical institutions and professionals

As a consequence of the interdisciplinary character of the profession and the close relation to the social sphere, teamwork involves cooperation with several other non-medical institutions. Most often it is the local Board of Guardians that assists in our work. These agencies are responsible for the appointment of a temporary guardian, social worker, guardian teacher, etc. There is also close cooperation with different foster homes, since many children who are placed in such institutions are psychologically disturbed.

As there is no school psychologist network in Hungary (although a few schools occasionally employ psychologists), we try to keep in close touch with school doctors and nurses. This is mostly done by giving lectures, conducting training or organizing psychoprophylactic days.

5. Graduate/postgraduate training and continuing medical education

Graduate training: The role of medical faculties

In Hungary there are 5 medical universities, and in 4 of them there is a formal basic teaching programe. In 1 university, in Budapest, there is postgraduate training. In the other 4 universities, there is no regular child psychiatry training. At Albert Szent-Gyorgyi Medical University in Szeged, the Department of Child and Adolescent Psychiatry has been working independently since January 1, 1998. Otherwise, there is no child psychiatry department within the university system. It is understandable, therefore, that child psychiatry as an independent subject is included in the curriculum only in Szeged; at other universities, it is merged with psychiatry or pediatrics and few lectures are given on the topic, the actual number depending on the head of the given department.

Naturally, in such cases there is no opportunity for clinical practice in the field of psychiatry either.

Postgraduate training, a joint effort

To become a specialist in child and adolescent psychiatry after the final medical examination, a doctor must first pass a basic examination in pediatrics, psychiatry or neurology. Having completed this, the candidate has to spend 2 practical years in child psychiatry, 1.5 years being spent in a department and 0.5 years in outpatient care. Depending on the basic examination, this is followed by 0.5 years in pediatrics or psychiatry practice (those with an initial examination in psychiatry have to spend the 6 months in pediatrics and vice versa). During the 2.5 years, psychotherapeutic training is also necessary, which is later followed by a test and oral examination. Having completed the practical phase, the candidate has to pass a week-long practical examination and later an oral examination before an examining committee, appointed by the National Specialist Examination Board.

Continuing medical education in child and adolescent psychiatry and psychotherapy

At the time being, there are no formal requirements for continuing medical education for specialists, although in several cities (e.g., Budapest and Szeged) regular courses are organized for specialists; however, these are not obligatory.

Training programs for other disciplines

Child and adolescent psychiatry is included in several specialist training programs. We regularly organize continuing training courses in the frame of pediatrics, psychiatry, clinical psychology and child neurology, and for family doctors.

We are often asked to supply further training courses for teachers and social workers. Every 1–2 years, we also organize courses for child psychiatric nurses. Child psychiatry additionally forms part of the curriculum of the postgraduate training of general nurses.

6. Research

Research fields and strategies

A broad range of research has been carried out in child and adolescent psychiatry in Hungary in the past 5 years. The publications have dealt considerably with organizational questions relating to child and adolescent mental hygiene and the difficulties involved in the training of medical specialists. Epidemiological surveys have been organized to determine the exact extent of child psychiatric morbidity. Researchers have examined the external and internal risk factors which play major roles in the development of psychiatric diseases and have dealt with the efficiency of drug and psychotherapy in connection with certain illnesses.

Research training and career development

For high-quality research in the future, it is necessary for the young researchers to be prepared for scientific work. Unfortunately, no such training is available for child psychiatrists in Hungary. In recent years, there have only been 3 Ph.D. degree theses in the field of child psychiatry. At present, there is no acknowledged Ph.D. program in child psychiatry and a thesis cannot be written in this field.

Funding

Research is carried out mostly at the universities; there are currently a number of governmental projects which cover the costs of research. Primarily the Ministry of Welfare and the Ministry of Education invite applications and evaluated them. The Hungarian Academy of Sciences and the National Social Security System Mental Hygiene Fund also help financially in certain areas of research.

Mainly central organizations finance prevention projects in the area of mental hygiene. Among the private foundations, the Soros Foundation is the most important in giving aid to child and adolescent psychiatry research.

Despite the diversity of funds, however, it can be said that child and adolescent psychiatry receives relatively small amounts for scientific research.

A greater potential for grants is afforded by joint research projects with foreign institutions. Such was the TEMPUS-JEP project, in which, in collaboration with the leading professors of the Child and Adolescent Psychiatry Departments in Glasgow and Würzburg (Profs. W. LI. Parry-Jones and A. Warnke), the Child and Adolescent Psychiatry Unit of Szeged Medical University was able to spend 600,000 ECU for the improvement of education.

One recent trend in Hungary can be considered very positive. As the national budget is quite small, the institutions tend to have quite low patient numbers, and hence many institutions cooperate in order to carry out research together, with the help and under the leadership of the partner institutions.

The Fogarty Foundation (USA) was founded for the specific purpose of financing an epidemiology project in childhood depression; this was managed by Professor Maria Kovács at Pittsburg University; and there is an ongoing project with the participation of 16 institutions, examining the genetic background of childhood depression. This project is directed and funded by NIMH (USA).

7. Future perspectives

The current flow of information and pace of life mean that a child now experiences more by the age of 18 than he or she would have throughout life 60–70 years ago. There are many more events in the lives of children, and the rapid rate of social change requires more and more survival strategies from the young generation. Thus, the morbidity level is increasing. As diseases are polyetiological, research must be approached from different angles, such as prevention and exploration of the pathological causes and therapy.

Research

Only in recent years in Hungary has high-quality research in the field of child psychiatry begun to rapidly develop. Thus, there is still a great deal to be done, such as the development of internationally accepted scientific tools, standardized questionnaires and interview techniques.

We have to educate a team which will provide scientific answers to all the questions relating to the discipline of child psychiatry and will formulate and carry out an appropriate research plan. The above-mentioned projects, funded with foreign assistance and with the guidance mentioned above, will help us a great deal. It is also necessary to locate financial sources to promote this research.

Training

It is important for all medical universities to acknowledge the inevitable role of the teaching of child psychiatry in medical training.

It is crucial for child and adolescent psychiatry to become a basic profession in Hungary, in line with the European norms. Accordingly, we have elaborated a curriculum, with the help of a TEMPUS project, which has not yet been approved by the National Medical Specialist Qualifications Committee.

In order to maintain and improve the knowledge of active medical specialists, it is essential to introduce a compulsory training system.

Improvement of services and care systems

There are many institutions of child and adolescent psychiatry in Hungary, but they do not form a nationwide network. They are randomly located around the country. Therefore, there are many locations where there is no patient care. It is important for the present child psychiatric outpatient network to be able to form at least one complete team in every county.

In Transdanubia, it is crucial to establish at least 2 inpatient departments, so that both patient care and regional specialist training can be raised to an adequate level. There are no temporary rehabilitation institutes; their establishment should therefore be a priority.

It is clear that there is a great deal still to be done in Hungary in the field of child and adolescent psychiatry. Without improvement of the present health-care system, the training of professionals, scientific research, and financial help, we cannot move forward. It is highly encouraging that the present small group of professionals is enthusiastic in their work, and we are gradually achieving developments in an increasing number of fields.

Selected references

Böszörményi G, Brunecker E (1980) Child and Adolescent Psychiatry. Medicina

Gádoros J (1992) A hazai gyermek és ifjúságpszichiátria. (Helyzetkép és javaslat) Psych Hung 7: 193–203

Magyar Statisztikai Évkönyv (1992 and 1993) Központi Statisztikai Hivatal Budapest

Parry Jones WLI, Vetró Á, Warnke A (1994) Teaching and training in child and adolescent psychiatry in Hungary. In: Sensky T, Katona C, Montgomery S (eds) Psychiatry in Europe. Gaskell

Vetró Á (1995) Quo vadis child and adolescent psychiatry. Gyermekgyógy 46: 102–108

Vetró Á, McGuinness D, Fedor I, Dombovári E, Baji I (1997) Epidemiological survey of behaviour problems among children of school age in Szeged. Psych Hung 12: 193–201

Vetró Á, Parry-Jones LI (eds) (1996) Textbook of Child and Adolescent Psychiatry. GyLE

Child and adolescent psychiatry in Iceland

H. Hannesdóttir

1. Definition, historical development, and current situation

Definition

Child psychiatry has only existed for the last 28 years in Iceland. For decades the main emphasis in the development of child psychiatry has been on promoting the clinical services but the speciality has not as yet been exactly defined by health authorities. Today the main emphasis is to promote the academic situation. The speciality was first inaugurated in medicine in 1970 but the speciality requirements have since then been twice modified in 1986 and 1997. In 1997 the speciality was called "Child and Adolescent Psychiatry" but earlier "Child Psychiatry".

At present there are ten child and adolescent psychiatrists in the country. Most of them have received their speciality training in the Nordic countries, two partly in U.S.A. and one partly in Britain. Four of the ten are not working in child and adolescent psychiatry and one is retired. At the moment only five child and adolescent psychiatrists are working in the speciality.

Historical development

The roots of child psychiatry go back to psychology, pediatrics, psychiatry, pedagogy, and the social sciences in Iceland. During the years 1960–67, a psychological department for children was established under the auspices of the Reykjavik Department of Public Health and under the management of a psychologist, adult psychiatrist, pediatrician and a social worker. The work of this department was primarily psychological investigation and individual evaluation of children, but it was also to give individual guidance to parents and to advise up-and-coming psychologists and educationalists. This mental health department, which was the first of its kind in Iceland, provided services for children and adolescents up to 15 years. There was no child psychiatrist in the country at this time. During the years 1967–76 this mental health department continued to be run by the Reykjavik Department of Public Health, with a "Healthy and Well Service" for children up to the age of five under the management of a pediatrician. During its existence from 1960–1976, 2,100 children were seen at this child guidance clinic. The first child psychiatric department in Iceland opened in August 1970 in Reykjavik. It had been evident for many years that there were indeterminable child psychiatric problems and a great need for such a service in the country. Special reports on these were sent to the Director General of Public Health from both pediatricians and psychiatrists. It was proposed that a child psychiatric department should be established under the auspices of the National University Hospital. In 1968 Social Affairs in Reykjavik began discussions between the city and state concerning the establishment of a psychiatric department for children and adolescents; the outcome of these discussions was that both parties agreed to establish such a department within the University Hospital for children with mental disorders.

In 1970 the first chief child psychiatrist was appointed. The service was in the early years connected to the department of pediatrics within the university hospital but functioned as an independent speciality; however, it came under the department of adult psychiatry division of the National University Hospital in 1983 and after that lost its independence both administratively and academically. The unit has been located from the beginning at a considerable distance from the main hospital and because of that the service has been more isolated. The unit consists now of an outpatient unit, inpatient unit for children younger than 12 years, and in 1987 an adolescent inpatient unit was established for adolescents up to the age of 18 years. Older adolescents receive inpatient treatment in the division of adult psychiatry or, if they have drug or alcohol problems, at the National Hospital for Drug and Alcohol Detoxification.

On May 3, 1980, the Icelandic Association of Child and Adolescent Psychiatry was established to promote the evolution and the development of the speciality and to organize its official annual meetings on training and research. The association is linked to the Icelandic Medical Association and has at the present time 16 members, ten of them are certified in child and adolescent psychiatry, three are females. At the present time three are in resident training in child and adolescent psychiatry abroad.

Current situation

Iceland is divided into health care districts. In each district there is a central hospital or health care facility for specialized health care but without child psychiatric or guidance services for children except in Reykjavik and Akureyri, the capital of the north in Iceland. Most health care districts have psychological services connected to the school authorities. Due to current economic recession, profound changes are taking place in Iceland to decrease the cost of services for general hospital care. One day in a hospital for child psychiatry can cost around four times that in adult psychiatry which has aroused interest among politicians and clinical staff in the effectiveness of child mental health services.

Medical treatment is socialized in Iceland; care at hospitals is free for children and adults. For outpatient services a limited amount of payment is requested. Infant mortality rate is low and longevity is high. Many needs for children and adolescents with mental problems have not been met in Iceland. Child and adolescent psychiatry must utilize its knowledge of the etiology of mental disorders to promote the health of children and strengthen the capacity of families and communities to reduce the incidence and prevalence of substance abuse, which is a serious problem in Iceland among adolescents.

An important milestone in child and adolescent psychiatry in Iceland was when the European Union of Medical Specialists (E.U.M.S.) acknowledged child and adolescent psychiatry/psychotherapy as a main speciality in medicine in October 1993 at a meeting in Copenhagen.

2. Classification systems, diagnostic and therapeutic methods

Classification systems

The International Classification of Diseases (ICD-10) is used in Iceland together with a history taken and various symptom checklists like the Child Behavior Check Lists by Achenbach and his family of check lists and traditional psychological tests. For research purposes, the DSM-IV, the American Psychiatric Associations' system, has also been used, especially for international scientific purposes.

Diagnostic methods

Teamwork among the specialists has been emphasized from the beginning of the service. Outpatient care has always been the primary mode of treatment for children and adolescents. Children are seen in the outpatient clinic for screening, diagnostic work-up, and treatment with their parents and often siblings. These consultations are usually carried out before it is considered whether admission to the inpatient wards is needed. Only 14.6 % of children from outpatient department were admitted to inpatient wards in recent years. Referrals are from daycare centers or primary schools, psychological services of the schools or the social welfare departments, MDs or parents.

The connection between the hospitals (state) and health care sector (community) is currently being challenged in Iceland.

Therapeutic methods

Clinical child psychiatry is relatively well established in Iceland but with limited consultative work in the pediatric wards, other child/adolescent caring institutions, and in the social sectors. An attempt is made in child psychiatry not to overlook important biophysical factors in the evaluation and treatment process by not focusing solely on socio-educational factors. The total needs of the child must always be considered first and foremost with emphasis on continuity of care during the treatment.

In crisis situations, intervention through support is often enough, with family counseling or therapy in the outpatient department. The main focus has been on services for children within their families following psychodynamic approaches and communities and schools through family work. The philosophy of work has been to consider individual needs and current problems – biophysical, intrapsychic, and within the family. Individual psychotherapy has been limited but most frequently administered with family counseling/therapy and/or psycho-educational treatment and art and music therapy. The role of psychoactive medication or psychopharmaca is explored and has been used more frequently in recent years if there seems to be an indication for this, especially as in ATDD, depression or severe, frequent aggressive outbursts.

The principal mode of treatment has been family-oriented therapy. The main focus is on the mode of interaction among family members. Most of the therapists use more than one approach or theory in their practice. Behavioral therapy, cognitive therapy, and hypnosis have been on the increase among all therapists, especially among psychologists, nurses, and social workers.

3. Structure and organization of services

Types of services and funding

The Department of Child and Adolescent Psychiatry is a department within the adult psychiatric division of the National University Hospital. It is the only one of its kind in Iceland. The population of Iceland is not more than 270,000 and around 65,000 are less than 16 years old. Around 4,500 children are born each year in Iceland. The department comprises an outpatient unit, an inpatient unit for four children younger than 12 years, and since 1987, a unit for eight adolescents younger than 18 years. Earlier a long-term day hospital unit for six children existed at the time, and the unit served autistic children from 1970 until March 1996. The average length of stay for inpatients services during the past ten years has been 65 days.

Total budget from the community and state to child and adolescent psychiatry in Iceland was in 1997 $ 1,937,000 but to adult psychiatry around $ 27,352,000.

Outpatient services

According to World Health Organization's proposal, there should be one child guidance clinic per 50,000 inhabitants. But this figure has not yet been reached in Iceland. Child psychiatry has not had high priority in the community or university hospital administration. For young children from age 0–5 years old, there are "well baby" clinics mainly connected to primary health care facilities for early detection and intervention. Unfortunately, child psychiatry has not been integrated into the well baby clinics as of yet to detect early mental health problems during infancy, such as in Finland and in many other countries.

The majority of consultations in child and adolescent psychiatry are carried out in the outpatient services, and the outpatient unit establishes the primary mode of treatment. In 1997, 3,530 visits were in the outpatient department at the University Hospital. There is a great shortage of facilities and outpatient service in the country and waiting lists for the service have been up to one year. During the past 24 years there has been family therapy orientation in the speciality beginning in the outpatient service.

Inpatient services and personnel

Those hospitalized are only a small number, on average 14.6 % (Hannesdóttir, Stefánsson 1995). During the past ten years 643 children were admitted to inpatient services in child and adolescent psychiatry in Reykjavik. Parents have not been admitted to the units together with their children except in a few exceptions. A staff of about 60 make up the service team (1997), which are multi-disciplinary, currently consisting of 2 child psychiatrists, 5 residents, 6 psychologists, 4 social workers, 17 nurses, one occupational therapist, and 2.5 secretaries. Duties and responsibilities of the various disciplines have been defined in a handbook. The patient to staff ratio in the inpatient services has been 1:2.8.

Today there is increased discussion about the coordination of mental health services for children. The need for child psychiatric beds has been estimated to be about 4 beds for 10,000 children. According to this, there has been a considerable shortage of beds in the speciality in the country. There has been an increased tendency in the past few years to look at prevention and treatment of mental disorders of children as an issue of general public health.

The low service utilization rate in child and adolescent psychiatry in Iceland (0.2 %) points towards great clinical needs that are not met when prevalence rates from epidemiological studies are compared to service utilization rates.

4. Cooperation with medical and non-medical disciplines

Cooperation with pediatrics and psychiatry

Of the two pediatric wards in Reykjavik no formal liaison or consulting services are being carried out by child and adolescent psychiatrists. In the two main pediatric wards in Reykjavik, psychological evaluations are more frequently asked for than child psychiatric consultations. Cooperation with regard to these fields will hopefully develop in the near future both in psychosomatic disorders and in neuropediatrics and in the field of prevention in the well baby clinics.

Since 1985, there has been an inpatient unit for school children with behavioral problems, which is directed by a social worker, attached to the department of adult psychiatry at the City Hospital in Reykjavik. This unit was in January, 1998 connected to the Child and Adolescent Unit at the University Hospital.

Clinical rounds and meetings have been jointly held with adult psychiatry of the University Hospital since 1983. The administration in child and adolescent psychiatry and the teaching of medical students have been under adult psychiatry.

Cooperation with non-medical institutions and professionals

Within the Government Agency of Child Protection and the Ministry of Social Affairs, a service has been given to adolescents between 12–15 years old with behavioral problems and delinquency for the past 30 years. The service is given by teachers, pedagogues, social workers, and psychologists and consists now of residential treatment homes for 45 adolescents. The service is primarily in charge of the day-to-day administration of 80 child protection committees in the country, according to law on child protection.

The Diagnostic Center for Mentally and Physically Handicapped Children is under The Social Ministry in Iceland. Since March 1996, this center has been primarily responsible for the diagnosis and treatment of autistic children and adolescents. However, since 1970, autistic children were taken care of by the Department of Child and Adolescent Psychiatry. Unfortunately, there is no integrated treatment or diagnostic workup between the Department of Child and Adolescent Psychiatry and the Center for Mentally and Physically Handicapped for autistic children.

Recently two communities developed a service for families with young problem children in Reykjavík run by a social worker. All these services have suffered from the absence of child and adolescent psychiatrists in their clinical work.

One child psychiatrist is developing services for children in the north of Iceland, Akureyri, within the district hospital in the department of pediatrics, on the initiative of the inhabitants in the district.

A few child and adolescent psychiatrists, working in the private sector part time both in Reykjavik and Akureyri, have played an important role in services in recent years. Private practice in child and adolescent psychiatry is partly paid by the state insurance and partly by the patient him/herself and is not restricted.

5. Graduate/postgraduate training and continuing medical education

Graduate training: The role of medical faculties

After six years of medical school, the postgraduate training definition to become a child and adolescent psychiatrist requires five years of training out of which three years are in child and adolescent psychiatry, one year in adult psychiatry, and one year in pediatrics according to rules and regulations on speciality training in medicine in Iceland from 1997.

The department of Child and Adolescent Psychiatry at the University Hospital has been responsible for teaching medical students in child and adolescent psychiatry and for training MDs from other specialities since 1974 under the leadership of the professor in adult psychiatry.

The speciality has never had a chair at the Medical Faculty of the University in spite of 24 years of teaching medical students by child psychiatrists through lectures. Child and adolescent psychiatry has, therefore, not been included in the medical school curriculum. No bedside teaching in child psychiatry exists currently for medical students. The teaching in the Faculty of Medicine runs parallel to the teaching of adult psychiatry and has been administered by the professor of adult psychiatry from the beginning, even the examinations in the speciality which sometimes have been multiple choice, oral or written examinations. New research work in child psychiatry from Iceland in recent years has not been presented to medical students in their teaching at the Medical Faculty of the University or used there in other ways to promote the development of the speciality. No formal teaching has been in child and adolescent psychiatry in the Department of Pediatrics at the University Hospital. Because of this urgent need to establish a chair in child and adolescent psychiatry, special reports have been sent several times to the Ministers of Health and Education, the Deans of the Medical School, the Rector of the University of Iceland, and the Director General of Public Health in the country to support and promote a teaching chair and formal teaching program at the university without any response.

Postgraduate training, a joint effort

No formal postgraduate or postdoctoral training programs have been available in the country because no academic professorship has been established in Iceland to lead and organize the speciality training. Training programs for other disciplines do not exist either in the country. The need to integrate teaching in child and adolescent psychiatry into various other fields of study has been advocated but is in no way fulfilled at present in Iceland.

Continuing medical education

Continuing medical education is not obligatory but important in Iceland because of the isolation of the country and its small population. Specialists can spend two weeks per year for continuing medical education and are reimbursed of expenses if they are employed by the community or state.

6. Research

Research fields and strategies

Research has been carried out since the 1960s, mostly individual projects, both clinical and high quality epidemiologic research. The first international research project in epidemiology was carried out from 1991–1994 and is the largest project. This project focuses on the mental health of children from 2 to 18 years, selected at random from the general population, using the Child Behavior Check Lists of Thomas Achenbach as a screening instrument (Hannesdóttir, Einarsdóttir 1995).

Several projects so far have been carried out in the country on a team basis on demographic data, diagnosis and classification, treatment methods, ATDD, children's sleep disorder, drug and alcohol abuse of adolescents, and on the prevalence of autism. Iceland participates currently in an European eating disorders project (COST B6). Most of this work is basic research in medicine in Iceland.

Research training and career development

An important turning point with regard to research took place in the beginning of the 1980s, when the first Nordic Child Psychiatry Research meeting was organized in Finland in 1982, and since then research meetings have been organized in all five countries every 2–3 years. These meetings have stimulated research in child and adolescent psychiatry in all five Nordic countries. One icelandic child and adolescent psychiatrist is finishing his dissertation, the first one in the speciality.

Of the five Nordic countries, academic and administrative structure is weakest in child and adolescent psychiatry in Iceland in spite of the increasing growth in research work, publications, and active participation in European and international conferences in the speciality.

Funding

Research fundings have been extremely limited, and research work in the field has mainly been on a voluntary basis in recent years. There is no special funding devoted to child and adolescent psychiatry in the country or connected to the two universities in Iceland.

Important research has been carried out on development, behavior, and psychopathology of school children in the departments of Social Science and Psychology at the University of Iceland in Reykjavik in the past. Hopefully, in the near future more interdisciplinary cooperation in research work between the medical disciplines and the psychological/social and behavioral sciences will appear.

7. Future perspectives

Research

The government has not yet decided upon a national policy in mental health for children and adolescents as to what has caused serious difficulties in the administration of child and adolescent psychiatry in Iceland for many years, with lack of ambition, independence of the discipline, and autonomy of the service given.

Health care administrators are missing the fact that adolescents are suffering from serious addictive disorders, probably the most common unmet mental health disorder with various comorbidities.

The future goals are first and foremost to put more influence on the government to gain a chair at the university to integrate teaching, training, and clinical work and to do more research work especially in the fields of genetics and results of the outcome of treatment. More coordinated community work is needed among all specialities taking care of children and adolescents through improved laws and legislation and by breaking down the walls between the ministries and the professional people to integrate the services.

Improvement of services and care systems

There is a considerable shortage of mental health service for guidance of children and parents, which in other countries is connected to outpatient services in the communities, pediatric departments, and primary care physicians.

The future of child and adolescent psychiatry in Iceland is uncertain in many ways, mainly due to lack of academic leadership and limited interest from the government, communities, and health authorities, to a shortage of organized services and policy for the whole country, and to the budgetary crisis faced by the Medical Faculty and the University Hospital. We need to break down the walls between ministries, communities, states, institutions and professionals to build up new services where professional people put their knowledge and experience together to advise children with mental health disorders, including drug and alcohol abuse care, without limits. It is important and necessary to follow closely and strengthen the relations between child psychiatry and neuro-pediatrics due to new research in the field. We must prevent isolation of the speciality, possibly through more collaboration between professors of child psychiatry by planning joint education, training, and services in child and adolescent psychiatry for all the Nordic countries because of their small populations, fairly similar culture and problem-types, and approaches and attitudes in the speciality.

Linkages of mental health specialists with primary health care, pediatric units, schools, the police, social service agencies, drug and alcohol treatment centers, and the juvenile court will provide an important function to improve the inter-organizational networks.

Infant psychiatry is a new and rapidly developing clinical and scientific field within child psychiatry in many countries but is not developed as of yet in Iceland.

The main future goals cover five different areas, all aiming at a better treatment for the patients: 1) To improve quality in the clinical daily work for patients and professionals; 2) to develop methods for measuring quality in treatment; 3) to improve education for students and specialists; 4) to promote basic and clinical research and development; 5) and to encourage more interdisciplinary work.

Iceland needs new models for administering clinical work and rethinking of mental health services for children and adolescents. We talk about "health care without limits" while at the same time service utilization rate is only 0.2 % and the adolescent's addiction disorder is drastically lacking recognition in Iceland.

The University Academy in the country has to recognize the scientific contribution of the discipline to utilize the important research work that has already been done in the speciality to promote further development in the field of mental health for children in Iceland.

Selected references

Achenbach TM, Edelbrook CS (1983) Manual for the Child Behaviour Checklist and revised child behaviour profile. Burlington, VT. University of Vermont

Barn- och ungdomspsykiatri under 90-talet. Kristianstad: Kristianstad: Boktryckeri AB, 1993. Danmark

Direktoratet for Köbenhavns Hospitalsvæsen (1987) Psykiatriplan for Köbenhavsn Kommune 1988–2000. Köbenhavn

European Union of Medical Specialists (1992) Compendium of Medical Specialist Training in the EC. U:E:M:S: secretariat, 20, Avenue de la Couronne, B-1050 Brussels

Hannesdóttir H (1993) Child and adolescent psychiatry in Iceland. The state of the art, past, present and future. Nord J Psychiatry 47: 9–13

Hannesdóttir H, Einarsdóttir S (1995) The Icelandic Child Mental Health Study. An epidemiological study of Icelandic children 2–18 years of age using the Child Behaviour Checklist as a screening instrument. Eur Child Adolesc Psychiatry 4: 237–248

Hannesdóttir H, Stefánsson JG (1995) Child and Adolescent Psychiatric Outpatients in Iceland. Demographic data and diagnosis. Nord J Psychiatry 49: 169–174

Piha J, Almqvist F (1994) Child psychiatry as an academic and clinical discipline in Finland. Nord J Psychiatry 48: 3–8

Psykisk barna- och ungdomsvård. Stockholm, SOU, 1957: 40

Rydelius PA (1993) Child and adolescent psychiatry in Sweden – from yesterday until today. Nord J Psychiatry 47: 395–404

Spurkland I (1993) Training in Child and Adolescent Psychiatry in Norway. ACPP Rev Newsletter 2: Vol 15: 3

Smedegaard N, Hansen N, Isager T (1993) Danish child psychiatry. Past, present, future. Nord J Psychiatry 47: 75–79

Statistics in Iceland (1991) Reykjavik, Iceland: Hagstofa Íslands

Stefánsson JG, Hannesdóttir H, Líndal E (1994) A Note on an Increasing Suicide Rate in Iceland. Arctic Med Res 53 (Suppl 2): 576–579

Sundhedsstyrelsen. 90'ernes psykiatri. Omstilling på psykiatriområdet. Delrapport. Köbenhavn, 1991

Sundhedsstyrelsen. 90'ernes psykiatri. Planlægning af psykiatrien. Hovedrapport. Köbenhavn, 1991

Sundhedsstyrelsen. 90 érnes psychiatri. Indsatsen for psykisk syge. En faglig redegorelse. Delarapport, 1991. Danmark

The University Hospitals Annual Reports, 1970–1997. Reykjavík, Iceland: The University Hospital, Skrifstofur Rikisspitala, Rauðararstigur 32, Reykjavik, Iceland

Tyrfingsson Th (1996) Annual Report from the National Center for Addiction Medicine, Vogur Hospital, Iceland

Vanvik IH, Spurkland I (1993) Child and adolescent psychiatry in Norway. Today and tomorrow. Nord J Psychiatry 47: 155–160

Child and adolescent psychiatry in Ireland

P. McCarthy

1. Definition, historical development, and current situation

Definition

"Child Psychiatry" in Ireland is understood to be that medical speciality that responds to the needs for prevention, treatment, and rehabilitation of children and adolescents who suffer from those psychiatric disorders that are relatively adequately described in both the ICD and DSM classification systems. This response is in a manner consistent with the standards of treatment of the Royal College of Psychiatrists.

Historical development

Child psychiatry in Ireland started in the late 1950's, when a number of Irish psychiatrists, having trained in child psychiatry in England, Scotland, and the United States, returned to develop services under the auspices of religious orders who had traditionally been involved in general hospital management, adult psychiatric hospitals, and services for the mentally handicapped. Their training had been a combination of very pragmatic dynamic and also psychoanalytically oriented psychotherapies.

The social services of the state, which were by the early 1970s beginning to accept more and more responsibility for children and families in the community at large, then commenced the development of child psychiatric services throughout the country. The numbers of consultant (specialist) child psychiatrists has risen from a figure of 5 in 1968 to that of 47 in 1998. The first 15 specialists received their training abroad, but many of the more recently appointed specialists have been Irish trained; the training scheme being under the direction of the Irish Psychiatric Training Committee, and being accredited by the Royal College of Psychiatrists (the College whose Membership embraces almost 100 % of all psychiatrists in both the United Kingdom and the Republic of Ireland).

Recent advances

The first university chair in child and adolescent psychiatry was established in Dublin University Trinity Medical School in 1997, and a second chair has been established in University College Dublin Medical School this present year (1998). These chairs come after (rather than before) the development of quite an active teaching and research involvement over the past 20 years. However, it is anticipated that they will catalyse much greater academic activities.

Current situation

The population of Ireland is 3.62 million in the Irish Republic and 1.65 million in the North of Ireland. Roughly 22 % of the population is aged under 14 years; but in certain areas of Dublin (which contains one third of the total population of the country) there are pockets of 140,000 total population where 31 % is under age 14. These variations have significant implications for service planning.

Twenty-six percent of the population (1,375,000) is below 16 years old. There is one child psychiatrist per 30,000 children under 16. Older adolescents (16 to 20 years of age) are largely served by the general adult psychiatric services; although significant numbers inevitably find themselves in the outpatient care of specialist child and adolescent psychiatrists.

For administrative purposes Ireland has always been divided into 32 counties. Of these 32 counties, 26 comprise the sovereign Republic of Ireland and the remaining 6 are Northern Ireland. For child psychiatrists, however, all are members of the same Royal College of Psychiatrists, and share the same post-graduate training and Continuing Medical Education (CME). The child and adolescent psychiatric trainees from all the major training schemes in the country, whether it be Cork, Galway, Belfast or Dublin, share many of the special training programmes, and colleagues in both jurisdictions are actively involved in the "Irish Division" of the Association of Child Psychology and Psychiatry (ACPP).

Everybody in Ireland is entitled to free state provided psychiatric treatment; but there is a medical insurance scheme which covers the cost of private inpatient treatment for those who wish. However, only one of the private hospitals provides a young adolescent inpatient unit (12 beds). All other inpatient needs for children and adolescents of less than 16 years are catered for in small state funded inpatient units; 2 in Dublin (14 and 8 beds), and 1 in Galway (15 beds). At the moment in Ireland it is pointless to differentiate between private and public (or state sponsored) child psychiatric services, as private facilities and resources are negligible. There is no private inpatient setting for children under the age of 14.

Private insurance provides only the most meagre cover for consultation and outpatient work. The result is that 95 % of specialists are in state sponsored salaried positions, and at least 95 % of all child psychiatric treatment is performed by these salaried state employed specialists. Newly trained specialists must apply for one of the state funded posts that becomes available.

The objectives of service provision tend to be categorised as follows:

- Treatment and rehabilitation programmes for those youngsters who develop mental illnesses such as schizophrenia, manic depression, Tourette syndrome, anorexia nervosa, etc.
- Services for children with autism, Asperger syndrome, and other pervasive developmental disorders.

- A range of services that are hopefully preventative and that are specifically directed at issues such as attachment disorders, post traumatic stress disorder, child sexual abuse, attention deficit hyperactivity disorders, and forensic assessments.

2. Classification systems, diagnostic and therapeutic methods

Classification systems

The ICD-10 classification system is used in all Irish child psychiatry departments and community child psychiatric clinics. This is done in a multiaxial framework mimicking that produced for the ICD-9 (Cox 1982).

Most departments also use the "presenting problem" schedule of the Association of Child Psychology and Psychiatry (ACPP) or the Scottish modification of same.

Diagnostic methods

All the usual psychological test batteries are used as required, e.g., I.Q. testing, perceptual testing, Achenbach questionnaires. Additionally, sleep EEGs, and brain scans are obtainable at relatively short notice (a few days) in all centres. Colleagues in paediatric neurology are available in the university hospitals, and cadres of neuropsychologists have been developing in these centres. Of particular interest has been the availability over the last 5 years of very well trained and sophisticated speech and language therapists, who not only bring us new descriptive terminology (e.g., "semantic pragmatic disorder" for what might be described as the language difficulty of children with Asperger's syndrome), but also batteries of language testing and assessments whose validity would appear to be very good, but whose usefulness in designing therapeutic interventive programmes is undoubted. The basic and essential clinical interviewing of child and family, however, remains the most valued diagnostic tool.

Therapeutic methods

Although, in Ireland, psychoanalytic concepts are well understood, and their value appreciated, very little psychoanalytic psychotherapy is in fact practiced by Irish psychiatrists. The reason for this is twofold:

- The demand for assessment and treatment in the public clinics is so great that the briefer psychotherapies, with target symptom relief, are used.
- The lack of medical insurance cover for outpatient work. Very few families can cope unaided with the cost of private long-term psychotherapy.

The fact that postgraduate M.Sc. degrees can now be acquired in quite intensive two year university programmes, in subjects such as "family therapy", "psychoanalytic psychotherapy", "child psychoanalytic psychotherapy", and "cognitive behaviour therapy", has had an increasing influence on the type of therapies practiced in Ireland. Most clinics have personnel, whether they be specialists in child and adolescent psychiatry, or psychiatric social work, or psychology, etc., who have M.Sc.'s in one or other of these therapeutic techniques. The treatment teams are always headed-up by a consultant (specialist) child and adolescent psychiatrist, who would not only prescribe and supervise medication where indicated, but who would also have psychotherapeutic expertise.

Of the therapies, family therapy, or a brief form of psychoanalytically orientated psychodynamic therapy, or cognitive behaviour therapy are those that are, selectively, more frequently availed of; however, antidepressants (particularly the SSRI's) and psychostimulants (particularly Ritalin) are being increasingly used to compliment such psychotherapy.

Multisystemic therapy, involving a variety of other agencies, is increasingly being developed in relation to the issue of "conduct disorder".

3. Structure and organization of services

Guidelines for services for children and adolescents with psychiatric disorders

The child and adolescent specialty in Ireland is expected to service children (from birth to the 16th birthday) whose I.Q. is above 60. A separate group of specialists (trained in mental handicap) cater to the needs of mentally handicapped children (both inpatient and outpatient) who attend special schools. The schools are under the control of the Government Department of Education.

Children with epilepsy and other neurological disorders are treated by paediatric neurologists, who may be in liaison, where indicated, with specialists in mental handicap or specialists in child and adolescent psychiatry.

The Republic's Department of Health has recently formally adopted a funded policy whereby six-bed child psychiatric inpatient units will be developed in 8 centres throughout the country, and 3 regional 14 bed adolescent units (for the age group 12–16) will be established immediately in Dublin city, Galway city (in the west), Cork city (in the south). These inpatient units will complement those few that exist at present. The inpatient needs for the 16–18 year old age group will be serviced by specialist facilities within the general adult psychiatric service, and which will be manned by specialists in adolescent psychiatry. They will develop treatment programmes for that age group, based on their inpatient settings. This planning is based on the pragmatic reality of what tends to have been developing in a number of progressive general adult hospitals already.

Types of services

Services are provided both in child psychiatric outpatient clinics based in the community and in paediatric hospital departments, where inpatient consultation and liaison services are also provided to paediatricians. Inpatient treatment units and specialist centres for children with pervasive developmental disorders and severe developmental disorders of speech and language, complete the range of services.

All services are over-burdened with referrals and have quite long waiting lists.

Outpatient services

These are provided by child psychiatrists and their multidisciplinary teams and are available, free of charge, to all sectors of society.

Quite apart from the medically oriented child psychiatric clinics, there are a small number of centres devoted to counselling and psychotherapy. Some are run privately (with small state funding subvention) and some by religious orders. There are, however, in addition state sponsored groups of psychologists and social workers in each of the health board areas, who provide counselling for schools in their areas, and some educational psychological assessments. They may also do group bereavement work. Some of the health boards have small specialist teams (3 or 4 persons) to investigate allegations of child sexual abuse. The total numbers of such professionals is roughly about 100. Their numbers are growing, however, as more people obtain the post-graduate M.Sc.'s in the various forms of therapy. Small numbers are developing private practices. However, the income from such practice is meagre, as patients do not get recompensed from medical insurance or state bodies.

Daypatient services

There are 3 different types of daypatient services operational in Ireland:

- Specialist centres for children with autism. There are five such centres in the country to which children are minibused from their homes each morning and returned late afternoon. One of the centres now provides an inservice training setting for staff who will be working in specialist programmes for low functioning autistic patients in mental handicap centres.
- There are three adolescent dayhospital units which each have 40 adolescents attending at any one time. Referral to such dayhospitals is via specialist child psychiatrists in child psychiatric clinics and departments. These dayhospitals are seen as being less expensive to run than inpatient units and to have advantages for certain patients, in that family and other important contacts are not lost.
- Day group therapy programmes in outpatient clinics. The state pays for taxis to bring these children from their homes to and from the clinics each day.

Inpatient services

There are 6 inpatient units in the country, four in the Republic and 2 in Belfast. One of those in Belfast and one in the Republic are specifically for adolescents. Plans, as described in Section 1 are for an enlarged inpatient provision country wide. Funding is already committed to these developments.

Complementary services and rehabilitation

- Each of the eight health board areas in the Republic has developed a range of group homes (6 to 8 youngsters) with house parents and supporting staff; also a range of short-term and also long-term fosterage placements. Collaborative day "Outreach" programmes (for disenchanted young adolescents who have opted out of the regular school system) have been developed by the educational authorities.
- The Department of Education provides residential places in a range of special schools for 130 youngsters aged 12 through 16 who have been referred to their care (and detention) through the court system because of continuous delinquent activity. The present philosophy is to continue using such educational facilities, but to now develop high supervision settings within the health sphere rather than further extension of the educational detention centres.
- A number of long-term residential workshops are available for older adolescents who have come through the childhood "autism" services. These are run by independent limited companies whose boards of directors include members of the Irish society for autistic children and professional and managerial persons from the state organizations. These have been very successful in improving the quality of life, both for young autistic adults, and also their families. This programme has helped with the down-sizing of the larger old mental institutions.

Personnel

The numbers and professional discipline of professionals within the child and adolescent psychiatric services are determined by negotiations, in response to need and demand.

Funding of services

At least 95 % of all funding comes to the child and adolescent psychiatric services from the Central Government Department of Health via the decentralized health board administrations. These latter administrations may then pay the salaries of personnel directly, or give a lump sum of money to a private organization, e.g., a religious order with a tradition in this line of work, who may then supplement it with monies from charitable donations.

Evaluation

The only evaluation studies that have so far been completed in Ireland are those on "parent-training". These have shown very clearly that when experienced mothers, following a short period of in-service training, spend two mornings per week in the homes of young disadvantaged parents who have poor child rearing competencies, the subsequent capacity of the children, at age 4 years to participate successfully in school is dramatically improved relative to control groups. This has been shown to be a very inexpensive and very worthwhile programme and has been extended to many communities throughout the country.

With the recent creation of Academic Departments of Child and Adolescent Psychiatry within the two medical schools, it is anticipated that more comprehensive evaluation studies of other activities will proceed.

4. Cooperation with medical and non-medical disciplines

Cooperation with paediatrics

All four of Ireland's paediatric hospitals have within them a Department of Child Psychiatry. However, none of them have an actual inpatient child psychiatric unit. The emphasis is upon consultation and liaison activity. Any child presenting in the A & E Department with self-injury is routinely admitted to a paediatric inpatient bed and not discharged until the child and family have been assessed (within 48 h) by the child psychiatrist.

There is specific involvement of the child psychiatric team in disorders such as juvenile diabetes, haemophilia, and fibro cystic disease; group work (with parents particularly) receive special attention. Excellent relationships have developed between the paediatricians and the child psychiatrists with regard to shared work in all the other somatoform disorders. In one of the paediatric hospitals, the child psychiatric team works very closely with the paediatric neurologists in the care of children with epileptic behavioural disorders, brain injury, and brain tumours. A specific 6 bed residential setting is planned for that activity in that particular hospital.

Both the child psychiatrists and hospital based paediatricians have been enthusiastic about the involvement of child psychiatry in the paediatric hospital setting. All such hospitals have "outreach" community child psychiatric clinics in suburbia.

Cooperation with psychiatry

At a training and professional level, there is much shared interaction between child and adolescent psychiatry and general adult psychiatry. Both have representatives on the executive council of the Irish Division of the Royal College of Psychiatrists, and child psychiatrists have, over time, held many of the senior posts within that organisation. The rotational training scheme for the generalist adult psychiatric trainees also involves a routine placement of 6 months or longer in the child psychiatric services. Libraries and tutorial facilities are shared. Child psychiatric departments also exist in a number of those general hospitals that contain general adult psychiatric 50 bed units.

The child psychiatric service will see newly referred children who have not as yet reached their 16th birthday. Although it may continue work with such children subsequently, those presenting for the first time who have already reached their 16th birthday are treated by the general adult psychiatric services. Neither this latter service nor the child psychiatric service are pleased with this arrangement. The planning at present is for the development of adolescent psychiatric programmes (with specialists in adolescent psychiatry) in the general adult service.

The situation is a little complicated by the new mental health legislation (to come into effect before the end of 1999), whereby there will be a different system of involuntary admission for treatment for those below and above their 18th birthday. Those under age 18 will only be involuntarily treated by order of the courts, whereas those above age 18 can be involuntarily admitted and treated by order of the psychiatrist.

The child psychiatric service tends to have retained an ongoing and active involvement in the programmes for autistic persons who have matured into adulthood, and it is child psychiatry rather than adult psychiatry who tends to be on the boards of management of those unique adult institutions for autism.

Cooperation with doctors in private practice

Eighty percent of young patients seen in child psychiatry clinics are referred there by doctors in general practice. The other 20 % of referrals come via social workers in the community services and similar agencies.

Roughly 70 % of the general practitioner's income is a government salary for the care and treatment of non-fee paying patients, but this issue is irrelevant in terms of referral to the child psychiatrist. All child psychiatric treatment is free to all persons in society. A very small percentage of patients specifically request private treatment, but very few child psychiatrists actually spend much time in private work. The necessary back-up resources and facilities are only available within their public service facilities.

Cooperation with non-medical institutions and professionals

Unlike Germany and some other European countries, all child guidance clinics are headed by a consultant (specialist) in child and adolescent psychiatry. It is assumed and accepted that such psychiatrists are largely involved in psychotherapy, and so they have not as yet tended to refer to themselves as doctors in "Child and Adolescent Psychiatry and Psychotherapy". This may change, however, with the increasing numbers of well-trained social workers and psychologists who are now offering private psychotherapy at a relatively low fee.

The child psychiatrist (and the 2 trainee child psychiatrists that are also usually on staff in such clinics) tend to consult a variety of other (non-medical) agencies, e.g., special schools for delinquent children, high supervision group homes, fosterage services, etc.

5. Graduate/postgraduate training and continuing medical education

Graduate training: The role of medical faculties

As mentioned in "Recent advances" (p 175), the first two chairs of child and adolescent psychiatry have been established in Dublin over the past two years. All the other medical schools have chairs of general psychiatry, and part time lectureships in child psychiatry which are held by specialists who are otherwise in largely full-time public service practice, usually those specialists whose attachment is to a paediatric hospital. It is hoped that further child psychiatric chairs will be created in the near future.

All of the six medical schools involve the child psychiatrists at three stages during the course of their six year undergraduate training. Medical students have an introductory series of lectures in developmental psychology during their second year in medical school, and then in their last two years they have a course of 8 seminars (each lasting half a day) in child psychiatry (during which time they would visit and meet with autistic children, children in inpatient units, etc.) and subsequently they attend a number of seminars while having their experience in pediatrics. This latter involvement would obviously centre around issues of somatoform disorders, overdose, crisis response, etc. In their written exam roughly 10 % of multiple choice questions are on issues of child and adolescent psychiatry.

Postgraduate training, a joint effort

The first child psychiatric experience of a trainee psychiatrist is usually during the 3 year long in service training course for sitting the membership examination of the Royal College of Psychiatrists. This is usually a six month placement in a child psychiatric clinic. It must be appreciated, too, that many postgraduate doctors will have spent a number of years in general practice, or other disciplines, e.g., paediatrics, neurology, before commencing the three year training course for membership of the Royal College of Psychiatrists.

Having obtained the membership, many such postgraduate doctors then obtain public salaried posts as "Registrars" (non-consultant/specialist) in child psychiatric clinics, where they work under the supervision of consultant specialists. Following on anything from 1 to 3 years experience therein, they then may become successful in applying for one of the few (9 training posts in Ireland) specialist training posts in child and adolescent psychiatry. This specialist training (Senior Registrar) lasts four years, and at the end of this time, without examination, the doctor may apply for a post of consultant/specialist when one such post becomes available (through retirement or through the creation of a new post).

Continuing medical education in child and adolescent psychiatry and psychotherapy

At the moment, such continuing medical education (CME), which in Ireland is referred to as continuing professional development (CPD), is not obligatory. However, the salaried contract does provide £1,000 Irish pounds per year for continuing educational expenses, and the contract also provides for 10 days of fully paid free time for educational purposes.

Training programmes for other disciplines

Most child psychiatrists are involved in the training programmes for nursing, speech and language therapy, occupational therapy, social work, and more recently, special teachers.

6. Research

Research fields and strategies

Most research in Ireland has been epidemiological, i.e., trying to estimate the incidence and prevalence of the ICD-9 and -10 categories of disorder in the population. This has been mainly with a view to being more informed when designing service provision. A great wealth of information, specific to the Irish population, urban and rural independently, has been acquired on such issues as conduct disorder, hyperkinetic syndrome, autism; however, information has also been gathered on the prevalence of maternal depression in the families of children presenting to child psychiatric clinics, family disadvantage in children presenting to paediatricians, etc. Large scale chromosomal studies have also been completed with reference to many different disorders. Some "follow-up" studies are now appearing on the value of group home and fosterage care of conduct disordered young adolescents.

There has not been any research done which has used the newer neurophysiological computerised technology.

Research training and career development

This is a significant element in the four year Senior Registrars training for specialist child psychiatry. Training in research methodology, the use of computer software programmes such as the SPSS, and then supervision of research projects occupies one full day per week of their four year training. It is hoped that, in this way, a cadre of well trained young specialists will be available for the developing academic departments of child and adolescent psychiatry in the medical schools.

Funding

Most funding comes through the health boards, but increasingly, other sources of funding have been materialising, and the two new Professors have been successful in securing some paediatric research monies, monies from the Government Department of Social Affairs and also from the Medical Research Bureau of Ireland. Participation in multi-centre E.C. projects has also been a feature of recent research.

7. Future perspectives

There are a number of "forces" operating within Irish society that will tend to shape the direction of Irish child and adolescent psychiatry in future years. Political forces would have the discipline largely involve itself in the fraught issues of "conduct disorder" and would put pressure on government agencies to organise services in that way. Parental groups on the other hand mount pressure, both on the profession and on the Government Health Department to develop more sophisticated services for specific groups, e.g., ADHD services, autism service, Tourette syndrome, anorexia nervosa. The profession itself would, of course, see itself as having an important part to play in the multisystemic development of approaches to conduct disorder, but to have a specific part to play in the more clear cut psychiatric disorders of childhood. Additionally, the professionals would emphasise the very important preventive roles they can play in the paediatric hospitals and neonatal units, i.e., prevention as it applies to PTSD, Attachment Disorders, etc.

Research

It is anticipated that the recently formed university medical school departments of child and adolescent psychiatry will forge co-operative links with their departments of sociology and psychology with a view to researching the usefulness of family interventive approaches in the field of "attachment disorder" and to study the usefulness of bringing an "attachment disorder" focus to the multisystems approach to work with severely conduct disordered adolescents.

Training

The training as it exists at the moment is considered to be very good, and the postgraduate doctors that one in fact sets out to train are nearly always doctors who are already quite mature both in paediatric and psychiatric knowledge. However, the numbers in training are too few. This comes back to the issue of "funding". Already in Ireland the situation has developed where, having put pressure on government to establish new salaried specialist posts throughout the country, we do not have the trained personnel available to take up such appointments.

Improvement of services and care systems

The planning, by the Central Department of Health, over the last few years, for the development of services throughout the country is essentially very sensible, and there is commitment to realise such plans. The main ingredients of future planning are

- Provision of more inpatient facilities country wide.
- Development of adolescent programmes (for the 16–18 year old age group) within the general adult services.
- The targeting of specific issues that relate to prevention, e.g., PTSD, attachment disorders, and ADHD.
- Other plans include the creation of autism specific programmes in the mental handicap services country wide, the adoption of computerised data gathering, the use of the ICD-10 multiaxial system and the ACPP presenting problem list, and finally, the development of a more specific child and adolescent forensic psychiatric service with a built-in university department of child psychiatry research component.

References

Available upon request from the author

Child and adolescent psychiatry in Italy

E. Caffo

1. Definition, historical development, and current situation

Psychiatry and child psychiatry have had in Italy a long history, which goes back to the 17th century, when the care of disturbed men, women, and children became a public health imperative. The reasons of the growing importance of these two disciplines had at the beginning more to do with needs of social control than with genuine scientific or medical reasons.

The objective of this contribution is to sketch the history of child psychiatry in Italy, underlying the role of the pioneers of this discipline and their relationships with other European experts active in the field. This clarification seems needed even in order to make possible a full understanding of the current status of the discipline.

Historical development

The development of child psychiatry in Italy was particularly impressive in the first few decades of this century, when a number of child specialists put forward theories and models of care which soon gained wide popularity in all of Europe. These pioneers were Maria Montessori (1870–1952), Sante De Sanctis (1862–1935), and Giuseppe F. Montesano (1868–1951).

Maria Montessori played a special historical role for both child psychiatry and education. At the end of the nineteenth century, she started to develop the pedagogic method for which she then became famous. In 1896, Montessori was the first woman ever to obtain a medical degree in Italy (at that time women were not accepted in the Faculty of Medicine). She then began her career at the University of Rome and in 1898 presented for the first time her method ("Sull'educazione morale" – "About moral education") at the Turin National Pedagogic Conference. Following that conference, Montessori, together with Montesano and Bonfigli, other two distinguished child psychiatrists, created in 1901 the "Lega Nazionale per la Protezione del Fanciullo" (National League for the Protection of Children). Although the League was soon dissolved (1905), this was one of the first attempts to create a scientific organization concerned with the care of children. In 1900, Montessori went to Paris and to London, and then she visited a number of European countries. She was particularly impressed by the work of the French child psychiatrist Seguin. She gradually developed her own pedagogic method, initially based on the "intuition that the question of the 'mentally deficient' was more pedagogic than medical". At that time the poor obstetric care, the deficient nutritional conditions, and a variety of other social and medical reasons, converged in raising the number of children with mental retardation.

Montessori stated that medicine had to be combined with education for the therapy of abnormal children: education of mentally retarded subjects did not have to be considered "specific", but had to be based on the same teaching principles suitable for normal subjects. At that time, Montessori was asked by the Minister of Education to train teachers for abnormal children: she founded the Scuola Magistrale Ortofrenica (Training College for Teachers of the Mentally Retarded) and classes for abnormal children established in Rome. After this experience, she decided to fully commit herself to pedagogy, and she enrolled in the Faculty of Philosophy. In 1907, Montessori was offered the opportunity to teach a class of normal children, in order to test the teaching method that would eventually spread all over in the world.

Sante De Sanctis, who was one of the first researchers to identify child schizophrenia (1905), wrote a well-known treatise, entitled "Neuropsichiatria infantile" in 1925. He also advocated the separation of child psychiatry from adult psychiatry. In 1915 the Istituto Medico-Pedagogico Treves (Treves Medical-Pedagogic Institute), later called the "Treves – De Sanctis", opened in Milan, and soon became an active research center. At the XVI Conference of the Italian Psychiatric Society, De Sanctis insisted on the formative autonomy of child psychiatry, which should "integrate its culture in neurology, psychiatry, pediatrics and psychology".

In 1925 Medea established Pro Infanzia Anormale (PIA – Pro Abnormal Children), with the aim of promoting child mental health concepts. The special classes spread and various medical-pedagogic institutes were established in Milan, Venice, Rome, Florence, and Salerno. In 1932 PIA organized the 3rd National Medical-Pedagogic Conference in Rome, where De Sanctis highlighted the two poles of child psychiatry (organic and psychosocial) and again proposed team work as the basis for the study of children. In 1934, B. Di Tullio contributed to the set up of Consultori di pedagogia emendativa (Corrective pedagogy surgeries) at the Youth Courts to tackle the psychological aspects of child deviance, and in 1936 he created the first Centro per lo studio della criminologia minorile (Center for the study of child criminology). Many initiatives for the mentally retarded were started, and the number of special classes in schools increased.

In contrast to De Sanctis, Giuseppe Montesano stressed the psychopedagogic aspect of child psychiatry and tried to give a scientific foundation to the field of mental retardation through the opening in Rome, in 1909, of the first special class for mentally retarded children; in 1911, Montesano established "L'assistenza dei Minorenni Anormali" (Treatment of abnormal children), a specialized pedagogic journal.

Child psychiatry in Italy came to a standstill in the mid-1930s, then regained momentum at the end of the Second World War. "New" child pathological conditions emerged, some due to the effects of the war, most notably infantile cerebral palsy and similar disorders. The Swiss influence became more and more visible: in 1946 the "Italian Swiss Health Center" organized a conference in Milan with the participation of Minkowski, Piaget, and Rey, followed several months later by the 1st International Conference ("Semaine Internationale d'Etudes pour l'Enfance de la Guerre") (SEPEG) in Lausanne, attended by a number of Italian child psychiatrists.

A year later, in 1947, Bollea and Venturini organized a national conference of the SEPEG in Rome, where the discussion focused on the structure and the functions of Centri Medico-Psico-Pedagogici (Medical-Psycho-Pedagogic Centers, CMPP) and the Opera Nazionale Maternità ed Infanzia (National Maternity and Children's Organization, ONMI) was created in Italy. In 1947 the first two CMPP were set up in Milan (with Porta and Berrini) and in Rome (with Bollea, who was helped by other prominent psychiatrists of the time, including Bartoleschi and Ossicini); in the space of one decade, the number of these facilities increased to more than two hundred. They were characterized by a team work orientation (each team normally including a neuropsychiatrist, a psychologist, a social worker, and/or a teacher); the emphasis on team work represented a great innovation for that time.

In the same year, 1947, Di Tullio established the Ente Morale per il Fanciullo (Moral Organization for the Care of the Young), with the aim of helping juvenile delinquents. The following year, Bollea and Venturini founded the Societa "Italiana per l'Assistenza Medico-Pedagogica ai Minorati fisici e psichici dell'Eta" evolutiva (SIAME – Italian Society for the Medical-Pedagogic treatment of the physically and mentally disabled during the development years) and organized various conferences. In 1948, at the Venice conference of the Italian Psychiatric Association, an Italian Child Psychiatry Committee was established, with Carlo De Sanctis as president and Bollea as general secretary.

During those years a special law for the care of children with cerebral palsy was approved, recognizing a number of special provisions for these children. In 1958, Italian child psychiatry gained international recognition for the first time: in Lisbon, Bollea was elected vice-president of the International Association of Child Psychiatry. Two years later, in 1960, he was also elected president of the European Committee of Child Psychiatry.

In 1953 the journal Infanzia Anormale (Abnormal Children), originally established in 1907 and then interrupted, was published again. In 1969, the name of the journal was changed to Neuropsichiatria Infantile (Child Neuropsychiatry), and in 1984 it finally took the more precise and appropriate name Psichiatria dell'infanzia e dell'adolescenza (Child and Adolescent Psychiatry).

In 1956 the first university chairs in child neuropsychiatry were assigned, and in the following years (1957–1963) the first residency programs were created in Rome, Genoa, and Pisa; one of the most prestigious was the one in Rome, run by Giovanni Bollea, who can be considered the real father of modern child psychiatry in Italy. Nowadays, there are more than twenty university chairs in child psychiatry and a dozen residency programs (Bollea 1980).

Recent advances: Child psychiatry or child neuropsychiatry?

Since its origin, in Italy child psychiatry has been called "child neuropsychiatry" in order to preserve the term originally used by De Santis, Montesano, and Montessori since 1902. At that time De Sanctis provided a rationale for this junction: he stated that "child psychiatry is the somato-psychic study of every disorder in the intelligence and behavior of a child between the age of 0 and 18" (the term "child" is now often replaced with "child and adolescent" or "of the development years" to better indicate the age range of the patients treated). This orientation was consistent with the biological foundations of the discipline and seen as the most scientific way to approach the study of psychiatric disorders. It should be stressed that a strong organic emphasis had some humanistic consequences, because it gave the status of "sick" to the mentally ill, often regarded as moral or sociopathic deviants.

Although with time, in line with the international trends, adult psychiatry was split from adult neurology, in the field of child psychiatry this unification remained alive. This had (and has) several consequences, both positive and negative. Among the positive consequences of this unification are the emphasis given to the bio-psychosocial unity of the sick child and the recognition that any disorder, in the development phase, has strong psychological correlates. On the other hand, in Italy, many have interpreted "child neuropsychiatry" as "child neurology", giving much more importance to the neurological component of the discipline. This problem will probably be solved in the framework of the needed homogenization of Italian rules with European rules.

In the post war period, the main areas of scientific interest for the Italian child psychiatry have been (1) behavioral disturbances, (2) child and youth delinquency, typical of the post war period, and (3) rehabilitation of the mentally retarded. In this sense, the Italian tradition of child neuropsychiatry has always encompassed genetic psychology and psychodynamics and has entailed psychomotor and functional rehabilitation in every form of organic, mental, and developmental disorder. Interestingly, while in adult psychiatry the influence of the English psychodynamic tradition was predominant, in child psychiatry the influence of the French psychoanalytical school was stronger: reference authors were, for many years, Lebovici, Diatkine, Mises, Soule, etc. In the diagnostic field, for many years the classification scheme proposed by Mises was predominant, and the ICDs were favored over the DSMs. However, with time, the DSM-III classification and orientation became increasingly popular, forcing child psychiatrists to adopt an empirical approach in diagnosis and classification (Guaraldi, Caffo 1986).

Italian child psychiatry has also been characterized by a limited use of psychotropic drugs as compared to other countries (e.g., the US) and by a widespread use of individual and family-oriented psychotherapies. As stated by Bollea (1960), "the true child psychiatrist basically has a humanistic and social mentality.... A clinical case is immediately seen and felt in the inseparableness of the patient from the humus in which he lives (p. 154). ... The child is a completely dependent being... and a knowledge of the environmental factor (family-school-society) is fundamental" (p. 155). As already indicated, the teamwork orientation is the most appropriate to deal with the complexity of clinical situations. Again Bollea (1960) underlined that in each team, run by a child psychiatrist, there is a sort of "horizontal hierarchy" (p. 154), in which various viewpoints are fairly considered: the attitude of a child psychiatrist must be to achieve a synthesis of the two poles – biological and social – to "perceive them dialectically fused" (p. 155).

Current situation

On December 31, 1996, the population of Italy was 57,333,000. Children up to the age of 5 constituted 4.8 % of the entire population (2,751,984). Children and adolescents from the age of 5 to 14 represented 10.1 % of the Italian population

(5,799,633). Adolescents from the age of 15 to 19 represented 6.1 % of the entire population (3,496,313). Children and adolescents in total represented about 21 % of the total population.

At the time being (1998), child and adolescent neuropsychiatric services are represented in almost every province of Italy. There are 23 university departments of Child Neuropsychiatry in Italy with 16 having postgraduate training. The curriculum to obtain the speciality as a child neuropsychiatrist and psychotherapist takes five years.

Twelve hundred child neuropsychiatrists are practising regularly all over the Italian territory as of December 1998. Half of them are women.

2. Classification systems, diagnostic and therapeutic methods

Classification systems

In Italy, classification systems have been used for a long time after other Northern European countries. The system more widely used in nearly all university departments and in most of the community services is the ICD-10 classification system. From a clinical point of view, the DSM-IV is the most often used.

Diagnostic methods

Diagnostic procedures which include physical examination, hematological and biochemical tests are routine when diagnosing a child or adolescent.

EEG recordings and neuroimaging tests are ordered in the event that organicity needs to be ruled out. Neuropsychology tests are usually done by neuropsychiatrists and psychologists when needed. Mother and child interactions and family diagnosis are crucial in the diagnostic evaluation. Developmental neurological signs are also an important part in the diagnosis of the child.

Therapeutic methods

Different modalities of treatment are used in Italy. The main orientation of the different departments is toward a psychodynamic approach. The use of different types of psychotherapy including the psychoanalytical and the family-type reflects the day-by-day life of a neuropsychiatrist practicing in Italy. The use of psychotropic medications has been not well accepted in the Italian child-psychiatric field especially for the ages of twelve and under.

In addition to the usual therapeutic approaches, psychomotor therapy and family therapy are used as conjunct therapies. At the end of the 1970s, a social policy decision was made to close inpatient services. At the present time, there are very few inpatient beds for children and adolescents.

3. Structure and organization of services

At the end of the 1970s, a social policy decision was made to close inpatient services. At the present time, there are very few inpatient beds for children and adolescents.

The general principle for delivery of child psychiatric services in Italy is to deliver services that are family-oriented, community-based, easily accessible, and in the main stream of general medical and pediatric practice. In this context, child psychiatrists usually have a psychosocial orientation: they provide specific child psychiatric assessment and treatments but also the linkage between the child and a variety of other services in the community. The general orientation has been basically psychoanalytic and psychosocial, although newer theories and methods have been implemented more recently.

The vast majority of child psychiatric care is delivered in outpatient facilities. There are a range of other services, such as those relating to schools or those for children with special needs. Particularly for younger children, supplementary services include physical, psychological, and psychoeducational treatments. Family support is provided for those families with severely handicapped children. These children are often served in special programs and centers in which parents may have an active role in guidance. Parents receive emotional support, information about caring for their child, and help in the day-to-day care of the child from professionals and other families.

Children with neurological problems, such as epilepsy, are treated in inpatient facilities that are pediatric in orientation. These may be in child neuropsychiatry or pediatric departments, depending on the particular hospital or academic department.

There are major regional differences in the types of services available, and a major national issue is where the children with the most severe disorders have to be treated, since no long-term residential or inpatient treatment centers exist.

In some parts of Italy, large residential centers provide care for children who have no intact families and for children with motor, cognitive, or emotional difficulties: formal assessment by child psychiatrists is uncommon in these facilities and the precise nature of the treatment is not always known.

In general, there are more services for young children than adolescents, and there are very few highly specialized services even for those with chronic psychiatric and neurological diseases. Today in Italy, there are 1,200 child psychiatrists with varied types of training emphasizing neurology, psychiatry, and psychosocial treatments to varying degrees. A recent proposal recommends one child psychiatrist for every 5,000 to 6,000 children. In addition, the same proposal recommends two to three psychologists for every 5,000 to 6,000 children, ten therapists for 10,000 children and adolescents, two psychotherapists for 10,000, six social workers, and six educators.

Child psychiatric services are provided with state funding. Only to a very limited extent, and exclusively for outpatient psychotherapy, do individuals pay for the treatment. Until the 1980s, children could be maintained in long-term treatment without formal assessment. Currently, there is increasing emphasis on careful assessment of quality. However, it is still the case that there is broad variation in quality.

4. Cooperation with medical and non-medical disciplines

Cooperation with pediatrics

Community and hospital child psychiatry facilities are in general part of departments of pediatrics. Pediatrics is part of the maternal and child care programs in medical schools in the community: care is provided for children from birth to adolescence and child psychiatrists work closely with pediatricians to deliver the care in these departments. In some hospitals, an overlapping exists between neuropsychiatrists and neuropediatricians (i.e., pediatricians with neurological but not psychiatric training). Child psychiatrists work in consultation-liaison with pediatrics and provide emergency services and emergency programs for children exposed to trauma, accidents, and domestic violence.

Community pediatricians work with the families and child psychiatrists work along with them providing services to families.

Cooperation with psychiatry

Child psychiatry has tried to maintain its autonomy from adult psychiatry. In some regions, child psychiatry has been included within the adult psychiatry department. In one sense, this will facilitate long-standing work of child psychiatrists in collaboration with adult psychiatrists in the care of children whose parents have psychiatric difficulties. On the other hand, these new laws may threaten the close and positive relationships between child psychiatry and pediatrics. At the present time, child psychiatrists in Italy are trying to determine the best ways of utilizing the resources from adult psychiatry while maintaining its long-standing historical relationships with pediatrics and maternal child care. An important area of overlap is the care of adolescents. Child psychiatrists are determining the best ways of dealing with the transition from adolescence to young adulthood, especially for those children with persistent and serious psychiatric problems, to assure that there is a continuity of care from child to adult psychiatry. The general orientation of Italian child psychiatry emphasizes the close collaboration between child psychiatrists, social workers, educators, and the traditional department. More recently, there has been a close relationship also with police departments. As a public service, child psychiatrists are very intimately involved with pediatricians and family practitioners. Unlike some other European countries, in Italy there is a strong tradition of child guidance clinics.

5. Graduate/postgraduate training and continuing medical education

Medical students receive 10 to 14 hours of lectures and training in child psychiatry during their pediatric rotation. Medical students with special interest in child psychiatry can have extensive experience in clinical work with children during their psychiatry and pediatrics training. To become a child psychiatrist, a medical graduate has a five-year curriculum. The requirements for training programs, with currently 14 medical schools, are decided on both a national and local basis. In general, during the five years, a trainee in child psychiatry has the following curriculum: approximately one year is spent in pediatrics, approximately one year in psychiatry and/or neurology, and three years are spent in child psychiatry. In addition to formal course work, major emphasis is placed on direct experience in a variety of clinical settings. A lot of flexibility is allowed to trainees in child psychiatry, depending on the special interest of the training program and available resources. By law, during the five years, trainees in child psychiatry also become fully trained as child psychotherapists.

Significant differences, however, could be observed among the different residence programs: some programs are much more heavily influenced by neurology, and the graduates tend to be neuropsychiatrists. Others are more influenced by psychotherapy and psychodynamics, and their graduates tend to be more involved in psychotherapy. A third major stream emphasizes an eclectic approach with heavy emphasis on psychosocial interventions. There is no compulsory continuing medical education, although many Italian child psychiatrists participate in local, regional and national meetings. The faculties of child psychiatry provide the training for specialists in physical or psychoeducational treatments as well as training in social work and psychology. In this way, child psychiatrists learn to collaborate with the other disciplines, and the other disciplines learn the special orientation of child psychiatry.

6. Research

Traditional research in Italy has emphasized clinical description of phenomenology including long-term follow-up of individual cases. Over recent decades, there have been two major streams of research: the first emphasizes children with neurological and developmental disorders including children with developmental disabilities and reading disabilities. The second major area of research has been the evaluation of treatment approaches, especially psychoanalytic, psychodynamic, and educational approaches. More recently, investigators in Italy have begun to become familiar with the major trends in systematic research in other parts of Europe and in the United States. Currently, there are no systematic training programs for research in child psychiatry. More recently, the Italian National Institute of Health has been developing a national strategy for career development and research infrastructure in mental health. There are only limited funds available from the federal government for research in psychiatry. In general, research is subsidized as part of clinical care and seen as closely related to evaluation of patients and of outcome of treatment. Some private funds are available for certain types of research. As part of the new national plan, attempts are being made to develop systematic research funding from Italian or European sources.

7. Future perspectives

Research

Italian child psychiatrists are increasingly interested in the advanced research methodology in use in Europe and in Northern America. To facilitate their learning above these methods, research study groups have been established in Italy and young Italian child psychiatrists are encouraged to visit foreign scientific institutions for shorter and longer periods of study. At the same time, the national leadership in child psychiatry is reassessing purposes and methods for training. As child psychiatry becomes more sophisticated, it is recognized that child psychiatric training has to adapt itself to allow child psychiatrists to make the best use of emerging methods and diagnoses and treatment.

Training

There are 14 residence programs and about 25 chairs of child psychiatry in medical faculties, corresponding to less than one chair for every two schools of medicine. Increasing the number of these programs is a major issue for the Italian child psychiatric community. A major policy issue is also, as reported above, the relationship between child neuropsychiatry and child psychiatry on one hand, and child neurology on the other. The advantages and disadvantages of having a field which spans child psychiatry and child neurology as currently exists in Italy is a matter of open discussion. Thinking about the subspecialization of child neuropsychiatry into child psychiatry on the one side and child neurology on the other relates to emerging bodies of knowledge and differences in treatment approaches taken by these two fields. There is broad difference in opinion about the best way of proceeding in the future.

Improvement of services and care systems

The development of more services for young children, for children with severe disorders, for children involved with emergencies and trauma, and the need for re-thinking the acute services that may be necessary for children in hospitals are becoming important issues for media and professionals (Cohen, Caffo 1998). Finally, leaders in Italian child psychiatry are reviewing traditional criteria for longer-term residential treatment and other types of approaches to the more seriously disturbed children. As reported above, there is still great paucity of services for adolescents, especially for adolescents who have comorbid substance abuse and psychiatric disturbances.

There has been a long-standing interest within child psychoanalysis in the first years of life in infant psychoanalytic understanding. There is now a development of more programs that use these and other approaches to intervene early for children of very high risk, especially those children who come from families with abuse and neglect, families burdened by mental illness and families suffering from physical illnesses. Italian child psychiatry rightfully takes pride in its involvement with the community and the entire nation. These interests are exemplified by helplines for children, public educational approaches, recruitment of volunteers in social and mental health programs, and dissemination of knowledge to pediatricians, family doctors, social workers, policy makers and others who intervene in the lives of children.

Selected references

Bollea G (1960) Evoluzione storica e attualitá della neuropsichiatria infantile. Infanzia Anormale 37: 141–163

Bollea G (1980) Compendio di psichiatria dell' età evolutiva. Bulzoni, Roma

Cohen JD, Caffo E (1998) Developmental Psychopathology: a framework for planning child mental health. Epidemiologia e Psichiatria Sociale 7 (3): 156–160

Cohen JD, Caffo E (1998) Developmental psychopathology and Child Mental Health Series: Risk and Protective Factors in Children, Families and Society. In: Yung GJ, Ferrari P (Eds) Designing Mental Health Services and Systems for Children and Adolescents: A Shrewed Investment (pp 3–13). Brunner/Mazel, Philadelphia

Guaraldi GP, Caffo E (Eds) (1986) II DSM-III in Età Evolutiva. Diagnosi e Classificatione dei disturbi psichici nell' infance e nell' adolescenza. Masson, Milano

Child and adolescent psychiatry in Latvia

A. Kishuro

1. Definition, historical development, and current situation

Definition

In Latvia, child and adolescent psychiatry is defined: "child and adolescent psychiatry is an independent medical discipline investigating etiopathogenesis of neurotic and psychical disorders in children and adolescents and their clinical manifestation, diagnosis, therapeutic methods, school and social adaptation". As can be seen, psychotherapy is not added, as a discipline it has been separated and remains independent for some reasons. Of course, it does not mean that psychotherapy is not used but the situation has to improve by joining efforts for better help.

Historical development

Until World War II, child and adolescent psychiatry was considered part of general psychiatry, so general psychiatrists were the specialists treating children more or less as "adults in miniature", following classic German and French schools and authors, as Latvia was part of the European society.

After World War II, in the Soviet Union, the leading Soviet psychiatric school was based on classic German psychiatric conceptions and research using biological approaches in diagnosis and treatment. Since 1950, in the Latvian Soviet Socialist Republic, child psychiatry was admitted as a sub-speciality in psychiatry.

Preparation and organization was carried out by Dr. Yevgeny Zaltsman, MD, who founded a section of child and adolescent psychiatry in the Psychiatrist Society in 1950 and took leadership as a chief child psychiatrist until 1997. His energy and scientific orientation allowed the development of education more specific to child and adolescent psychiatrists, which was closely linked with the development of child and adolescent psychiatry in the Soviet Union.

So, Latvian child and adolescent psychiatry (CAP) has developed from several traditions:

- A neuropsychiatric tradition, coming mostly from German "classical" psychiatry, followed by the Soviet psychiatric school, still continues;
- A tradition in pediatric education; this could be considered as a possibility to organize psychosomatic services;

- The recent attempts to develop a psychodynamic-psychoanalytic approach as an additional tool for the job;
- The empirical-epidemiological tradition developed in the Soviet Union had more influence than research in England and the United States for understandable reasons.

After re-establishment of the Republic of Latvia, child and adolescent psychiatry is still an informal section in the Latvian Psychiatric Association, which means that there is no need for special certification in CAP; the accent is on competence and experience in the job within child and adolescent psychiatry.

Recent advances

Funding of the treatment of psychiatrically disturbed children and adolescents is mixed – in some departments it is free (covered by the state budget), in some insurance covers it, and in some both are responsible.

The social security system is responsible for severely mentally ill and handicapped children and adolescents until the age of 18, covering medication expenses and funds for rehabilitation and living.

Current situation

In 1997, there were approximately 2,400,000 inhabitants in Latvia, including approximately 500,000 children and adolescents, which is about approximately 20 % of the total population. In the capital Riga are about 940,000 inhabitants including approximately 170,000 children and adolescents.

At the end of 1997, child and adolescent psychiatry was represented by 5 inpatient departments with 10 to 50 beds each, 4 larger outpatient departments, and child psychiatrists skilled in child psychiatry in some regions in the countryside or small towns. Overall, the system employs 26 child and adolescent psychiatrists and an uncertain number of psychotherapists – about 8–15 (it depends on funding as psychotherapists are fully privately employed). Thus, there is one child and adolescent psychiatrist per 20–30,000 children and adolescents. Most of them are involved both in outpatient and inpatient services.

Touching private practice, there are only some attempts in this field, compared to psychotherapy, where all the services are private, without funding from the state or from insurance.

Among the enormous number of needs include: the establishment of at least one chair or department of CAP in the Latvian Medical Academy or Medical Faculty of Latvian University, as we do not have a single one. Education is still done voluntarily by the staff from the Department of Psychiatry, Latvian Medical Academy.

2. Classification systems, diagnostic and therapeutic methods

Classification systems

In Latvia, the ICD-10 classification system is widely used in daily practice since February 1, 1997. DSM-IV is used more or less for scientific purposes for better understanding and explaining the situation. All psychiatric units including CAP and academic structures use basic case documentation, including history, symptoms, multiaxial ICD-10 diagnosis, and a description of therapeutic measures carried out or recommended.

Diagnostic methods

In diagnostics, a wide range of diagnostic procedures are available – neurological examination, EEG recording, CT, MR imaging, as well as laboratory methods, and additional pediatric examination in cooperation with other disciplines. The use of neuropsychological methods is becoming more important in diagnostics.

Therapeutic methods

In the field of therapy, the biological approach is used in more or less all serious cases, mostly in inpatient wards. In addition, psychiatrists in outpatient departments use in parallel an eclectic therapeutic approach, called "working with the patient in a psychotherapeutic way". Psychotherapists use more specific methods including psychodynamic and behavioral and family therapy techniques.

3. Structure and organization of services

Guidelines for services for children and adolescents with psychiatric disorders

Neither concepts nor guidelines for child and adolescent psychiatry exist in Latvia; the system created in the Soviet Union is still used. Some of the general principles similar to those in Germany are mentioned in the new Psychiatric Law, which is in a working stage, but it does not contain a special chapter on CAP.

Types of services

Generally main two types of services are developed: inpatient and outpatient departments. Initial attempts to arrange complementary services and rehabilitation have been made.

Outpatient services

The majority of outpatient departments are located in larger cities, totally 4, not only for inhabitants of these cities, but also neighboring areas of the countryside.

The existence of a well-developed community-based child and adolescent psychiatric care system is needed, as there are still some regions in more remote locations without CAP specialists. Private practice psychotherapists are mostly located in the capital of Latvia, where approximately 40 % of the overall population lives.

With regard to child guidance and early detection and intervention, pediatric services and family doctors are taking care of these.

Daypatient services

A daypatient medical care system in child and adolescent psychiatry is not developed in Latvia.

Inpatient services

At present, 4 inpatient service departments exist, including one so-called "university department", where some voluntarily consultation service is done by an assistant professor from the department of psychiatry.

Child and adolescent psychiatric patients fill approximately 160 beds throughout the country – 15 beds per 15,000 inhabitants. It can be explained by the lack of daycare and rehabilitation services as well as other poorly developed complementary services.

Complementary services and rehabilitation

As mentioned above, rehabilitation services are not developed in Latvia. Care for long lasting and chronically ill psychiatric patients is provided by two hospitals for chronic patients, located in the countryside; these are for the most severely psychiatrically handicapped children, whose parents are not capable of caring for them, others are kept in their families. Those handicapped patients, who do not need special psychiatric treatment, can be kept either in families or "children homes" under the care of educated personnel.

The large number of children kept in long-term inpatient establishments can be explained by the large number of "pseudoorphans" coming from asocial families, refusing to take care for their children. On the other hand, these families had economic situations pushing parents to hand care of the children over to the state.

"Transition homes", group homes, foster homes/family nursing exist in projects. Some foster homes/family nursing establishments exist for the "non-psychiatric" part of population.

During recent years a few establishments, similar to youth centers in Germany, started as places where psychically and otherwise handicapped adolescents can spend time during the day, working on an occupation, rehabilitation, or education. The need for such centers located as close as possible to patients' homes, all around the country, together with those three centers started in the capital is rather high.

Personnel

The needs in staff of child and adolescent psychiatry are not defined; rules are more or less the same as in the Soviet Union. In addition, there is a growing tendency to cut existing staff. The number of staff in wards depends on finances in the defined area, but during the last 5–6 years the number of "new" additional staff and team members as psychologists, special teachers, and social workers has been growing; however, the lack of these specialists is still felt.

Funding of services

In Latvia, inpatient and outpatient services are paid from the state budget (local authority) or insurance or both sources at the same time. The situation is not certain. Responsibility for chronically ill and mentally handicapped children and adolescents is assumed by the social welfare system, supporting needs for medication and small additional funds for other purposes.

Evaluation

No serious studies have been done to evaluate psychiatric services; however, recent foreign experience studies and the pressure to re-organize psychiatric services, emphasizing outpatient care, may change the situation toward more community-based services, closer to users, as well as hospital admissions.

4. Cooperation with medical and non-medical disciplines

Cooperation with pediatrics

In hospitals having a child and adolescent psychiatric inpatient ward, CAP experts are widely consulting in neighboring departments, as the field of psychosomatics for children and adolescents is not developed in the country. Psychiatrists may be invited to consult in wards and departments in other clinics, cooperating with pediatrics in fields such as chronic somatic illnesses, intensive care, neurology, including brain damage, and metabolic disorders. The need to develop cooperation in the field of early detection and intervention is high.

Cooperation with psychiatry

Departments of CAP are in a different situation – two of them belong to psychiatric clinics close to adult departments, one close to a general psychiatric department inside a regional hospital, and one, in the capital, belongs to a pediatric hospital located far from the general psychiatric hospital.

Child and adolescent psychiatry shares diagnostic approaches with general psychiatry, but deals with the same age group as pediatrics. The association with general psychiatry is more common than with pediatrics. Child and adolescent psychiatrists are working closely with general psychiatry concerning the adolescent group 16 to 20 years of age, family psychiatry regarding ill children with ill parents or a mixture, and longitudinal observing and treating perspective, which is not well developed except some long-lasting family cases.

Cooperation with doctors in private practice

Undoubtedly, this type of cooperation is not well developed, it works more in the direction toward CAP, not the reverse. An explanation is that only few specialists are in private practice; more commonly they are with state or private medical companies employing specialists. It means that the system works poorly, as the primary health care system is insufficiently developed; thus, the process is still going on.

Cooperation with non-medical institutions and professionals

Close cooperation has been developed with different types of special schools – for children with learning disabilities, speech or language disorders, behavioral and conduct disorders, for mentally handicapped children, consulting psychiatric and psychological problems.

Cooperation with increasing numbers of psychotherapists is still developing, still mostly "one way", as mentioned above. Finally, consulting services are delivered to different "children's homes" all over the country.

5. Graduate/postgraduate training and continuing medical education

Graduate training: The role of medical faculties

There are two universities where one can study medical science – the Latvian Medical Academy, dealing with all fields of medical science only, and the Latvian University with a newly opened medical faculty (since 1998).

During studies in the Latvian Medical Academy, pediatric students have 20 hours dedicated to child and adolescent psychiatry, general physicians 10 hours during a 6-year course. During the few last years, new study programs have been developed in connection with ICD-10 and the process is still going on and increasing.

Postgraduate training, a joint effort

To become a specialist in CAP after graduation from the medical faculty, the candidate or resident has to spend at least 3 years studying in the department of psychiatry. The program consists in the 1st year of only general psychiatry, the 2nd year of child psychiatry, adult neurology, drug abuse, psychotherapy in equal parts, and the 3rd year of practical work under supervision in outpatient and inpatient wards. After that, candidates have the right to take a so-called "approbation" exam to receive a certificate for independent practice in psychiatry in general. There is no special certification in CAP, but CAP specialists are preferably of pediatric origin.

Continuing medical education in child and adolescent psychiatry and psychotherapy

There are no formal rules for continuing medical education; the process depends on each specialist when and where to take part in various educational events at home or abroad.

Training programs for other disciplines

CAP specialists occasionally take part in training processes in different disciplines as invited lecturers; however, it is an uncertain situation which needs to be improved.

6. Research

Research fields and strategies

Research in child and adolescent psychiatry is a narrow field and includes only two main directions:

- Classification of disorders and behavioral disturbances using ICD-10;
- Evaluation of therapeutic methods, including medication.

Research training and career development

This very important part of research is poorly developed.

Funding

No special funding for research purposes in the field of CAP is available from either the state or other sources.

7. Future perspectives

The future perspectives of child and adolescent psychiatry in general, specialist training, and research are uncertain at present, depending on the financial situation in the country, prestige of CAP professionals, and on higher appreciation for the importance of child psychiatrists and other specialists during the process of growing-up and educating a healthy society in the future. It is rather important to describe and evaluate the present situation in the field of CAP, to find out needs of the society, to create guidelines for development in the future, and in connection with that to build child and adolescent psychiatry on a new, modern level.

Selected references

State Mental health Care center (1997) Situation in psychiatry for 1997

Child and adolescent psychiatry in Lithuania

D. Puras

1. Definition, historical development, and current situation

Child and adolescent psychiatry (CAP) in Lithuania has been developing before the end of the 1980 under the strong influence of the Soviet school of child psychiatry. There have been several sites for spreading the knowledge within the field of CAP in the former Soviet Union, with some differences in interpretation of classification systems and treatment modalities (Moscow, St. Petersburg, Kiev). However, in general, Soviet child psychiatry was mainly influenced by child neurology and general psychiatry. The biological model of interpretation and management of most disorders in childhood and adolescence was prevailing in the Soviet child psychiatry. There was an ideological taboo to claim that social problems cannot be considered as one of the causes for mental, emotional or behavioral disorders, as they were supposed to have been solved by the political system. This intervention of communist ideology into the field led to the overemphasis of organic and endogenous factors both in diagnostic interpretations and management of all possible disorders in the field of mental health.

Until the 1970s the official title of the speciality was "child psychoneurology". In the middle of the 1970s the specialized training of child psychiatrists started and the official separation of child psychoneurology into child neurology and child psychiatry occurred throughout the Soviet Union (in Lithuania this happened in 1976). However, ideologically, child psychiatry remained under strong influence of both child neurology and general psychiatry. Those child psychiatrists in Lithuania, and, generally, throughout the former Soviet Union, who were more influenced by the Moscow school of general psychiatry, were preferrably using the diagnosis of childhood schizophrenia for the cases of autistic disorder, obsessive-compulsive disorders, anorexia nervosa, etc. Another group of professionals, those who were more influenced by the school of child neurology, tended to see emotional and behavioral disorders in childhood and adolescence as a consequence of a hypothetical organic brain damage during the early period of development (pregnancy, labor, the first years of life).

The situation in Lithuanian child and adolescent psychiatry started to change dramatically toward the end of the 1980s, as a result of the democratic changes in the society and restoration of the independent state. Three factors contributed to the radical changes in the situation of child and adolescent psychiatry:

- As there was no more ideological control over information in the field of mental health, mass media immediately raised the broad spectrum of social problems which had been closed for the general public for the fifty years of Soviet regime.

Many of these problems have been directly connected with children's mental health (mentally handicapped children, abandoned children, drug and alcohol abuse among adolescents, child abuse in families and institutions).

- The "iron curtain" was raised, and the professionals had for the first time the opportunity to be introduced to the experience of democratic and developed countries in the field of services and therapeutic approaches in the field of CAP.
- Independent professional associations and nongovernmental organizations of citizens were developed, with proposals of radical changes in the system of care for children with developmental, emotional, and psychosocial disorders.

The first years of changes resulted in the following achievements:

- The University Center for Children with Developmental Disorders was established in 1991 by the Ministry of Health, as a model clinical and training institution.
- The Lithuanian Psychiatric Association was founded in 1990, with a chapter for child psychiatry, which grew into the Lithuanian Society for Child and Adolescent Psychiatry in 1996.
- Reform of training of medical specialists, which had a goal to gradually reach international standards in the field of the training of medical doctors, including child and adolescent psychiatrists, commenced in 1991.

However, the new achievements were followed by new problems for the field of child and adolescent psychiatry. In the new market of medical specialities and struggle for limited resources of funding, there was a growing danger to lose the competition to the traditionally stronger specialities, such as pediatrics, child neurology, and general psychiatry. The situation of uncertain perspective for child and adolescent psychiatry as an independent medical speciality with a broad spectrum of services has remained through the subsequent years of this decade. This uncertainty was the main motivation for the active representatives of child and adolescent psychiatry to constantly seek new allies among medical and nonmedical specialities, special education, social welfare and child protection agencies, as well as newly founded nongovernmental organizations.

2. Classification systems, diagnostic and therapeutic methods

As a result of dramatic social and political changes at the end of the 1980s and beginning of the 1990s, Lithuanian child and adolescent psychiatry became open to the variety of diagnostic and therapeutic attitudes, which originated from different countries and schools.

Lithuanian child and adolescent psychiatry, as a part of health care system, adopted ICD-10, which has been used since 1997 as an official classification of diseases in Lithuania. There is also a great interest in DSM-IV, especially among professionals who are involved in research.

Much more controversial was the development of new therapeutic approaches, as it was influenced by a large variety of schools from different countries. This might be a partly reflection of a historical tradition that culturally and geopolitically influenced Lithuania during the last centuries including very different countries – Western, Northern, Eastern and Central Europe, United States. After the 50 years of forced domination by the communist ideology, the influence from the east (Russia and other countries of the former USSR), though decreased significantly, never stopped to exist. However, until the end of the 1980s the only opportunity for postgraduate training was the lectures, seminars, and courses of Soviet trainers; since 1990 training seminars and workshops have been organized with participation of lecturers from nearly all European and North American countries. The philosophy of the University Center for Children with Developmental Disorders has been from the very beginning to remain open to all possible approaches in the field and to resist the attempt of any school or therapeutic approach to become dominating over the others, so that the optimal balance within the biopsychosocial paradigm could become a firm basis for Lithuanian child and adolescent psychiatry.

This was not easy to achieve, because after many years of overemphasis of biological approaches, the psychodynamic model was becoming extremely popular among young professionals, and there was an obvious tendency to take the other extreme in the development of mental health services for children and families. A group of young and ambitious psychotherapists, which succeeded in founding the Vilnius Center for Clinical Psychotherapy, clearly accepted the psychodynamic approach as the basis for everyday practice of psychotherapists and other mental health professionals. In this new situation, the philosophy of the University Center for Children with Developmental Disorders was to accept the psychodynamic approach as one of the basic approaches, but not as the only alternative for the former biological paradigm, and to keep looking for more socially and community oriented approaches, which could be helpful in everyday work with children and families at risk.

3. Structure and organization of services

Lithuania has a population (as of January 1, 1997) of 3,707,213 inhabitants. There are 997,202 children and adolescents (0–18 years of age), i.e., 26.9 % of the population.

The first child psychiatric inpatient department was opened in 1962. The number of child and adolescent psychiatrists has been gradually increasing and in 1997 there were 50 certified child and adolescent psychiatrists. Additionally, 18 medical doctors are in the child and adolescent psychiatry residency training at Vilnius University.

Traditionally, the following three types of services existed in Lithuanian child and adolescent psychiatry during the Soviet period:

- *outpatient services* – as a part of general psychiatric policlinics (dispensaries) in larger cities, there has been a district child psychiatrist per 20,000 children;
- *inpatient services* – there was a tradition to have inpatient units for children with 40 to 60 beds each, in general psychiatric hospitals; the total number of

child psychiatric beds was approaching 200 (for about children's population of 1 million);

- *three large institutions* for severely and moderately mentally retarded children (under the Ministry of Social Welfare);
- *a large network of special schools* (more than 40 of them throughout Lithuania), most of them – residential institutions – for children with mild mental retardation (many of these children have been only labeled as mentally retarded, and their real problem was usually social deprivation due to the social problems in families).

All the services for children with psychiatric disorders and mental retardation in the former system were funded by the state budget. The health care budget was responsible for inpatient and outpatient psychiatric services; social welfare provided funds for the psychoneurological institutions for moderately and severely mentally disabled children. The system of education was funding special boarding schools for mildly mentally retarded children.

Currently the health, social, and educational services are undergoing changes in the transitional period to the market economy. In 1997, the Health Insurance Law was introduced, with "per capita" funding for primary health care, and limited pay for outpatient and inpatient services at the secondary and tertiary level. Initially, mental health was not on the list of primary health care services, as it was supposed that general practitioners will be responsible for the whole area of primary health care, including mental health. But psychiatrists, child and adolescent psychiatrists, and NGOs interested in mental health protested against discrimination of mental health services. According to the Mental Health Act, which was adopted by the Lithuanian Parliament in 1995, every municipality has to establish a mental health center – a team of mental health professionals who will provide outpatient mental health care services at the primary level to the local inhabitants. A psychiatrist, child and adolescent psychiatrist, psychologist, and social worker are included on the list of obligatory team members. At the end of 1997 the Ministry of Health and the Council of Obligatory Health Insurance agreed to introduce amendments to the initial documents, and very limited funding (approximately 0.7 USD for each inhabitant per year) was additionally allocated for the primary mental health care. The process of developing community based mental health centers started, and the main concern of child and adolescent psychiatrists is now to lobby for the autonomy of services for children and adolescents within primary mental health care. The alternate option, rather popular among national and local authorities, is that general psychiatrists could take care of all age groups, including children and adolescents, in the primary mental health care.

One more problem caused by the introduction of Health Insurance was that outpatient services covered by insurance have been restricted to one consultation of any medical specialist once per three months. The philosophy behind this decision was to give priority to the general practitioners, and the medical specialists would only consult the patient when there is a need. In the initial list of specialists, a general psychiatrist was the only representative of mental health professionals. However, after protests from the side of child and adolescent psychiatrists, they were included on the list of medical specialists who would be paid for consultation. But two main problems remain unsolved. The first is how outpatient treatment (e.g., psychotherapy) will be paid. Another problem is that all non-medical professionals (such as, psychologists, speech therapists, clinical social workers) have been excluded from the lists of professionals whose services could be paid by insurance.

The official position held by psychiatrists, child and adolescent psychiatrists, other mental health professionals, and NGOs of consumers of mental health services or their relatives is that mental health services are again in danger of being neglected by the new system of funding of health services. One of the proposals to the government, which was recently made, was to officially recognize the need of mixed funding for mental health services, i.e., to fund mental health services from health insurance and from the budget.

4. Cooperation with medical and non-medical disciplines

Within the medical specialities, child and adolescent psychiatry has been making attempts to become independent from general psychiatry and to maintain good relations with the traditionally strong disciplines of pediatrics and child neurology. Reasonable success has been achieved in this development. In the list of specialties, child and adolescent psychiatry now exists as an independent specialty, but is still within the branch of specialties "Psychiatry". In the field of service delivery, there has been a clear movement to separate from general psychiatry and to develop independent services or to be affiliated with pediatric services. Thus, the National Child Development Center with a clinical unit for child psychiatry is an independent non-profit health care facility. Two inpatient child psychiatric units have been recently opened within general or pediatric hospitals (Kaunas Medical Academy Clinic and Šiauliai Children's Hospital).

Another trend was to initiate the coalition with non-medical professionals – psychologists, social workers, special educators, NGOs of parents and children's rights protection organizations, and to raise the problems of adequate services for children and families on the political level. The political reality which was clearly defined from the beginning of the 1990s was that the following two problems are important to the government – namely changes in the services for children with disabilites and prevention of child abuse. This was why the strategy of the University Center for Children with Developmental Disorders (since 1997: National Child Development Center) was to emphasize issues of early intervention for developmental disorders and prevention of child abuse as the main issues in the field of children's mental health and developmental disorders. This led to the development of the National Health Program for Children with Developmental Disorders, which was approved by the Lithuanian Government in 1996 and incorporates the development of psychiatric services for children and adolescents.

5. Graduate/postgraduate training and continuing medical education

There are two sites where medical doctors are trained in Lithuania: Kaunas Medical Academy and Medical Faculty of Vilnius University. Child and adolescent psychiatry has been a recognized discipline in Vilnius University, which has a long tradition of training pediatricians in the independent undergraduate program for six years of medical studies.

Before 1991 child psychiatry was taught as a course within the Department of Nervous and Mental Diseases. In 1991, during the reform of university clinics and departments, child psychiatry separated from the new Clinic (Department) of Psychiatry and, thus, a new university department was founded. From 1991 to 1996 it was called the Children's Mental Health Center. Since 1997, the official name of this university department is Clinic of Social Pediatrics and Child Psychiatry. There is currently one position of associate professor and Head of the University Clinic and two full staff positions of assistant professors (these are shared by eight experienced specialists in child and adolescent psychiatry and clinical child psychology who work in the National Child Development Center).

In 1991, Lithuania started the training of medical specialists in residency programs. This was a step forward, as the Soviet system of training of medical doctors was one year of specialization (internship) added to six years of studies in the medical faculty. Thus, the certificate of child psychiatrist was received prior to the year 1991 after one year of specialization in child psychiatry.

Since 1991 a residency training program of child and adolescent psychiatrists has been run at Vilnius University, under the supervision of the Children's Mental Health Center (currently – Clinic of Social Pediatrics and Child Psychiatry). The three year training program includes general psychiatry, psychotherapy, child neurology in addition to training in child and adolescent psychiatry. There are also alternative options for a tertiary two year residency program in child and adolescent psychiatry for those medical doctors who have completed their residency program in general psychiatry or pediatrics.

6. Research

From 1995 to 1997 four young professionals (three child and adolescent psychiatrists and one pediatrician) received four-year grants for research at the Clinic of Social Pediatrics and Child Psychiatry, Vilnius University. Their research includes infant mental health, spectrum of autistic disorders, and prevention of suicidal attempts in children and adolescents. Generally, the research is oriented toward assessment of needs for community-based services, including prevalence of disorders and evaluation of the effectiveness of different services. Until recently, no resources from the state budget have been available for research in the field of child and adolescent psychiatry. During recent years, some national programs have been launched by the government, e.g., the national program for prevention of juvenile delinquency and the national program for integration of the disabled persons. Development of services is a priority for these programs, but there is a possibility that some research projects will be funded by aforementioned programs.

7. Future perspectives

Lithuania is a country which has a clear ambitious goal after a forced break of fifty years to again join the community of developed and democratic nations. The first eight years of independence and democracy demonstrated that despite unfavorable heritage of totalitarian regime and low socioeconomic standards, there is considerable progress in the development of the civil democratic society. Politicians are paying more attention every year to the protection of children's rights, support for families, and improvement of mental health services. In this situation, child and adolescent psychiatrists and other mental health professionals have to cooperate with all interested organizations and with each other in order to lobby for a better quality of services for disturbed children and adolescents.

Selected references

Puras D (1994) Treatment approaches in Lithuanian child psychiatry: Changing the attitudes. Nordic Journal of Psychiatry 48: 397–400

Puras D (1997) Lithuanian psychiatry – a need for mental health coalition. European Psychiatry. The Journal of the Association of European Psychiatrists 12 (Supplement 2): 162

United Nations Development Programme (1997) Lithuanian Human Development Report. Living standards and choices – 1997. Vilnius

Child and adolescent psychiatry in Luxembourg

C. Frisch-Desmarez

1. Definition, historical development, and current situation

Definition

It is important to emphasize at the outset that we accept the tenets of present-day child psychiatry, such as that psychopathology has multifactorial etiologies and that children, adolescents, and families require a global, multi-disciplinary, psycho-medico-social approach that includes a psychotherapeutic dimension. We also consider that the scope of child psychiatry covers the whole field of psycho-medico-juridico-social issues, so that it includes children in difficulties at school as well as those who are victims of cruelty or present a psychotic pathology.

Historical development

It was only in 1988 that the first child psychiatrist was appointed in Luxembourg. Until then, psychiatry for children was conducted by psychiatrists for adults. They would see children and their families, usually in private consultation, and few actual therapies were undertaken. A large proportion of infant and juvenile psychiatry was conducted by neurologists.

However, since 1973, several guidance services have been set up (Thoma 1998). These are distinctive in that, unlike other European countries, they come under "Éducation Différenciée" (Special Education), which means that their primary concern is with children in difficulty at school (Ministère de l'éducation Nationale 1993). These services began with a very small number of professionals, often only one psychologist for an entire region, and even today some still lack a multi-disciplinary team. After their creation, the psychologists who worked in them found themselves faced with problems that were far more extensive than simply educational difficulties, and they began to cover the wider field of psychiatry for children of primary school age. On their own personal initiative, professionals working in these services underwent training in various therapeutic techniques in Belgium, France, or Germany. Until the arrival of the first child psychiatrist, collaboration between the guidance services and psychiatry was very ad hoc. Certain psychiatrists with more of an interest in family work eventually provided consultation, collaborating with some of the psychologists from the services. But, even today, once again in contrast with other European countries, there seems little prospect of integrating a child psychiatrist into these teams, despite the broader range of psychopathological problems with which they have to deal and even though there is a prospect of widening still further the scope of their mission (Loi du 30 juin 1990, Memorial luxembourgeois).

The project of creating a child psychiatry service at the pediatric clinic (Centre Hospitalier de Luxembourg) was first debated early in the 1980s. But for various reasons, principally the lack of motivation to give priority to its budget, the project was repeatedly postponed from one year to the next and was only started in 1995 (Vervier & Schmitz 1995; Vervier, Schmitz & Keutgens 1995). Even today, it is still merely an outpatient service. However, its team is multidisciplinary and includes one and a half full-time child psychiatrists. It is developing liaison child psychiatry and working in close collaboration with the pediatric service.

Ten years ago, a number of early intervention services were set up. These were aimed at children under four years of age who presented developmental delays or imbalances. These services were composed of professionals from different disciplines (remedial teachers, movement therapists, speech therapists, etc.). Some of these services worked in close collaboration with the child psychiatrists.

Recent advances

In 1990, the Luxembourg health ministry asked Professor Häfner of Mannheim, Germany, to report on the condition of psychiatry in Luxembourg. From this there emerged a whole series of points that did not take sufficient account of the specificities of Luxembourg and proposed to apply measures to our country that were specific to Germany. This report (Rössler, Salize, Häfner 1993) was wholly inadequate at the level of child psychiatry and was later supplemented by Professors Rössler and Salize, in collaboration with Professor Häfner. This report contained more details about the creation of a psychiatric service for children and adolescents in Luxembourg, but also left little room for a psychotherapeutic approach or for our own particular psychiatric culture of Francophone origin. The publication of these reports was a very important event because their conclusions still influence the Luxembourg health ministry's whole policy in psychiatric matters, pushing it in a rather hospital-centered direction. A "counter-report" by an outside expert from Belgium or France was called for by professionals, but this demand has not yet turned into action (Achten et al. 1998).

There are several reports on the child psychiatry network in Luxembourg, written between 1992 and 1995. These are the reports by Professor Häfner (Germany), supplemented by his colleagues Rössler and Salize (1993), Rohmann-Estgen (1993), Vervier & Schmitz (1997), Frisch-Desmarez (1997), and the final report of a working group on child psychiatry completed in November 1993 (Achten et al. 1998). This working group was set up by the health ministry in the light of Professor Häfner's report.

Current situation

Luxembourg has a population of about 400,000 people at present of whom around 96,000 are under eighteen years of age. It is an independent Grand Duchy, ruled by a democratic parliamentary government under the aegis of a constitutional monarchy.

Children only enter the educational system at four years of age, which means that many situations of psychiatric risk may be detected very late. The language spoken by the population is the Luxembourg dialect and children learn to read and write in German. French is introduced at school at eight years of age. About 31 % of the population is foreign, mainly of European origin.

It is important to note that Luxembourg does not possess a complete university system, although there is a university center that teaches first-year studies in certain faculties. This means that students in medicine and psychology are obliged to go to other European Community countries to pursue further studies. The basic medical training of child psychiatrists is mostly done either in Belgium, France, or Germany. As a result, a range of very disparate approaches are taken to child psychiatry in Luxembourg.

There are at present (early 1998) four child psychiatrists in the Grand Duchy of Luxembourg: two and a half work in private practice and collaborate with different institutions for children and adolescents, and one and a half work in the child psychiatry service of the pediatric clinic. The rest of the domain of child psychiatry falls in the responsibility of the psychologists and various therapists. Apart from the guidance services, there are a certain number of services with an educational orientation and services belonging to various associations that offer consultations to children, adolescents, and their families.

2. Classification systems, diagnostic and therapeutic methods

The diagnostic classifications used in Luxembourg are either the French classification of R. Misès or the DSM-IV.

3. Structure and organization of services

3.1 Guidelines for services for children and adolescents with psychiatric disorders

A school structure is already in place for autistic and psychotic children, and also for children with speech disturbances, as well as two small schools for children with non-specific behavioral disturbances and others for handicapped children. In the other "differentiated teaching" (special educational) structures, children are mixed together. There is also no specific structure for the hospitalization of adolescents whose pathology (suicide attempts, severe eating disorders) requires emergency admission. It still sometimes happens that, when no other solution can be found, very young adolescents are admitted to the hospital as emergencies at the Neuropsychiatric Hospital of Ettelbruck, which is a classic psychiatric hospital for adults and has not yet been able to divest itself completely of asylum practices. If such adolescents are violent, they may also be sent to prison. It should also be emphasized that solitary confinement is a measure taken with some adolescents if they become "unmanageable" in an institution.

In these services, a child psychiatrist could function by taking an overall view of the functioning of the personalities of different family members and ensuring a global and coordinated therapeutic approach to their problems.

The Grand Duchy has a very high placement rate for children and adolescents (1 %, counting institutional and family placements together). A National Placements Arbitration Commission gives direction in various situations (Centre National d'Aide au Placement, CNAP 1997; Ministère de la famille 1993; Ministère de la famille 1996). Very recently, it was decided that before making a placement order, apart from when one was made by the courts, children must undergo a psycho-pedagogic examination. But nearly 80 % of institutional placements are judicial placements (Association des Directeurs de Centres d'Accueil, ADCA 1998; Pregno 1998). These figures are extremely high, especially for an economically privileged country, but they are a consequence of other deficiencies in the coordination of resources (ADCA 1998). There are in fact numerous social assistance, socio-pedagogic, and psychological services which could in principle avoid this sort of immediate judicial measure. But lack of coordination and long-term thinking about cohesion among these various types of aid prevent it from happening. The lack of training in many of the professionals involved shows up above all in their difficulty in taking a global approach to the psychic problems of children, adolescents, and their families.

Outpatient services

The child psychiatry consultation service at the children's hospital (Centre Hospitalier de Luxembourg)

This service is composed of a multidisciplinary team that responds to a wide range of demands in the field of child psychiatry. It includes psychiatrists, psychologists, therapists, and care givers for children and their families, within a consultative framework. This team also collaborates closely with the pediatric service and the service for mistreated children.

The therapy center "La passerelle" (SANEM)

This is a small center that has room for eight to ten children aged beween five and twelve years. It is the only day center in the country with therapeutic aims that takes children on either a full- or a part-time basis. This structure caters to children with psychoaffective and conduct disorders as well as neurotic or pre-psychotic pathologies. The team comprises special teachers and one and a half full-time psychologists. Here, the child psychiatrist has a consulting role.

The consultation service "Le relais"

"Le relais" can offer a therapeutic program for young people who are breaking down socially, at school, or even in their families. It is aimed at young people and adolescents aged 14 to 22 with psychic problems, psychoses, problems with dependency, and conduct disorders. It is a service that functions without a child psychiatrist despite the severity of the psychopathological disorders commonly presented by the young people to whom it caters.

The polyvalent medico-social and psycho-pedagogic services of the sector

Given the central place they occupy in the network of medico-social care, these services are regularly faced with complex family and individual problems.

Educational psychology and advisory services

These are psychology services for school children in post-primary education. They are integrated schools, are accessible to students, and are attuned to their needs. They play a very important role both at the level of educational guidance and also in steering some children toward outside therapeutic help. Some members of these teams have had more indepth training and can also intervene as individual or family therapists.

Family planning centers

These centers offer consultation to adolescents who want to talk about sexual problems. For a very long time, these were the only places where they could go to talk in confidence about sexual abuse. A woman gynaecologist prompted the development of these centers and initiated a policy of openness about adolescents' sexuality.

The central social aid centers (SCAS)

The central social assistance services (including the youth protection section, the social defence section, and the guardianship section) often see adults who are not in a fit state to care for their children, and children who present with dangerous behaviors (aggression, sexual abuse, running away, etc.).

The youth protection section of SCAS must carry out the social investigations required by the courts, the number of which is continually rising.

The second task of the youth protection section of SCAS is to take responsibility for educational help in families for which such help has been stipulated by the youth tribunal.

The Luxembourg association for the prevention of cruelty to children (ALUPSE)

ALUPSE is a non-profit association concerned specifically with the mistreatment of children in the Grand Duchy of Luxembourg (Seligmann 1998).

Telephone helplines for children and adolescents

A telephone helpline for young people has been in existence since 1992, on the initative of several associations. This helpline is aimed at children or adolescents in crisis who do not always have access to a third party with whom they can talk about their difficulties.

Drug abuse (Jugend-an drogenhëllef)

This is an outpatient service that cares for drug abusers, and young people can approach it directly. The team is also involved in prevention and collaborates with various institutions.

New Life (Neit Liewen/Nouvelle vie)

This is a service for pregnant women in distress, and helps them to prepare either to accept or to part with their baby.

The list above is not exhaustive, and other associations may have a psychological consultation service open to the public.

Inpatient services

The Syrdallschlass therapy center at Manternach (drug abuse) and the therapy center at Useldange (alcohol)

Only a very small number of adolescents can be treated at these two specialized centers.

Pediatric services in the hospitals at Esch, Ettelbruck, and the Centre Hospitalier de Luxembourg

Only two of these hospitals offer psychopediatric liaison.

Reception centers

There are more than 400 places for young people in the country's various reception centers and FADEPS (reception and crisis aid hostels). In general, children can stay from three to six months at the FADEPS, which take children who are in socio-familial crisis (Andrich-Duval 1993). These centers play a big role in caring for children who often come from pathological and very dysfunctional families and frequently exhibit serious mental disorders. The psychopathology encountered at these centers really calls for the presence of a child psychiatrist in the same way as an emergency ward.

Complementary services

Special education (differentiated education)

The differentiated education sector is aimed at children who are unable to undertake traditional education in Luxembourg. Several special school structures exist to respond to certain rather specific needs, such as speech disturbances, behavioral disorders, or psychotic or autistic symptoms, but they are small and can only take in a few children.

Children placed abroad

No official figures exist, but after a count made at various ministries, it seems that each year thirty to forty children either native to Luxembourg or whose families reside here go for treatment to specialized residential institutions abroad (mainly in Belgium, Germany, and France) for serious psychic difficulties (anorexia, psychoses, conduct disorders, etc.) (Vervier & Schmitz 1995). They often remain there for longer than a year. Children who are sent in this direction are usually over eight years old, the majority being adolescents more than twelve years of age.

4. Cooperation with medical and non-medical disciplines

At the moment, changes are being made to include child psychiatrists in some multidisciplinary teams (outpatient and institutional), although these are consultative positions and, therefore, without real power over decisions about therapeutic orientation. Child psychiatrists are still not recognized by many professionals in the roles that they ought to have as referents, guarantors, and coordinators of therapists and therapeutic projects (Achten, Agreby, Frisch-Desmarez et al. 1998; (see also Historical development section).

5. Graduate/postgraduate training and continuing medical education

Luxembourg does not possess a complete university system. This means that students in medicine and psychology are obliged to go to other European Community countries to pursue further studies. The basic medical training of child psychiatrists is mostly done either in Belgium, France, or Germany.

6. Research

In Luxembourg we do not have any biological or pharmacological research in child psychiatry. However, there are several research projects in the Centre Hospitalier in the field of new born children and infancy. Other projects concern the field of hyperactivity and learning disabilities.

7. Future perspectives

Improvement of services and care systems

A plan exists to create the following at the children's hospital (CHL):

- A crisis center
  This would be for children under twelve years of age and would provide a crisis unit with a residential sector. Continuity of care would be ensured by a day center and the provision of child psychiatric consultation.

- A daycare center
  The team would be multidisciplinary and directed by a child psychiatrist. This project would be for children presenting neurotic or pre-psychotic pathologies, or perhaps for ones whose schooling was breaking down or were in family crisis. It is not intended for children with more severe psychopathological problems such as psychoses or major developmental imbalances (Vervier & Schmitz 1997). There are also plans to create a hospital structure for adolescents. It seems important to make separate hospital arrangements for children and for adolescents, primarily because of infrastructural incompatibility.

Conclusions

Luxembourg is a country without its own tradition of mental health care for children and adolescents, coming very much within the sphere of influence of Germany, Belgium, and France. It is now time to form a synthesis of all these "imported" elements so as to develop a new model of child psychiatry proper to the Grand Duchy.

As described above, and the list is certainly not exhaustive, Luxembourg is a country with a wealth of structures in the field of child psychiatry in the broadest sense, but with very few child psychiatrists. Those who exist are included in certain teams but most often in a consultative capacity except in the outpatient child psychiatry service at the Centre Hospitalier de Luxembourg. Having child psychiatrists even as consultants is certainly progress when compared with the situation ten years ago when there were no child psychiatrists at all in the Grand Duchy. However, despite some change in attitudes, for many psychologists or other institutional therapists, and above all for the public authorities, their role remains unclear. Consulting a child psychiatrist is still regarded as a serious step to take, with the implication that the child or adolescent in question must have a very serious psychiatric pathology to require it. The whole wider field of child psychiatry in which child psychiatrists could play essential roles in ensuring care and as referents for the continuity of therapeutic projects is still largely unexplored.

In effect, what is lacking most is a policy for care provision and an overall, long-term view of the whole of infant and juvenile mental health that might promote development of a more global approach to the question. At present, most of these services function in a disjointed way, without a spirit of coordinating care and without a priority concern for training the professionals who work at ground level. We even end up with situations that are not improved by intervention but are actually aggravated by the absence of a long-term strategy and the lack of coordination among the various services.

Collaboration between the law courts and child psychiatry is something else that deserves to be strengthed. The youth tribunal has very insufficient means at its disposal, which often results in decisions having to be made under emergency pressure, pre-empting any chance of intervention by a child psychiatrist. Expert opinion in cases of abused, mistreated, or neglected children or in situations of divorce is relatively seldom sought at all, and rarely in a context of collaboration with child psychiatrists. Lack of means cannot, however, explain everything in this overlapping domain of justice and child psychiatry. Here, too, a policy of collaboration would need to be thought about as something for the long term and not as an ad-hoc reaction to situations as they arise.

In conclusion, we would, therefore, say that the Grand Duchy is a country rich in European influences and in potential of its own. During the last ten years there have been enormous developments in care for children in psychic difficulties. But there is still a lack of real political will for change in the vast domain of child psychiatry. So long as the function of child psychiatry is not recognized as having a central place in the provision of psychic care for children, adolescents, and families, Luxembourg will continue to lag behind other European countries.

Selected references

Achten E, Agreby J, Frisch-Desmarez C, Pregno G, Seligmann R, Rohmann-Estgen MJ, Schmitz R (1998) Appel aux responsables politiques pour une prise de conscience des problèmes et des difficultés que rencontrent de nombreux enfants et adolescents. In: Pregno G (ed) Les enfants, orphelins de droits, pp 331–334. Le Phare, Luxembourg

ADCA (1998) Rapport officiel sur l'accueil de jour et de nuit des mineurs. Working paper, ed. by l'Association Des Centres d' Accueil, Luxembourg
Andrich-Duval S (1993) Concept des Foyers d'Accueil et de Dépannage (FADEP) au Luxembourg, Working paper, Luxembourg
CNAP (1997) Texte de coordination adopté à l'assemblée générale sur les amendements du Centre National d'Arbitrage et de Placement, Luxembourg
Frisch-Desmarez C (1997) Psychiatrie de l'enfant et de l'adolescent, Revue Agora, 1: 28-31, Luxembourg
Häfner (1993) Report on psychiatry in Luxembourg. Ed. by Ministry of Health, Luxembourg
Mémorial du Grand-Duché de Luxembourg A no. 30 (1990) Loi sur l' organisation des Services de Guidance de l'Enfance, 30 June 1990. Ed. by government, Luxembourg
Ministère de l'Education Nationale (1993) Les institutions spécialisées. Monography ed. by Ministry of Education, Luxembourg
Ministère de la Famille et de la Solidarité (1993) Convention des centres d'accueil, Ministry of family, Luxembourg
Ministère de la Famille (1996) Les droits de l'enfant au Grand-Duché de Luxembourg: Rapport initial du Grand-Duché de Luxembourg. Monography ed. by Ministry of Family, Luxembourg
Misès R, Fortineau J, Jeammet P, Lane IL, Mazet P, Plantade A, Quémada N (1988) Classification francaise des troubles menteaux de l'enfant et de l'adolescent. Psychiatrie de l'Enfant 31: 67–134
Pregno G (1998) Les centres d'accueil pour enfants et adolescents: A la recherche de leur identité. In: Pregno G (ed) Les enfants, orphelins de droits, pp 257–272, Le Phare, Luxembourg
Rohmann-Estgen MJ (1993) Konzeption einer Kinder- und Jugendpsychiatrischen Klinik. Working paper, Luxemburg
Rössler W, Salize HJ, Häfner H (1993) Gemeindepsychiatrie, Grundlagen und Leitlinien. Planungsstudie Luxemburg. Verlag Integrative Psychiatrie, Wien
Seligmann R (1998) L'association Luxembourgeoise de la prévention des sévices à l'enfant. Situation actuelle et perspectives, Discussion paper, Luxembourg
Thoma AM (1998) Le Service de Guidance de l'Enfance de l'Education différenciée. Discussion paper, Luxembourg
Vervier JF, Schmitz R (1997) Projet d'aménagement du Centre de Soins Pédopsychiatriques du Jour. Report, Centre Hospitalier Luxembourg
Vervier JF, Schmitz R (1995) Rapport du Service de Pédopsychiatrie CHL. Report, Centre Hospitalier, Luxembourg
Vervier JF, Schmitz R, Keutgens B (1995) "Projet d'un service national de psychiatrie de l'enfant et de l'adolescent, première étape: développement d'une structure hospitalière et ambulatoire pour enfants au centre hospitalier de Luxembourg", Report, Centre Hospitalier Luxembourg

Child and adolescent psychiatry in the Netherlands

H. van Engeland

Definition, historical development, and current situation

Definition

The field of child and adolescent psychiatry covers diagnosis, treatment, prevention, and rehabilitation of psychiatric disturbances in children and adolescents from birth up to the age of eighteen. Child and adolescent psychiatry is not a separate specialism but a super specialism. This means that the postgraduate training for child psychiatrists takes a total of 5 ½ years; 3 ½ years being devoted to general psychiatry and two years to child and adolescent psychiatry. Training is given only in recognized training centers. These centers are inspected every five years by a visitation committee that monitors the standards of training.

Historical development

Toward the end of the nineteenth century, the society in the Netherlands, as in the rest of Europe, began to realize that children had their own needs and demands. This led to the introduction of the Child Laws, compulsory education, and the establishment of children's hospitals. Psychiatry, too, began to take an interest in children. Mrs. N. C. Bakker, the wife of the future professor H. C. Rümke, opened a separate outpatient clinic for children in the Valerius Clinic in Amsterdam in 1919. Mrs. O. van Andel-Ripke did the same at the psychiatric-neurological university clinic in Utrecht in 1920. Influenced by the American Child Guidance Movement, the first child guidance center providing help for children with behavioral difficulties was established in Amsterdam in 1928 under the leadership of Mrs. N. C. Thibaut. This initiative was quickly followed in other large cities. The child guidance centers, which worked along multidisciplinary lines, later played a major role in the development of child and adolescent psychiatry. The pioneers of child psychiatry, Th. Hart de Ruiter, L. N. J. Kamp, and E. C. M. Freyling Schreuder, all worked part-time in such centers. In 1984, after a reorganization of the area of mental healthcare in the Netherlands, the child guidance centers were disbanded and their work was incorporated into the activities of the RIAGG (the Regional Institutions of Ambulatory Mental Health Care).

In the 1930s, outpatient clinics for children were created as part of the university psychiatric clinics (F. Grewel in Amsterdam 1931, E. D. E. A. Carp in Leiden 1936, and H. C. Rümke in Utrecht 1938). At the same time, the first university child psychiatry facilities were established (by Grewel in Amsterdam from 1936 to 1938, by Carp in Leiden from 1937 to 1946, and by Rümke, in collaboration with Kamp, in Utrecht from 1940 up to the present day). The outbreak of the Second World War and the German occupation of the Netherlands all but put a stop to the further growth of child psychiatry in the Dutch universities. After the war, a number of teaching posts were recognized (L. N. J. Kamp in Utrecht and A. D. van Krevelen in Leiden 1950; Grewel in Amsterdam 1954). Soon after, the first full university lecturers in child and adolescent psychiatry were appointed (Hart de Ruiter in Groningen, 1951; van Krevelen in Leiden and Kamp in Utrecht, 1956). In 1956, in Groningen, Dr. Hart de Ruiter became the first professor of child psychiatry. The appointment of Kamp in Utrecht followed in 1964 and, at present, seven of the eight medical faculties in the Netherlands have a chair of child and adolescent psychiatry.

Child and adolescent psychiatrists also began to organize themselves within their professional organization, the Dutch Society of Psychiatry founded in 1877. In 1948, the Child and Adolescent Psychiatry Section was set up with L. N. J. Kamp as its first chairman. The section organizes study groups, conferences, and congresses and, at present, with a membership of 250, it is the official platform of child and adolescent psychiatry in the Netherlands. In spite of several attempts, child and adolescent psychiatry has never been recognized as an independent medical specialism. However, since 1987, it is possible to become registered as a child and adolescent psychiatrist after completion of a two-year training.

The Child and Adolescent Psychiatry Section is a member of the International Association of Child and Adolescent Psychiatry and Allied Professions (IACAPAP), of the European Society of Child and Adolescent Psychiatry (ESCAP), and of the World Association of Infant Mental Health (WAIMH). In 1960, the section organized the IACAPAP congress in Scheveningen, chaired by Professor D. A. van Krevelen and in 1995 it organized the 10th ESCAP congress in Utrecht, chaired by Professor H. van Engeland.

The publication of "The Dutch Textbook of Special Child Psychiatry" by D. A. van Krevelen in 1950 was an important milestone in the development of child psychiatry in the Netherlands. In 1972, "Hoofdlijnen van de Kinderpsychiatrie" (Main Themes of Child Psychiatry) by Th. Hart de Ruiter and L. N. J. Kamp was published, a book that had an enormous influence on the generation of child and adolescent psychiatrists of that time. In the 1980s, "The Manual of Child and Adolescent Psychiatry" by J. A. R. Sanders-Woudstra and H. de Witte gained great influence. Recently, "Child and Adolescent Psychiatry" by F. Verhey and F. C. Verhulst, and "Psychopharmacology in Children" by R. Minderaa and C. Ketelaars were published. All of these books figure prominently in the medical curricula as well as in the training of psychologists, remedial educationalists, and social workers. Because Dutch is spoken in few countries, it took a long time before child psychiatry in the Netherlands had its own journal. This was at last the case in the 1980s. In a fruitful cooperation with the fields of remedial education and developmental psychology, the journals "Tijdschrift voor orthopedagogiek en kinderpsychiatrie" (Journal for Remedial Education and Child Psychiatry) and "Kind en adolescent" (Child and Adolescent) were established. However, these days, the most important scientific work of the Dutch child psychiatrists is published in the major, English-language, international journals.

The school of thought on which the Dutch child and adolescent psychiatry is based has three traditions:

- the *neuropsychiatric tradition* whose prominent proponents were Grewel and van Krevelen and which has its roots in neurology as well as psychiatry. The strongly neuropsychologically and neurobiologically oriented child and adolescent psychiatry as practiced in the university departments in Utrecht by H. van Engeland, in Groningen by R. Minderaa, and in Amsterdam by B. Gunning developed from this tradition.
- the *psychoanalytical, psychodynamic tradition* which was, for the most part, developed by Hart de Ruiter, Kamp, and Freijling-Schreuder and which was greatly influenced by American psychoanalytic traditions and the Child Guidance Movement.
- the *epidemiological approach*, introduced by F. C. Verhulst and mainly practised in Rotterdam by Verhulst and his group.

At the present time, the working methods of most child and adolescent psychiatrists and psychiatric centers can be described as eclectic. Besides a psychodynamic approach, behavioral therapy and especially family therapy have developed strongly. All Dutch child and adolescent psychiatrists undergo a long and thorough training in psychotherapy and all Dutch psychiatrists are themselves required to undergo learning therapy for a minimum of 50 hours. Since the 1990s, pharmacotherapy is an established part of the program of most centers.

Current situation

In December 1997, there were 16 million inhabitants in the Netherlands of whom 4 million were children up to the age of nineteen. Seven of the eight medical faculties have a chair in child and adolescent psychiatry and all have active research programs. Rotterdam (epidemiology) and Utrecht (neuropsychiatry and neurobiology) have, at the moment, the largest research centers, each with a research input of about five full-time employees and 10 to 20 PhD students.

There are 26 child and adolescent psychiatric institutions in the Netherlands, (including the seven university departments for child and adolescent psychiatry) where all facets of child and adolescent psychiatry are practiced. Since 1984, throughout the country 51 Regional Institutes for Ambulatory Mental Health Services (RIAGGs) have been active, each with a catchment area of 150,000 to 400,000 inhabitants. Each RIAGG has a youth care team where the child psychiatrist works together in a multidisciplinary team with the psychologist, remedial teacher, social-psychiatric nurse, social worker, and pediatrician. A total of 57 child and adolescent psychiatrists have their own private practices in which they practice all facets of child and adolescent psychiatry. A survey organized by the Child and Adolescent Psychiatry Section, which was carried out in 1997, showed that there are 257 child and adolescent psychiatrists in the Netherlands. Approximately half of them work in child and adolescent psychiatry as well as in adult psychiatry. Most are employed in psychiatric hospitals, child and adolescent psychiatric institutions or university hospitals, and many of them are working on a part-time basis. It is estimated that in the Netherlands, there are 156 full-time equivalents child and adolescent psychiatry available. Most of them are men but especially among the younger generation, many female colleagues are now being found. The profession is attracting an increasing number of women.

2. Classification systems, diagnostic and therapeutic methods

Classification systems

All of the institutions for child and adolescent psychiatry in the Netherlands use a diagnostic classification system: DSM-IV is the most popular. A few academic departments also use a basic documentation system for all the cases that they treat. Such a system contains demographic data, lists of symptoms, case history data, and a DSM-IV diagnosis. Since 1 January 1998, all RIAGG teams are required to classify their patients according to DSM-IV or ICD-10. However, in daily practice the implementation of this requirement sometimes presents problems, largely because the members of the multidisciplinary RIAGG youth teams do not possess the necessary knowledge to carry out this classification.

Diagnostic methods

The entire spectrum of diagnostic procedures is available and is used. This applies mainly to standardized interviews, neuropsychological diagnostics, systematized observation techniques, and family diagnostics. As far as laboratory techniques are concerned (EEG, neurochemistry, and neuro-imaging), child psychiatry is forced to enlist the cooperation of adjacent disciplines. In practice, this means that these more specialized diagnostics are only found in the university centers for child and adolescent psychiatry.

Therapeutic methods

In regard to the therapeutic interventions, we in the Netherlands have a wide range of methods at our disposal. Most institutions have the services of well-trained psychotherapists (psychoanalytical/psychodynamic; behavioral therapy and family therapy). During recent years, the expertise in the field of pharmacotherapy has developed rapidly in the large child psychiatry centers. Although some centers can be characterized by their strongly psychodynamically oriented approach, the method of most centers is eclectic.

3. Structure and organization of services

Table 1 gives an overview of the various types of child and adolescent psychiatry services in the Netherlands. During the past 10 years, the government has deliberately stimulated the development of child and adolescent psychiatric services. In spite of these governmental efforts, there is still a shortage of clinical services for adolescents, and the capacity in the outpatient/ambulatory care remains insufficient. This leads to unacceptably long waiting lists. The number of daycare places has increased considerably during recent years but, here too, more capacity is needed to meet future requirements. There are insufficient special facilities for chronic child and adolescent psychiatric patients; systematic rehabilitation programs and programs for child drug abusers and delinquent adolescents (forensic child and adolescent psychiatry) are almost completely non-existent.

Most outpatient consultations are carried out by the youth care teams of RIAGG. The annual incidence for the child and adolescent mental healthcare institutions varies from 1.5 to 2.3 %.

At the moment in the Netherlands, we have 26 institutions for child and adolescent psychiatry (including the seven university child and adolescence psychiatric departments) that all have outpatient, clinical as well as daycare facilities. In recent years, the distribution of the facilities throughout the country has improved considerably but the situation is not yet ideal. The majority of daycare clinics are linked to a clinical facility. The daycare clinics provide primary as well as secondary daycare. Primary daycare treatment means that the child can receive daycare treatment after an ambulant psychiatric examination has indicated that this is necessary. Secondary daycare means that clinical treatment is continued in a daycare program.

Table 1. Services for psychiatrically disturbed children and adolescents in the Netherlands

I Outpatient services
1. Child and adolescent psychiatrists in private practice
2. Child and adolescent psychotherapists (psychologists and pedagogues specially trained in child and adolescent psychotherapy) in private practice
3. Youth care teams of Regional Institutions for Ambulatory Mental Health Care
4. Outpatient departments of child and adolescent psychiatry institutions
II Daycare services
1. Medical daycare centers (only for preschool children and functioning independent from child and adolescent psychiatry)
2. Daycare centers integrated in departments for child and adolescent psychiatry
III Inpatient services
1. Inpatient services at university hospitals
2. Inpatient services at psychiatric hospitals
3. Inpatient services at independent institutes for child and adolescent psychiatry
IV Complementary services
1. Rehabilitation services for special groups of patients (e.g., children with epilepsy, children with severe head injuries)
2. Different types of residential settings for children and adolescents
3. Therapeutic foster families

Complementary services and rehabilitation

If the child's treatment has been completed within the mental healthcare service, but the child cannot be reintegrated into the family from which it came (either because of his or her long-term, chronic disturbed psychiatric condition or because the family environment is unable to offer sufficient support), the child can then be placed in a youth care institution. In the framework of the "Youth Care Act" (1982), the youth care institutions are funded by the government and provide the following facilities: family homes/units, special-educational institutions, sheltered living accommodation, therapeutic foster homes, and boarding schools that provide vocational training. In these institutions the accent is on remedial education, special education, and vocational counseling.

Funding of services

All child and adolescent psychiatric facilities (including the type of ambulant care that is provided by the RIAGG youth care teams) is financed from the Exceptional Medical Expenses Act. This states that this care is available to the population free of charge. The care for the chronic child psychiatric patients is mainly carried out by the youth care system and is financed in the framework of youth care legislation.

Evaluation

Up to the present day, no systematic investigation has been carried out into the (cost) effectiveness of the area mental healthcare institutions for the youth. We do, however, have at our disposal various follow-up studies, which make clear that a considerable number of the clinically and daycare treated children and adolescents are chronically disturbed and, therefore, require long-term care.

4. Cooperation with medical and non-medical disciplines

Cooperation with pediatrics

Most of the children's departments in general hospitals and all children's hospitals have their own "psychosocial teams" consisting of psychologists, educationalists, and social workers who can be called in by the pediatrician to deal with the psychosocial problems of the sick child. Most children's hospitals also have a liaison with a child and adolescent psychiatry department in order to treat pediatric patients with psychiatric disorders.

Cooperation with psychiatry

Most of the child/adolescent psychiatric departments in the Netherlands are part of a psychiatric hospital. Only a few departments are associated with a children's hospital. Child and adolescent psychiatry shares a diagnostic approach with general psychiatry, but deals with the same age group as pediatrics. In daily practice, there are three (intensive) areas of common ground with general psychiatry: psychiatry of the adolescent and the young adult, family psychiatry, and the longitudinal perspective. It is a fact that many psychiatric disturbances in children and adolescents persist until far into adulthood, demanding the development of care programs and a continuity of care in cooperation with general psychiatry. This is an important field for the future.

Cooperation with non-medical institutions and professionals

Within child and adolescent mental healthcare there are, on the one hand, the child and adolescent psychiatric institutions in the more narrow sense, where child psychiatry is the dominant discipline and where child psychiatrists bear the final responsibility for diagnosis and treatment. On the other hand, there are the RIAGG youth care teams in which the child and adolescent psychiatrist is a member but does not occupy the dominant position in the team. Although all of those who are engaged in the field of child and adolescent mental healthcare are convinced of the necessity of good cooperation between the medical and psychosocial disciplines, in practice, this leaves much to be desired. The introduction of the compulsory use of the DSM-IV/ICD-10 classification system within the RIAGGs will, hopefully, lead to better cooperation between the disciplines because there will then be, at least in the area of diagnostic classification, a common language.

The most important non-medical health care institutions with which child and adolescent psychiatrists have to cooperate are the institutions for youth care. These are child protection agencies, foster home/family nursing organizations, family guardianship associations and foundations who deliver residential treatment focussing on scholastic, vocational, and social rehabilitation. As of 1 January 1999, all these youth care institutions were amalgated into the "Bureau for Youth Care" (Bureau Jeugdzorg). It is hoped that this governmental action will lead to a better coordination of the field of youth care and to a better cooperation between the "Bureau for Youth Care" on the one hand and the medical mental health care institutions on the other hand. Discussions about how to implement this governmental act "Direction in Youth Care" (Regie in de Jeugdzorg) are not yet finalized. One of the most difficult issues in this discussion is how to create a fruitful and efficient collaboration between youth care and medical mental health care.

Many cases are referred to the child and adolescent psychiatrists by school psychologists and school doctors. Schools for special education in particular often call in the help of the diagnostic and treatment facilities of child and adolescent psychiatry. These cases mostly concern children with learning difficulties, speech/language difficulties, and behavioral disturbances. Also, the carers of the mentally handicapped often request further diagnostic and treatment advice for mentally retarded children who have psychiatric disturbances. The shortage of child psychiatrists means that, only too often, the questions remain unanswered.

Finally, in the Netherlands there are approximately 200 highly qualified child and adolescent psychotherapists who run their own private practices. These are, for the most part, psychologists and orthopedagogues who carry out psychotherapy on children when there is a psychiatric indication. Except for a small contribution from the patients themselves, the help is free and is financed from the funds of the Exceptional Medical Expenses Act.

5. Graduate/postgraduate training and continuing medical education

Graduate training: The role of medical faculties

In 1997, child and adolescent psychiatry was represented by a separate department or chair in 7 out of 8 medical faculties in the Netherlands. Thus, in one medical faculty (Maastricht), there is no formal teaching program in child and adolescent psychiatry for medical students.

At those medical faculties with a department of child and adolescent psychiatry, the curriculum of child and adolescent psychiatry for medical students is integrated into general psychiatry and/or pediatrics. Child and adolescent psychiatry is also included in bedside teaching. As far as the questions for the multiple choice examinations are concerned, approximately 15–20 % of the questions in psychiatry belong to the field of child and adolescent psychiatry.

Postgraduate training, a joint effort

Child and adolescent psychiatry is not a separate medical specialism; it is considered to be a super specialization in the field of psychiatry. So, to become a child and adolescent psychiatrist, one has first to finalize training in general psychiatry, which takes 4 ½ years. The last year of this training can be spent on child and adolescent psychiatry. Whenever a trainee decides to become a child and adolescent psychiatrist, he has to take another year of training in child and adolescent psychiatry. This implies that child and adolescent psychiatrists have an extended training curriculum. Of the two years of training in child and adolescent psychiatry, a substantial part of the training curriculum is concentrated on psychotherapy. Furthermore, the candidates must at least have extensive knowledge, experience, and proficiency in the following subjects: psychopathology of childhood and adolescence, diagnostic classification of childhood psychiatric disorders, developmental psychopathology, methodology of psychological testing and rating of psychological findings, neurobiological foundations of psychopathology; pediatric psychopharmacology, rating of laboratory values, expert opinion, indication for and techniques of behavior therapy, psychodynamic psychotherapy and family therapy, specific regulations of social legislation as well as legal norms of patient-doctor relationships, child protection measures, quality assurance in medical practice.

Training in child and adolescent psychiatry can only be given in recognized training centers. These centers are inspected every 5 years by a visitation committee that monitors the standards of training. Generally speaking in most training departments 1 ½ years of training is spent in outpatient services; half a year is spent in inpatient services.

After having completed the requirements for the specialist training no formal examination has to be passed. The trainee has to send in a logbook of his training activities as well as the judgement of his supervisor to the "specialisten registratie commissie" (Specialists Registration Committee). This registration committee will then approve the trainee's application to become a child and adolescent psychiatrist.

Continuing medical education in child and adolescent psychiatry and psychotherapy

A licence for practising psychiatry (and this applies to child and adolescent psychiatry as well) is given for a time period of 5 years. After that period, psychiatrists have to give an overview of their continuing medical education activities (following special courses, attending congresses, research activities, administrative activities as well as the amount of time actually spent on face to face contact with patients). If the Specialist Registration Committee approves these continuing medical eduation activities, a licence for another 5 years is given.

Training programs for other disciplines

Child and adolescent psychiatrists are included in several training programs for other medical and non-medical specialists. The main programs are carried out in the field of psychotherapy for psychologists, pedagogues, and nurses.

6. Research

Research fields and strategies

During the past two decades high quality research had been carried out in Dutch child and adolescent psychiatry in 5 areas:

- *epidemiology*: the focus is on studies in prevalence and incidence of child psychiatric disorders, the natural course of disorders over years, and the use of mental health services.

- *ethological research*: the focus is on mother/child interactions and peer interactions, mainly in children with pervasive developmental disorders and in children with disumptive disorders.
- *neuro-physiological research*: the focus is on evoked response studies and brain mapping in children suffering from autism and attention deficit hyperactivity disorders. The influence of psychopharmacological drugs on brain activity in autistic and ADHD children was studied recently.
- *neuro-chemistry*: the focus is on studies of the noradrenergic, the serotonergic, and the opioid neurotransmitter system. Pharmacological intervention studies in children with autism, ADHD, and Gilles de la Tourette were recently carried out.
- *genetics*: recently behavioral genetic studies (twin studies by means of questionnaires) were carried out and very recently studies in the molecular genetics of autism and attention deficit hyperactivity disorder were started.

Research in child and adolescent psychiatry is carried out in all university departments. Rotterdam (epidemiology) and Utrecht (neuropsychiatry and neurobiology) have at the moment the largest research centers. In line with a world wide trend, Dutch research in child and adolescent psychiatry can be characterized by three tendencies: (1) an increased consideration of the biological basis of psychological disorders at all ages, (2) a thorough consideration of the principles of the development (developmental psychopathology, and developmental neurochemistry), and (3) the introduction of evidence-based therapeutic interventions. Main topics are standardized diagnosis, and development of guidelines for treatment and outcome evaluation.

Therapy outcome evaluation is difficult to carry out and is only rarely done. Until now, most Dutch therapy outcome studies were focussed on the effectiveness of pharmacological therapies. Psychotherapy outcome research is needed and can be considered to be a challenge for the future.

Research training and career development

An up to date research training is the most important precondition for high quality research in the future. Nevertheless, trainees in child and adolescent psychiatry in the Netherlands are insufficiently trained in carrying out research programs. The result is that no more than 5 % of all child and adolescent psychiatrists did a PhD thesis. So in spite of the high quality research in child and adolescent psychiatry in the Netherlands produced at the moment, the future does not look good. What we need is regular research training seminars and PhD programs for psychiatrists who want to specialize in child and adolescent psychiatry.

Funding

Most of the research carried out in child and adolescent psychiatry is funded by the universities. The Dutch Science Foundation (NWO) also supports part of the research programs; however, child and adolescent psychiatry benefits only at a relatively modest level from the Science Foundation, mainly by single project funding.

Another important research funding organization is the Ministry of Health. In the recent past, special fundings for research in epidemiology and in addiction research was given, being a great help in the further development of research in child psychiatry in the Netherlands. Thirdly, a number of foundations are important for research funding, most prominently the National Foundation for Mental Health and the Korczak Foundation.

7. Future perspectives

The future perspectives of child and adolescent psychiatry in the Netherlands cannot be seen independently from the development of mental health care in general and from the further development of the "direction in youth care" program. Predicting the future of child and adolescent psychiatry in the Netherlands is very difficult. Formulating the needs for the future is perhaps a better strategy.

Research

The etiology and pathogenenis of many mental and behavioral disorders in children and adolescents are not yet understood. On the other hand, the available findings are not generally known and, therefore, not used in diagnosis, treatment, and prevention. So, for the future more emphasis should be put on:

- stimulating basic and clinical research,
- spreading the available knowledge to mental health care and youth care workers, and
- advocating child and adolescent mental health research among decision makers in politics and in the public.

Recently professors of child and adolescent psychiatry in the Netherlands in a joint effort wrote a "memorandum" for future research in child and adolescent psychiatry in the Netherlands. As far as the advocacy of child mental health is concerned, new efforts and negotiations with politicians, the Ministry of Health, and health insurance companies have to be initiated.

Training

As far as undergraduate training is concerned, there is a urgent need to establish a department of child and adolescent psychiatry at the medical faculty of Maastricht. With regard to postgraduate training, new regulations, more in line with the new European Curriculum being discussed in all countries of the European Union and the EFTA countries is necessary. Continuing medical education, specially focussed on the reconfirmation of licences for child and adolescent psychiatrists is necessary.

At the moment, a shortage of child and adolescent psychiatrists in the Netherlands exists. The profession is attracting an increasing number of women, implicating that for the future more and more child and adolescent psychiatrists will take part-time jobs. So, for the future the shortage of child and adolescent psychiatrists will even become worse. An extra effort to expand the number of trainees in child and adolescent psychiatry is urgently needed.

Improvement of services and care systems

In spite of the governmental support to stimulate the development of new services for child and adolescent psychiatry, there is still a need for future extra stimulation. At the moment the capacity of outpatient/ambulatory care remains insufficient, leading to unacceptably long waiting lists. Special facilities for forensic child and adolescent psychiatry and for the treatment of addicted children and adolescents are almost non-existent, and there is a shortage of clinical services for adolescents.

Hopefully, the governmental program "Directions in Youth Care" (Regie in de Jeugdzorg) will provide opportunities for a better coordination between child and adolescent mental health care institutions and youth care facilities. Of special importance is the creation of continuity of care for children and adolescents with severe and persistent mental health problems (chronically psychotic youngsters; youngsters with severe disruptive behavior disorders). Especially these categories of chronic child and adolescent psychiatric cases, who cannot be integrated in their original families after having finished child psychiatric treatment, are in need for enduring support, remedial education, and vocational counseling. Special programs to be carried out in youth care institutions need to be established. Many psychiatric disturbances of children and adolescents persist far into adulthood, demanding the development of care programs and a continuity of care in cooperation with general psychiatry. This also is an important field for the future.

In spite of the fact that politicians in the Netherlands at the moment are inclined to reduce mental health care budgets, hopefully, the above mentioned necessary developments will be initiated and stepwise realized.

Selected references

De beroepsuitoefening van de Kinder en Jeugdpsychiater: het verlsag van een enquete (1996) Sectie Kinder en jeugdpsychiatrie van de Nederlandse Vereniging voor Pschiatrie

De Goei L (1992) In de kinderschoenen: ontstaan en ontwikkeling van de universitaire kinderpsychiatrie in Nederland (1936–1978). NCGV: Utrecht

De Goei L, van't Hof S, Hutschenmakers G (1997) Curium 1955–1995. Bladzijden uit de geschiedenis van de Nederlandse Kinder- en Jeugdpsychiatrie. NCGV: Utrecht

Engeland H van, Hoeing J (1984) Geestelijke Gezondheidszorg voor kinderen: een inventarisatie. Rapport uitgegeven door de Geneeskundige Hoofdinspectie voor de Geestelijke Volksgezondheid. NHIGV: Utrecht

Hart de Ruyter Th, Kamp LNJ (1972) Hoofdlijnen van de Kinderpsychiatrie. Van Loghum Slaterus Deventer

Konijn C, Swets-Gronert F (1990) Jeugdhulpverlening in de RIAGG. NCGV: Utrecht

Minderaa RB, Ketelaars CEJ (1998) Psychofarmaca bij kinderen. Van Gorcum, Assen
Sanders-Woudstra JAR, De Witte HFI (1985) Leerboek Kinder en Jeugd Psychiatrie. Van Gorcum, Assen
Van Krevelen DA (1950) Nederlands leerboek der Speciële Kinderpsychiatrie. H. E. Stenfert Kroese, Leiden
Verhey F, Verhulst FC (1996) Kinder- en Jeugdpsychiatrie. Van Gorcum, Assen

Child and adolescent psychiatry in Norway

I. Spurkland, I. H. Vandvik

1. Definition, historical development, and current situation

Definition

In Norway, the field of Child and Adolescent Psychiatry (CAP) comprises preventive work, diagnostic evaluations, and treatment of children and adolescents with psychiatric disorders age 0–18 years. Assessment of the child's interaction with his/her family and the social network is a matter of course. Collaboration with other professionals both within and outside the psychiatric institutions and in various sectors is an essential part of the professional work. Consultation and/or advice to others who meet children and their families are important elements, e.g., primary healthcare (physicians, health nurses, midwives, physiotherapists) somatic hospitals, child habilitation, school pedagogical and psychological services, and child protection services.

Historical development and recent advances

Mental health care for children in Norway goes back to 1941 with the establishment of Mentalhygienisk rådgivningskontor (Child Guidance Clinic). The first child psychiatric department was opened at the National Hospital of Norway in 1950. Child psychiatry has been a speciality for medical doctors with specified requirements for training and service since 1951, and the Norwegian Association for Child and Adolescent Psychiatry was established in 1957. The Directorate of Health is responsible for certifying new specialists in all medical disciplines, but has delegated the task to the board of the Norwegian Medical Association. The speciality committees apply the regulations that govern specialization, and they evaluate and recommend applicants for specialist approval to the board, which is the decision-making body.

Norwegian child and adolescent psychiatry has roots in somatic medicine, in care for the developmentally retarded, in the mental hygiene and child guidance movement, in psychoanalysis, and in the care for socially disadvantaged and criminal children and adolescents. Multiprofessional teamwork has always been a prerequisite in child and adolescent psychiatry. The organization of services has a main emphasis on outpatient treatment and small treatment homes with a professional liaison to the outpatient clinics. Family theory and family work have always been important. However, in the 1950s professional thinking was influenced by seeing children as patients independent of their families. Accordingly, child psychiatry offered individual therapy to the child parallel to parent counseling. In the 1960s, emphasis was put on changing the parents' understanding and attitudes, implying that parental attitudes were the main reason for problems of children. In the 1970s we had strong ideological debates. Family therapy entered the field with a new understanding of systemic interactions. At the same time individual psychology put more emphasis on interdependent relationships as a basis for development. In the 1980s, empirically based knowledge tuned down the ideological debates. With the gradual development of neuropsychology/neuropsychiatry, the professional field has increasingly turned toward a more biological/individual understanding, and in the 1990s the professional profile is complex and more closely related to empirical than ideological theory, and there is also less professional splitting in the field. A psychodynamic understanding of child development has always been central in Norwegian child psychiatry. In addition, communication theories, systemic and cognitive theory, and biological models are used. There is now an increased awareness of "resilience" and children's "coping".

Current situation

The professional work with children and families now combines diverse theories, empirical data and methods. The difficulties of children and families and their resources should be considered based on a bio-psycho-social model. In treatment, the therapeutic interventions are combined with interventions from professionals both within and outside child psychiatry.

2. Classification systems, diagnostic and therapeutic methods

Classification systems

In Norway, the ICD-10 classification system has been the official one since 1997 and the basis for the nationwide statistics. In child and adolescent psychiatry, the multiaxial framework is used in order to increase validity and reliability. In research it is quite common also to use DSM-IV, especially for publishing in American journals.

Diagnostic methods

A broad spectrum of psychological and somatic diagnostic procedures is used. The basic theoretical framework is psychodynamic, together with a comprehension of the importance of family psychology and interaction of the family members, both for making a diagnosis and for the decision of treatment. Verbal and non-verbal communication adapted to the child's level of development is the child psychiatrist's most important instrument. Verbal communication is used as a method in relation to individuals, families, and groups during the whole assessment and treatment process. It is also more and more common to use different structured and semistructured interviews and questionnaires in clinical work. Neuropsychology has an increased importance in child and adolescent psychiatry. Cooperation with other disciplines is necessary when it comes to different laboratory methods and other somatic techniques.

Therapeutic methods

Various therapeutic methods are used. Most of the child and adolescent units have an eclectic approach. They are using individual therapy, different kinds of family/parent therapy, group therapy, parent counseling, and consultation to other health personnel. The use of cognitive and behavioral techniques is increasing. To a limited degree, psychopharmacotherapy is also used. Prevention and health promotion are also tasks for the child and adolescent psychiatrist, primarily as collaborator in the development of adequate preventive methods.

3. Structure and organization of services

Guidelines for services for children and adolescents with psychiatric disorders

The services for children and adolescents with psychiatric disorders are based on outpatient clinics as close to the patient's local environment as possible. The service should also be equally distributed in the country, a goal very difficult to fulfill in a large country like Norway with a scattered population. According to the report before the parliament (no. 41 (1987-88)), it was stated that each of the 19 counties in Norway should establish:

- one "resource outpatient clinic" which should support the building up of local outpatient clinics and institutions in the country
- one outpatient clinic in the area of each local hospital
- one specialized kindergarten for evaluation and trial of therapeutic methods for preschool children
- one child psychiatric treatment home or department for children 7–12 years of age
- one treatment home for autistic children and adolescents
- one treatment home or department for adolescents 13–18 years of age
- one emergency psychiatric department for adolescents
- one family inpatient unit

It was a governmental goal that 2 % of the child and adolescent population should have access to CAP services. This goal was reached in 1997, and in a recent report on psychiatry before the parliament (no. 25 (1997)) the new goal was set to be 5 %, which is more realistic according to general epidemiological findings.

Types of services

Most of the child and adolescent services are based on public outpatient clinics. There are only a handful of private practitioners, mostly due to a strong team tradition and a lack of specialists. Private practitioners are mostly working with patients in need of long-term psychotherapy. There is a shortage of CAP facilities in most parts of the country, particularly in the north. This is true also for rehabilitation programs and programs for chronic patients. In report no. 25, the government describes long-range planning for increasing the resources in both general psychiatry and child and adolescent psychiatry. There seems to be joint political agreement upon this plan.

Outpatient services

Each county has now established a resource outpatient clinic, and most of them also smaller local ones. To be approved as a CAP outpatient clinic, it is a condition that there are positions for a child and adolescent psychiatrist, a clinical psychologist, a social worker, and a clinical pedagogue, all trained in child and adolescent psychiatry. However, due to lack, particularly of child and adolescent psychiatrists, outpatient clinics have been approved even if this position has been vacant. In accordance with law regulations of 1975, both child and adolescent psychiatrists and clinical psychologists can be the head of outpatient clinics.

Daypatient and inpatient services

There exist approximately 300 treatment places (beds or day treatment facilities) in the whole country. There are few units having exclusively inpatient facilities. Mostly the beds are used in a flexible way, according to the need of the particular patient, changing between daypatient and inpatient status. There is a lack of inpatient facilities, specially for adolescents. Probably twice the number of what we have today would be more in line with actual needs. In order to increase the effectiveness of the treatment, there has been an increasing tendency to hospitalize the family for shorter periods together with the patient.

Inpatient family units

Since 1971, inpatient family treatment has been a tradition in Norway. There are several reasons for this tradition. The two most important ones were an increased interest in family therapeutic work and the recognition of the negative aspects of committing a lone child for treatment often far from home. In a large country as ours with a scattered population, the geographical reason was also important. However, the experience so far is so good that these units are regarded as very useful in their own right. On the average, the inpatient stay is four weeks, and there are pre-care visits, as well as post-care visits to the family's home and to the referring parties as a routine. One half of the counties have now established family units.

Complementary services and rehabilitation

Complementary services are provided by the social welfare system, by preference at a local level, i.e., they are community-based. These can be children's homes and foster homes. For a small number of chronic patients, it is necessary to build special units for one particular child with consultation from CAP. The habilitation system (within pediatrics) is responsible for the long-term follow-up of children and adolescents with pervasive developmental disorders.

Personnel

There is a lack of specialists within all professional categories. This is especially marked for child and adolescents psychiatrists. There are probably several reasons. Maybe the teaching during the medical studies is not good enough and does not create sufficient interest and curiosity. Doctors are in the minority vis-à-vis the other professions in the field, and this can be a difficult position, especially for a young doctor. The cooperation with other institutional bodies which is mandatory in child and adolescent psychiatry, may give doctors who are more action-oriented, a feeling of ineffectiveness.

There is also a drain of specialists from the child and adolescent psychiatry to neighboring disciplines, such as adult psychiatry and pediatrics. One reason frequently mentioned is that the shortage of senior personnel leads to a heavy workload, and that the multi-professionality may make fertile ground for conflicts. The salary level makes child psychiatry less attractive than other fields of medicine even though we now have a "recruitment supplement" to the salary. There is little opportunity for private practice when you are employed in a public clinic or institution, and most of the positions are in the outpatient system, with no extra remuneration for day and night duty. During recent years, the biological aspects of the bio-psycho-social model have gained a stronger basis. This may hopefully have a positive bearing on a physician's interest to stay in the field.

The positive side of the otherwise negative specialist drain is that child and adolescent psychiatry is known to offer well-organized, thorough training which also proves useful when working in other fields of medicine.

Funding of services

Medical services, including child and adolescent psychiatry, are paid by the state and the counties through the health insurance system. We have a compulsory health insurance system where everyone takes part. The long-term follow-up in the communities may also be paid by the social welfare system.

Evaluation

There is a lack of evaluation studies with regard to child and adolescent psychiatry. However, there is now increasing interest in such studies, and there are some ongoing projects. Some institutions do use Achenbach's questionnaires (CBCL, TRF, and YSR) routinely in clinical practice and for evaluation purposes.

The child and adolescent institutions have for many years been obliged to give the Directorate of Health information about their activities and types of patient care. This registration had many weaknesses. As a consequence, a data program, BUP data (CAP data) has been developed. Since 1990, the child and adolescent institutions have been using the program both for statistics and as an information system in daily work. This is now a nationwide system and can be used for planning of child and adolescent psychiatric services, both on a national and a county level. In addition, the system makes it possible to computerize all information about the patients instead of using paper records.

Further development makes it probable that BUP data can be a good tool in quality assurance.

4. Cooperation with medical and non-medical disciplines

Cooperation with pediatrics

With advances in medical and technical knowledge, children who previously died now survive and are treated. Some of them develop severe emotional problems in addition to the physical disease. These children have special needs for a close relationship between child psychiatry and pediatrics. Although the relationship between pediatrics and child psychiatry does exist in most of the regional and central hospitals, which have pediatric departments, both the quality and the quantity of liaison work appear to need further development. A recent study found that scarce psychosocial resources are spent in pediatrics and concluded that prevention and early intervention of mental and psychosocial disorders related to physical illness have not generally been given high priority in our country. Both specialists in child and adolescent psychiatry and clinical psychologists are engaged within consultation-liaison (C-L) services, but only a small number are working full-time, the rest work part-time, generally less then one day a week. Few child psychiatrists and psychologists in training gain experience from C-L services in pediatrics.

The types of patients most frequently referred to child psychiatry are cases of sexual abuse, physical neglect, and anorexia nervosa. Only two departments have a consultant from child and adolescent psychiatry working in their neonatal unit, but several reported that such work was included as part of the child psychiatric consultation service. A flexible approach with both individualized treatment and milieu interventions is needed. In Norway, we have no specialized treatment units for children with severe psychopathology in association with severe somatic diseases. Such functions need to be developed on a regional basis by close collaboration between pediatrics and child psychiatry.

Cooperation with psychiatry

The administrative association between child psychiatry and adult psychiatry varies in Norway. Mostly they have separate administrative units within the same hospital. In some regions adolescent psychiatric patients in need of acute hospitalization are hospitalized in the psychiatric wards; in other regions, the department of psychiatry has a separate unit for adolescents. In addition, there are psychiatric teams for adolescents and young adults with drug problems. These teams have also preventive tasks.

Children of parents with serious and/or lasting psychiatric disorders represent a group at risk for emotional and behavioral disorders. According to report no. 25, the psychiatric institutions are encouraged to establish routines for identification of needs of children of psychiatric patients and to take responsibility for establishing a good working relationship with child and adolescent psychiatry, child protection services, and the primary health care system.

During recent years, some counties have transferred the child psychiatric services from the health care system to the administrative units for family and child protection services. From a child psychiatric viewpoint this is most unfortunate and has made it even more difficult to recruit physicians for training and services in child psychiatry.

Cooperation with doctors in private practice

In Norway, we have only a handful of child and adolescent psychiatrists in private practice. In addition some child and adolescent psychiatrists and clinical psychologists working in hospitals and outpatient units run a more limited private practice in their spare time. The trend now is to stimulate the counties to establish contracts with specialists in psychiatry and clinical psychology so that they may be included in the general plans for the specialist health services. Referral of a child/family to child and adolescent psychiatry can be done by a general practitioner, pediatrician or specialist in any other field.

Cooperation with non-medical institutions and professionals

The most important non-medical collaborators are within the child protection services. A high percentage (30 %) of children referred to child and adolescent psychiatry have been or will be in need of services from the child protection services. Other cooperating services include school psychological services and different types of special schools. We have no separate child guidance clinics. But due to the shortage of child and adolescent psychiatrists, several of the outpatient child and adolescent psychiatric units lack these specialists and are staffed by psychologists, social workers, and clinical pedagogues.

5. Graduate/postgraduate training and continuing medical education

Graduate training: The role of medical faculties

Certification as a physician is a prerequisite for specializing. The medical studies take six years after graduation from upper secondary school (General Certificate of Education – Advanced Level). The studies include both theoretical and practical training.

During these six years, exams are consecutive and with more comprehensive exams at the end. After passing the exams, one is licensed to practice medicine in a hospital for one year and under supervision as a general practitioner for 6 months. These 18 months are compulsory before one is eligible for authorization as a full-fledged physician by the Directorate of Health. In Norway we have four universities, in Oslo, Bergen, Trondheim, and Tromsø, all with medical faculties. They all have a teaching program in child and adolescent psychiatry, although limited.

In Oslo this will change, because from 1996 the medical studies are re-organized toward problem-based learning. The students will now hopefully gain psychological understanding to different health problems from the very first day. The curriculum of child psychiatry is integrated into general psychiatry. The majority of students will have their practical training within general psychiatry and only one in five students will have bedside teaching in child psychiatry during the study. This is due both to a lack of facilities and lack of time.

Postgraduate training, a joint effort

The training program for becoming a specialist in child and adolescent psychiatry requires a minimum of five and a half years, including three years in child and adolescent, one year in adult psychiatry, and six months in pediatrics. The last year can be used to supplement one's training in either of the above-mentioned disciplines, or one may choose to train at another institution relevant to the field of child and adolescent psychiatry, such as a neurological department, maternal and child health center, an institution for handicapped children, etc. One may also do research in child and adolescent psychiatry during this year.

Two of the three years in child and adolescent psychiatry must be spent in an outpatient clinic. Of the total specialization period, at least two years must be spent in an inpatient unit, one of which must be a psychiatric institution for children and adolescents.

The training program in child and adolescent psychiatry includes at least two hours a week of individual supervision of at least 210 hours. A minimum of 40 hours must involve supervision of psychodynamically oriented psychotherapy of children.

The most important part of the specialist training is the daily clinical work, performed under supervision of a senior child and adolescent psychiatrist. In addition to the clinical work, the institution is obliged to provide a regular in-house theoretical training program for a minimum of four hours a week, covering a variety of areas. Special importance will be attached to developmental aspects, diagnostics, individual psychotherapy for children and adolescents, and the comprehension of family interaction.

The training program includes 180 hours of compulsory courses administered by the Speciality Committee. The courses are distributed as following:

- 60 hours of developmental psychology
- 20 hours of family psychology
- 40 hours of psychobiological comprehension of disorders in children
- 20 hours of neuropsychiatry
- 40 hours of other relevant courses of choice, approved by the Speciality Committee in child and adolescent psychiatry

After 1992, a course in administration is also required. This has come into force for all medical specialities.

These compulsory courses are since 1997 organized in 5 residential seminars, each lasting one week.

For the documentation of the content of the training, a logbook has been worked out. This is, however, not yet official, but serves as reminder for both supervisor and trainee. There are no formal exams. Within the Norwegian Medical Association formal examination for all medical specialities is a topic of discussion, but so far there is no general agreement.

Continuing medical education in child and adolescent psychiatry and psychotherapy

At the time being, there are no formal requirements for continuing medical education. The law regulations state that it is a duty for every doctor to keep updated in his field. The speciality committee is discussing how this can best be formalized. The Medical Association has created funding for financial support to attend seminars for the purpose of CME.

Training programs for other disciplines

Child and adolescents psychiatrists have joint training programs with other professions, e.g., with psychologists in psychotherapy and family therapy. Family therapy courses also include social workers.

6. Research

Research fields and strategies

Norwegian child psychiatric research has a rather short history. Early research was based on follow-up studies and more action-oriented research related to the baby welfare clinics. From 1982-1990 the Medical Research Council had a recruitment and training program for clinical psychiatric research. The coordinator of the program was a specialist both in psychiatry and child and adolescent psychiatry; thus, CAP was included. The program has now been prolonged as a research program for Mental Health, and clinical psychological and neuropsychological research has been included. In addition, a Council for Psychiatric Health was established in 1992, funded by a nation-wide TV-appeal. This has increased the possibilities for funding of psychiatric research. The last 10–15 years have seen a marked increase of child psychiatric research. Since 1991, there have been 8 doctoral dissertations (February 1999), 5 more are about to be finished. The four Regional Centers which are associated with the Medical Faculties have established chairs in child psychiatry, but so far, only 2 of them are occupied. All the regional centers have research fellows in CAP.

Important areas for present and future research include assessment, diagnosis and classification, outcome studies, epidemiology, genetics and temperament research, treatment research, neuropsychiatry and psychosocial aspects of somatic diseases/ somatic symptoms. The Norwegian Association for Child and Adolescent Psychiatry is represented in the Nordic working group for child and adolescent psychiatric research which arranges research conferences every second year.

No clear limits exist between research, evaluation, and quality assurance. The specialist health services are asked to implement quality assurance. Guidelines for CAP were published by the Norwegian Medical Association (1996). This was partly a result of the Norwegian Association for Child and Adolescent Psychiatry's work to assure quality of clinical practice in child psychiatry.

Research training and career development

Regional child psychiatric centers have been established in the 5 health regions with research and teaching as main responsibilities. All the Norwegian universities now have compulsory research training programs as a prerequisite for accepting a doctoral thesis. We presently have vacant academic positions at all the universities.

Funding

According to the report before the Parliament no. 25 (1997), further development of the regional centers with better funding of research fellows and postdoctoral grants will offer new possibilities for research.

7. Future perspectives

The report before the Parliament (no. 25 (1997)) suggests that more resources shall be allocated to all parts of psychiatric work, including research and evaluation of working methods. It is also suggested that CAP like the other medical specialities should be administratively associated with the central county hospitals. The aim is to increase the capacity of CAP so that 5 % of the population 0–18 years can receive psychiatric health services from specialists. To strengthen the outpatient units, it is advised to concentrate on increasing the staff of the outpatient units, to gain a more comprehensive staff of physicians, both of people in training and specialists, and to give opportunities for more time for clinical tasks. The physicians in training should also be encouraged to do small research projects as part of their training.

More differentiated day and inpatient services are necessary both as a part of quality assurance and for professional development and patient services.

The government has now set up a working group to examine the use of resources within CAP in order to assess the quality and quantity of the service.

Selected references

Årbok for BUP 1996 (Yearbook for CAP) Institusjonsforeningen, Oslo

General plan for the Norwegian association for Child and Adolescent Psychiatry 1998–2007. The board of NCAP 1996/97, Report from the Norwegian Medical Association, Oslo

Spurkland I (1993) Training in child and adolescent psychiatry in Norway. ACCP Review & Newsletter 15 (2): 78–79

Vandvik IH, Spurkland I (1993) Child and adolescent psychiatry in Norway today and tomorrow. Nord J Psychiatry 47: 155–160

Vandvik IH (1994) Collaboration between child psychiatry and paediatrics: the state of the relationship in Norway. Acta Pædiatr 83: 884–7

Child and adolescent psychiatry in Portugal

M. J. Vidigal, C. Marques, A. Matos

1. Definition, historical development, and current situation

Definition

Child and adolescent psychiatry in Portugal includes diagnosis, treatment, prevention, and rehabilitation of psychiatric and psychosomatic disorders, psychological, and social development disturbances during childhood and adolescence. But it also deals with problems which fall into the scope of other specialities: psychopathology of the pregnant woman, mother-child psychiatry, psychopathology of parent-child relationship, family psychopathology. This action must be developed by an interdisciplinary team including child psychiatrists, psychologists, social workers, nurses, nursery school teachers, and other therapists in order to obtain a better rationalization and profitability of efforts.

These goals are still far from being achieved, and they have obviously been changing since 1959 when the speciality became independent and was called Child Neuropsychiatry. In 1974 (when a political change occurred in Portugal, from an extreme right wing government into a democracy), it finally changed the name to Pedopsychiatry and since 1995 into Child and Adolescent Psychiatry. The designation psychotherapy was not added because it was refused by the Medical Association and due to the "advice" of the General Psychiatry College.

In spite of its early birth, it still lacked stimulation for the training of specialists, and it had a slow and discontinuous growth, having difficulties in being recognized for itself since there was a general tendency to regard it as a subordinate branch of general psychiatry.

António Coimbra de Matos defended a dynamic and intense training in child and adolescent psychiatry and he had the idea of creating in July 1989 the Portuguese Association for Child and Adolescent Psychiatry, with the aim of joining the child psychiatrists (specialists and trainees). Its first president was Margarida Mendo. In 1995, during the London Congress, this association was admitted to ESCAP.

The Portuguese Association for Child and Adolescent Psychiatry has organized every year, since 1990, a congress in different towns of the country addressed to all specialists and to all those whose work is connected with childhood and adolescence.

Historical development

Portugal has been influenced by what was happening in other countries, mainly Europe and, in the last few years, also America. First, the speciality was addressed to the education of mentally and sensorial handicapped children and then to the children with behavioral disturbances and also to the assistance of juvenile delinquency through an Act of 1871.

A reference must be made to the Portuguese Jewish physician Jacob Rodrigues Pereira, who started in the XVIII century in Paris, teaching the deaf-mute.

All the knowledge received from other sciences such as pedagogy, psychiatry, pediatrics, neurology, psychology as well as other social sciences and law, has contributed to the foundation of an independent speciality, specific as to its aims and method.

First stage: This was marked by the interest and development of pedagogy and re-education, then by psychometry and finally by a medical approach.

António Aurélio da Costa Ferreira was the first in Portugal who tried to solve the problems of mentally handicapped children through humane pedagogical medical therapy, founding in 1911 an agricultural community which reached considerable development (it was closed in 1920 due to lack of funds). In 1914, the first Portuguese Medical-Pedagogical Institute was created, where re-education of mentally handicapped children and adolescents (those able to be rehabilitated) was undertaken. This institute was named after him a few years later. In 1920, the first bulletin of the institute was issued.

Professor Vitor Fontes came next. Through his work, developed both at a national and international level, he followed the evolution of the international scientific knowledge of child medical-pedagogical treatment. One of his main concerns was to help the country recover from the developmental delay which was due to its isolation, resulting from immobilization principles the political system then defended. Vitor Fontes collaborated in the organization of many institutions for mentally handicapped children, and he intensified the campaign, through writings and conferences, in favor of the non-adjusted and handicapped children for which he received the 1954 Pestalozzi Prize (golden medal) of the Pestalozzi Foundation of New York. He modernized the António Aurélio da Costa Ferreira Institute (closed in 1989 due to new government guidelines). He founded the Parents School (it was open for almost 10 years), he organized a library on psychiatric, pedagogical, and psychology topics (the first in the country), and he published for 20 years the magazine "The Portuguese Child". He succeeded in creating special classes in the regular primary schools (1942), not forgetting teachers training.

Following the IV Psychiatry Congress, held in Lisbon, Vitor Fontes succeeded in creating the speciality of Child Neuropsychiatry in 1959.

Recent advances

Second stage: The next stage is somehow coincident with the first stage because it had already started during the 1940s. It represented a turning point in child mental health, and it was João dos Santos who pushed forward this change since he had participated in psychoanalytical, genetical psychology, and mental hygiene movements of child and adolescent psychiatry. João dos Santos (who has worked with Vitor Fontes) represented the transitional stage between the pedagogical medicine model and a new approach in pedagogy, with the application of psychoanalytical models. For political reasons João dos Santos was forced to leave the country; however, in France (1946–1950), he continued the training he had started in Portugal with Vitor Fontes and Barahona Fernandes. He worked in departments led by Henri Wallon, Heuyer, Ajuriaguerra, Lebovici, and Henri Ey.

When he returned to Portugal, his main concern was the training of the technical staff, which almost did not exist. Mental health was the main purpose of his work: he developed an important work which allowed the child and adolescent psychiatry to expand beyond the boundaries of mental handicaps (and related diseases) and be implemented in schools, families and communities, as well as in public health and mental hygiene.

He opened up the way for a completely new program in Portugal when he integrated mental health care in two mother and child health centers (in the 1950s and the 1960s), organizing primary prevention programs for detection of children's early emotional disturbances and health early detection on high risk populations with specific pathological characteristics. This program was never supported by the health authorities although it was not expensive, reached a broad scope of the population, and was completely integrated in the community. His indirect action (and later his followers) was close to the Caplan model in the USA.

In the meantime, during the 1940s, the psychiatric services had been restructured and child mental health outpatient services were created in the three main cities of the country (Lisbon, OPorto, and Coimbra); inpatient services for children were also created in the general psychiatric hospitals of these cities, which quickly turned into patient warehouses since they had no qualified staff. This situation was publicly denounced by João dos Santos who refused to work in such conditions because he did not accept the asylum system that promoted the inpatient admission of severe mentally handicapped children and refused such possibility to other patients who could be rehabilitated. Meanwhile, when João dos Santos returned from France, many of these children were already adolescents and the situation was chaotic as he had forecasted.

Since the model of psychiatric treatment centralized exclusively in hospitals proved to be inefficient, a Mental Health Law was enacted in 1963 in order to issue the principles for the "Sector Psychiatry". It included the creation of a state mental health center net all over the country, one center in the main city of each district (18 in continental Portugal, 3 in Azores and 1 in Madeira), intended to be closer to the community and to decentralize the assistential activity, until then developed only in the main psychiatric hospitals. In 1964, Child Mental Health Centers (the word Juvenile was added only in 1978) were created in Lisbon, OPorto, and Coimbra, which were organized and led, respectively, by João dos Santos, Celeste

Malpique, and Maria de Lurdes Carvalho dos Santos. These centers were technically, financially, and administratively autonomous.

In Lisbon, João dos Santos (being the Director of the Center) and his main collaborators (Margarida Mendo, who conducted the Child's Clinic, and António Coimbra de Matos, who organized and was responsible for mentally handicapped children rehabilitation) performed high quality work, in spite of the enormous budget problems and the high number of patients they had to treat. Meanwhile, the rehabilitation service evolved, pushed forward by Coimbra de Matos, into a specialized service for adolescents suffering from several pathologies, and it was named then Youth Clinic (1987).

The centers developed gradually always with very low budgets and an insufficient number of specialists and technical staff regarding their needs. In 1980, the Ist World Baby Mental Health Congress was held in Portugal having had a great impact; in 1983, an outpatient unit to address infancy mental health was created.

That same year graduate training in child and adolescent psychiatry was introduced in state mental health services and these services were restructured, which resulted in benefits for child mental health centers.

In 1992 the government enacted a law eliminating the juvenile and child mental health centers (Lisbon, OPorto, and Coimbra). As replacements, departments of child and adolescent psychiatry were created in the general or pediatric hospitals of these cities. With this integration, child psychiatry services lost their financial and administrative autonomy and many administrative officers as well as members of the technical staff had to be dismissed. This situation has led to the collapse of specific areas of intervention and of most of the community-based work.

Current situation

According to the last census (1991), Portugal has 9,867,147 inhabitants, 2,654,144 of which are children and adolescents from 0–18 years old (26.9 % of the total population).

In January 1998, the number of child and adolescent psychiatrists is as follows:

- In the Medical Association: 99 (all graduates) – 57 in the southern region, 34 in the northern region, and 8 in the rest of the country, almost exclusively concentrated in the main cities of Lisbon, OPorto, and Coimbra. These 99 graduates correspond to one child and adolescent psychiatrist per 26,810 inhabitants from 0 – 18.
- The Portuguese Association for Child and Adolescent Psychiatry (APPIA) has 125 members, trainees included. Nevertheless, not all of them work as child and adolescent psychiatrists. Only 39 specialists work in state hospitals.

Although small, the number of specialists working exclusively in private practice will probably increase, because those who finish training nowadays have limited access to public practice.

2. Classification systems, diagnostic and therapeutic methods

Classification systems

In Portugal, the ICD-9 classification system is still the classification used for official statistical purposes in psychiatry and in child psychiatry hospital services. Nevertheless, this system is only used for codification of mental disorders on a statistical basis.

For clinical and research purposes the large majority of services uses DSM-IV; ICD-10 is also used by some teams.

Internal classification systems following a psycho-dynamic approach were developed in several child psychiatry services and are considered of some use in daily clinical practice.

Diagnostic methods

In most departments clinical data are gathered through a semi-structured interview, and diagnosis is based on this information along with the psychiatric observation of the child and his family. Some teams use also video recordings of several situations considered important for diagnosis. In infancy, mother-child interactions are a special focus of attention and, therefore, systematically recorded.

A whole range of psychological tests and speech and pedagogic evaluations are also used. Most services do not have diagnostic procedures such as laboratory methods, imaging techniques or EEG recordings in an autonomous way. Since all services are comprised in a general or a pediatric hospital, cooperation with these other diagnostic fields is possible and works reasonably well.

Therapeutic methods

In this field, the orientation is considerably different and varies from one service to another. Although most teams are fairly eclectic, some of them tend to use mainly a psycho-dynamic approach, while others apply psychodrama and family therapy on a more frequent basis. Group therapy (either for child and parents), family counseling, therapeutic consultations, and also, when indicated, a pharmacological approach are some other intervention methods.

In most teams, the integration of the whole spectrum of therapies predominates. However, the absence of psychiatric inpatient units for children and adolescents makes it difficult to treat some disorders successfully.

3. Structure and organization of services

Guidelines of services for children and adolescents with psychiatric disorders

The state health care in Portugal covers the whole country. There are central hospitals in the three main cities (Lisbon, OPorto, and Coimbra) and district hospitals in the rest of the country. There is also a net of general medical practice centers throughout the country. The five medicine faculties do not include child and adolescent psychiatry in their curriculum.

Insurance has almost no expression in the private sector, which is only a complement for the state sector, and the patients are partly reimbursed for their medical expenses only in very few cases.

The general and child and adolescent psychiatry services were integrated in 1992 in the hospital care system as any other medical speciality.

The three Juvenile and Child Mental Health Centers of Lisbon, OPorto, and Coimbra were changed into Child and Adolescent Psychiatry Departments and integrated in central hospitals (pediatric or general); they are led by child and adolescent psychiatrists. Most of the district hospitals do not include child psychiatrists in their staff and, thus, besides the three main cities, the specialists distribution in the country is insufficient. Although there is an official planning for the assignment of child and adolescent psychiatrists in general psychiatry services, this planning has not been followed, either because no vacancies are opened or there are not enough specialists. In district hospitals, child and adolescent psychiatrists, although technically autonomous, are submitted to a general psychiatrist.

Presently, and following the former tradition, community-based work has been developed, but it is harder every time to do it, since hospitals are not prepared for that kind of work. We hope that in the future this work will be developed through a more rationalized distribution of the child and adolescent psychiatrists in the country.

Types of services

There is a need for a new balance between outpatient/day hospitals/inpatient facilities, and specialized units for children and adolescents with serious psychiatric disorders should be developed, as well as rehabilitation services.

Outpatient services

The distribution of child and adolescent psychiatrists in the country is not equitable. The lack is mostly felt outside the main urban centers (Lisbon, OPorto, and Coimbra). Furthermore, these city departments are not able to assist a very large number of patients, who sometimes live far from the centers and who are obliged to consult these city departments due to the lack of specialists outside the urban areas.

Assistance is based on outpatient services. In Lisbon there are four services working by sectors that are attended by children and adolescents of all age groups; one addresses children from 0 – 3 years old and another addresses the adolescent group. In OPorto and Coimbra there are also outpatient services for children and specific consultations for adolescents.

Daypatient services

There is one day hospital in Lisbon for adolescents. In OPorto and Coimbra there are two day hospitals for children and adolescents.

Inpatient services

The only one is located in OPorto.

Complementary services and rehabilitation

The complementary services include a rehabilitation service in Lisbon and liaison services in the three departments of Lisbon, OPorto, and Coimbra.

Funding of services

Support from outside the hospital system is not granted by the Ministry for Health but by the Ministry for Education, by social security, and mainly by private associations to which child and adolescent psychiatry services appeal: special education schools; centers for the education of mentally and physically handicapped children and adolescents; centers for sensorial handicapped children; centers for pre-professional training.

Besides the Association of Parents and Friends of Children with Autism and Mental Handicap, there are no specific services addressed to children and adolescents with serious psychiatric disorders.

It is almost impossible to integrate, outside the family, in a proper environment (transitional homes, group homes, youth centers, family nursing) children and adolescents with chronic psychiatric disorders, serious behavior problems or addiction problems.

Evaluation

So far, the Ministry of Health did not implement any evaluation of child and adolescent psychiatry services, although the medical association is planning to put forward service evaluation programs.

4. Cooperation with medical and non-medical disciplines

Cooperation with pediatrics

In Portugal, the majority of child psychiatry services are included in pediatric hospitals and, therefore, therapeutic cooperation between the two disciplines should be intense. Although the integration of Child and Adolescent Mental Health Centers in pediatric hospitals occurred in 1992, the articulation is not very good.

In the last 2 or 3 years some improvement has been reached and collaboration strengthened. Some hospitals enlarged their liaison services, and neuropediatrics, neonatology, chronic somatic diseases, and psychosomatic disorders are some of the areas in which cooperation is now possible.

Nevertheless, many pediatric services still do not have psychiatric liaison or consulting services, and many "frontier" areas are not the subject of collaborative team work as they should be. An important lack of articulation between the two disciplines is felt in the field of early diagnosis and prevention of mental illness.

Cooperation with psychiatry

More recently, some child psychiatrists have been placed in general psychiatry departments (mainly in district hospitals). Although cooperation between the two disciplines is usually good, many problems arise since the child psychiatrist works alone, without the support of a mental health team specialized in child and adolescent disorders, which makes it extremely difficult to cope with the broad spectrum of more complex situations.

In spite of the disadvantages of working in such conditions, one of the advantages of this interdisciplinary proximity is the articulation in the treatment of children and parents (in particular children of parents with psychiatric disorders).

Cooperation with doctors in private practice

In Portugal, the use of private practice implies the payment of these services by the patient, which restrains the use of these facilities. Our medical system still gives priority to public attendance, and in child and adolescent psychiatry the existing services are clearly not capable of meeting the population's needs.

Cooperation with non-medical institutions and professionals

One of the most important fields of cooperation with non-medical institutions are the public and private special schools attended by children with different psychological and psychiatric disorders (development delays, learning disabilities, behavioral disturbances, mental retardation, etc.).

Child psychiatrists also cooperate with institutions for socially deprived children and other institutions addressed to children with several handicaps (sensorial, motor, mental, neurological). Another area of collaboration is judicial counseling.

5. Graduate/postgraduate training and continuing medical education

Graduate training: The role of medical faculties

As of 1998 child psychiatry is not part of the curriculum (as a separate chair) in the five medical faculties of Portugal.

Postgraduate training, a joint effort

To be a child and adolescent psychiatrist in Portugal, one must have a medical degree and 18 months practice training, which is the normal curriculum to become a physician. Then one must go through a global examination at the national level to have access to any speciality.

The training in child and adolescent psychiatry takes four years. It includes three years in child and adolescent psychiatry (exclusively in Departments of Child and Adolescent Psychiatry in Lisbon, OPorto, and Coimbra), six months in general psychiatry, and six months in pediatrics (including training in child neurology). Substantial practice is required in psychotherapy. In Lisbon and OPorto, candidates must attend a pediatric emergency service.

The different components of the training curriculum are the following:

- History and present situation of child and adolescent psychiatry
- Normality and pathology: psycho-affective development and psychopathology in infancy, childhood, and adolescence
- Anamnesis and clinical evaluation of the child and adolescent; complementary evaluation techniques: neurological and psychological examinations; indication for and methods of speech, language, psycho-pedagogic and motoricity evaluations; indication for and methods of laboratory and imaging procedures and EEG recording
- Psychopathology: main psychiatric syndromes; nosology and differential diagnosis; classification systems
- Treatment: organization of a therapy plan; psychotherapies (psychoanalytical, cognitive, behavioral and systemic); family and group therapies; psychodrama; pharmacological therapy; other family and psychosocial interventions; management of emergency interventions; rehabilitation
- Other subjects: epidemiology; services organization; investigation methods; judicial counseling; prevention in mental health; the child psychiatrist in

different work settings: hospital, health center, courts, schools, and other institutions.

After finishing the four year training, an oral exam must be passed. Candidates are evaluated by a national jury. The examination includes 3 tests: curriculum discussion, observation of a patient with further discussion, and a theoretical test. The approved candidates receive the certificate for hospital and private practice of child and adolescent psychiatry.

Continuing medical education in child and adolescent psychiatry and psychotherapy

There are no formal requirements for continuing medical education in Portugal although the Medical Association intends to implement them for all medical specialities.

Child and adolescent psychiatrists participate in several regular seminars, namely on psychotherapy.

Training programs for other disciplines

Child and adolescent psychiatrists participate in several training programs for other medical and non-medical specialists. To be a general psychiatrist, candidates must go through six months of training in child and adolescent psychiatry. Pediatricians, general practitioners, psychologists, teachers, nurses, and social workers also attend training programs in the departments of child and adolescent psychiatry.

6. Research

Research fields and strategies

Research is being carried out in Portugal mainly regarding the following areas: mother-infant interaction, family communication, interaction and communication in child and adolescent groups; diagnostic classification in infancy; eating disorders; children of parents with psychiatric disorders.

This research is in line with the following main trends:

- Study of developmental psychology and psychopathology.
- Study of the etiology of psychiatric disorders in childhood and adolescence; detection of disturbed relational patterns in autism and other pervasive developmental disorders, schizophrenia and other psychotic disorders, specific developmental disorders, mood disorders, and eating disorders.

- Multi-level research on stability/change in psychiatric disorders in children and adolescents.
- Study of behavior disorders.
- Research on psychotherapy and new testing methods for child and adolescent groups.

Funding

There is no public or private funding for research in the departments of child and adolescent psychiatry, although there are projects, namely of epidemiological research.

The research at medical faculties and psychology schools is mainly in the field of psychopathological disorders in adulthood.

7. Future perspectives

Research

The purpose of the Portuguese Association for Child and Adolescent Psychiatry (APPIA) is to

- stimulate the research in psychology and psychopathology of childhood and adolescence;
- co-operate with the other members of ESCAP, other medical professionals, and members of allied professions;
- share the available knowledge with people and institutions belonging to the health care system and to the public in general;
- share experiences with other people and institutions the work of which is addressed to children, adolescents and their families, namely schools and judicial institutions.

Training

Our intended purpose is

- the introduction of a formal learning of child and adolescent psychiatry in the medical college curriculum;
- the improvement of training conditions for the future specialists in the three Departments of Child and Adolescent Psychiatry (Lisbon, OPorto, and Coimbra).

Improvement of services and care systems

There is no governmental program for mental health care in Portugal. The APPIA has been proposing a distribution of child and adolescent psychiatrists that might cover the whole country, because there are not enough specialists in state hospitals. We have undertaken a study showing the needs for child and adolescent psychiatrists in our country but the Ministry for Health did not implement it nor any other one.

Our aims are to

- participate, together with governmental health departments, in the definition of health care programs for children and adolescents;
- promote a national distribution of child and adolescent psychiatrists covering the whole country;
- create small inpatient units in Lisbon and Coimbra, day hospitals and also improve community-based work;
- create specialized services for specific pathologies in the central departments of Lisbon, OPorto, and Coimbra; and
- improve the co-ordination of the different medical and non-medical services that are addressed to children and adolescents with psychiatric problems.

Several of our colleagues contributed to the initial development of child and adolescent psychiatry in Portugal. Many of us are now making strong efforts in order to improve it; we are certain that many more among us will contribute for a better future of our speciality and to improve the health care of mentally disturbed children and adolescents in our country.

Child and adolescent psychiatry in Romania

T. Mircea

1. Definition, historical development, and current situation

Definition

According to the evolutional tendencies and to the understanding at European and worldwide levels of "psychiatry and psychotherapy of child and adolescent", the expert committee from the Health Department in Romania suggested in 1997 to change the specialty's name from "psychiatry of the child and adolescent" to "psychiatry and psychotherapy of the child and adolescent". Until 1996, the specialty functioned under the title "infantile neuro-psychiatry". These facts also had consequences in defining the area. By 1996, the practicing of the specialty unfolded both in neurology and in psychiatry (the psychotherapeutical treatments having no official certification). After 1990, the separation process between these two specialties (pediatric neurology and child and adolescent psychiatry) started, with systematic training according to the international requirements in the psychotherapeutical treatment methods.

At the moment, the field of "child and adolescent psychiatry and psychotherapy" is defined as "a specialized medical practice for diagnosing, treating, preventing, and habilitation/rehabilitation of psychiatric, psycho-organic, psychosomatic diseases or disorders as well as psychological and social behavior disturbances which are modifying the acquisitioning and exerting of specific human skills, resulting in a hindrance of a harmonious integration in the family and community and a hindrance of a good quality of life with the whole realization of the human qualitative potential throughout the first 18 years of development".

Historical development

The development of some caretaking services of children with deficiencies started in Romania already at the end of the 19th century, but officially the sanitary law in 1930 explicitly enforced "treatment and taking care of psychic diseases in specialized hospitals or in health houses". At the same time, at the University for Medicine in Cluj, the first "Handbook for Neuro-Mental Pathology" was published by Professor C. I. Urechia, which approached the specific neuro-psychiatric pathology of childhood in chapters 7 and 8. In this first period the scientific information was eclectic, all great European scientific currents being assumed, studied, and applied as orientative models. After the 2nd World War, the Soviet influence put its imprint (with small exceptions) both on the organization of infantile neuro-psychiatric services and on the theoretical orientation. In the same period (1948) the discipline of child neuro-psychiatry was established in the university educational system and established the first clinical medical services, which were functioning, at the beginning, either integrated in the pediatric clinics or close with the psychiatric clinics. The establishment of the pediatric faculties (from 1961 to 1989) made it possible to distinguish the specialty of child and adolescent psychiatry in the university education, further post-university preparation being done for child neuro-psychiatric specialization.

The infantile neuro-psychiatry scientific society existed under an umbrella represented by the Union of the Medical Sciences Societies (USSM); its journal, "Journal for Neurology, Psychiatry, Neurosurgery", also published articles, research, and scientific theses from the child and adolescent neuropsychiatry field.

After 1990, the "Society of Child and Adolescent Neurology and Psychiatry in Romania", a society which is reuniting professionals, physicians, and medium personnel (nurses) together with the associated professionals (psychologists, retrieve-specialists, social assistants, etc.), was established. A total of 21 national congresses for child and adolescent neurology and psychiatry have been organized and have had in the recent years international participation.

Publications in the child and adolescent psychiatry field, close to the university courses, have outlined the Romanian specialists' evolutional tendencies, especially in the neuropsychological approaches and the behaviorist orientation, the psycho-analytical approach being rare and non-systematic.

In 1989, the number of the child neuropsychiatry experts was almost 130; at the present, there are over 200 and with the associated professionals almost 300. Experts with psycho-pedagogical profiles from the different educational institutes for children with different deficiency degrees are not included in this number.

Recent advances

The changes in the civil society during the last 8 years have contributed to the evolution and progress of child and adolescent psychiatry and psychotherapy. The existing hospital-like institutions from the beginning of the 1950s were replaced by consulting panels with outpatient characteristics in the 1960s; in the 1970s the mental health centers (with daypatient services) were established, and in some university centers, medical-psycho-pedagogical complexes with retrieval services existed. After 1990, the most important changes consisted of the orientation toward outpatient services, the imposing of psychotherapy as a title, and the official recognition of the formation according to the international requirements. Also, new psychiatric services were founded (for example, the crisis centers for adolescents, hot-lines, non-governmental organizations which have interest in the child's and teenager's protection).

The precarious economic situation, the insufficient budget provided for health, and the borderline position of child and adolescent psychiatry in comparison with other medical disciplines make it difficult to achieve the progress desired by the experts.

Current situation

The population of Romania was established to be, at the last census, 22,810,035 inhabitants, of which approximately 4,800,000 are between 0 and 18 years or around 21 % of the entire population. From the administrative and territorial point of view, there are 41 regions with at least 1–2 physicians specialized in child neuropsychiatry.

In the university centers, the specialists number is larger (Bucharest, 32; Cluj, 15; Timisoara, 11) compared to other regions, but of the 11 medical universities only 3 have the child and adolescent psychiatric discipline. These are Bucharest, Cluj, and Timisoarar, which are also the centers for postgraduate medical specialties.

For every neuropsychiatric professional, there are around 24,000 children and teenagers (or 1/100,000 inhabitants), and the lack of the associated professionals and the associated services reduces the quality and complexity of the medical efficiency.

At this time, Romania has around 200 child and adolescent neuropsychiatrists, and it is expected from now on that the new graduating specialists be differentiated only as psychiatrists-psychotherapists CA.

2. Classification systems, diagnostic and therapeutic methods

Classification systems

In Romania, the official classification is ICD-10. In the university and post-university educational system, the DSM-IV classification is also used, especially for scientific research purposes.

Diagnostic methods

The diagnostic methods are based on clinical and paraclinical examination of the patient. From the paraclinical methods the complementary ones are psycho-diagnoses, the retrieval evaluation, psycho-pedagogy, and complementary neuro-radiological examination, e.g., EEG, EMG.

Therapeutic methods

Therapeutic methods are based on medication, associated with other interventions, such as relaxation methods, psycho-motor retrieval, psycho-pedagogic retrieval, and some kinds of psychotherapeutical approach (non-directive, behavior therapy, family counseling).

3. Structure and organization of services

Guidelines for services for children and adolescents with psychiatric disorders

The centralized character of the state had, as a result, a uniform partition of services for children and adolescents; however, there were huge differences between their competence and efficacy.

In Romania, 1971 was marked by the reorganization of the neuro-psychiatric assistance system, creating the major institutions which are necessary for complex care. They were divided into four different governmental departments, which had as result a fragmentation and dilution of the expert's influence in these institutions. The neuro-psychiatry professionals could exercise their jobs only in the institutions connected with the Health Department, the relationship with other departments being systematic only in isolated situations.

In the Health Department network, there were

- outpatient service – founded as Mental Health Laboratory, and then Mental Health Center,
- university clinic departments/hospital departments (in some towns as a part from the Pediatric Hospital),
- hospitals/departments for prolonged care,
- hospitals for chronic neuro-psychiatric diseases, and
- sanatorium for patients with neuro-motor deficiencies.

In the Labor and Social Protection Department, there were

- special professional schools for retrievable children with psychic deficiencies older than 14 years,
- special schools for children with sensorial deficiencies (deaf, visual problems),
- special schools/homes for partially retrievable children with psychic deficiencies under 16 years of age,
- special schools/homes for partially retrievable children with psychic deficiencies over 16 years of age,
- special hospital/homes for unretrievable persons with deficiencies,
- schools for moral reeducation for pre-delinquents under 14 years, and
- centers to receive minor children.

In the Education Department, there were

- kindergartens for retrievable children with sensorial and psychomotor deficiencies,
- general-help schools for retrievable children with psychic deficiencies,
- general schools for retrievable children with sensorial deficiencies, and
- general education high schools for teen-agers with sensorial deficiencies.

In the Internal Affairs Department, there were

- special camps for reeducation of children with behavior disorders and delinquents over 14 years.

(The above information was extracted from the National Neuropsychiatric Commission Report, 1971, appendix written by Dr. Eliza Ionescu, who organized and established in Timisoara the most modern and complex neuropsychiatric service at that time in Romania. This service included a clinical department, daypatient service, psychopedagogical recover base, and a Mental Health Laboratory.)

It seemed that these institutions could entirely cover the assistance needs in child and adolescent psychiatry but the lack of qualified personnel, the poor material base, and, in most situations, the nonexistence of complementary services and of the associated professions were a result of a poorly functioning system. The present state of the child and adolescent psychiatric and psychotherapeutic services has not radically changed, but, on the existing structure, the medical assistance has been modernized.

Types of services

We can say that even now there are units coordinated by the Health Department (clinic departments, hospitals for acute and long-term pathology, mental health centers with daypatient services – integrated or independent –, consulting panels for outpatients and private panels). The complementary assistance services for patients with handicaps are coordinated by the Handicap Inspectorate, which assumed some of the Education Department units (special schools, assistance institutions). In addition to this, new assistance and activities have been initiated by the NGOs, both in some prevention actions and in the long-term assistance for the patient in the family or community. Available in these services provided by the NGOs is the support of the professional and scientific competence by the experts in the field involved in these activities.

Outpatient services

Outpatient services are represented by the consulting panels in the outpatient service from the regional diagnostic centers (one for each region = 41 cabinets) and by the consultations in outpatient system provided by the mental health centers (which exists generally in universities and larger towns – approximately 20). Also included here are the consulting services, which are provided by private panels (we do not have enough information about the number of psychiatric consultations). These panels do not exist in all regions, and the population's accessibility to them is unsatisfying. Centers for early detection and intervention are established only in Bucuresti and Timisoara; in the future they are also going to function in other university centers.

Daypatient services

These exist in all university centers (11 units) and in some big towns where Mental Health Centers exist. They assure complementary services to the hospital departments (integrated) or they are independent (in daypatient system).

Inpatient services

There are 20 inpatient services, which include 7 university departments. Generally speaking, there is a non-uniform distribution of the units, and only half of the regions are covered with inpatient services (in larger towns). There are 4 beds per 100,000 people between 0–18 years of age.

Complementary services and rehabilitation

They are represented mainly by the special schools for children with handicaps and NGOs, which established protection and resocialization institutions for children with handicaps by developing social assistance services for children from the less popular social categories (street children, abandoned, neglected, abused).

Personnel

For many institutions, a handicap in their functioning is the insufficient number of professionals (physicians, psychologists, retrieval personnel) and the nonexistence of auxiliary personnel (nurses and infirmiers) specifically trained for the psychiatry profession.

Funding of services

Until 1998, the public health services were funded by the state (generally with less than 3 % of the BIP). A modification in the public health reform by introducing the assurance systems is desired.

Evaluation

We do not have any evaluation of the child and adolescent psychiatric services.

4. Cooperation with medical and non-medical disciplines

Cooperation with pediatrics

Usually, collaboration with pediatric services exists both in the university clinics and in the regional services with child and adolescent neuro-psychiatric services. It is a custom to apply inter- or pluridisciplinary consultation for psychosomatic disorders, convulsions, perinatal suffering (neonatology), etc.

Cooperation with psychiatry

The relationships with psychiatric services for adults consist of

- transferring the chronic patient's observation schedule from the child assistance evidence into adult evidence,
- evidence of psychotic patient's children, their monitoring or their treatment (where needed),
- following the evolution of the ex-patient's disease during the adult period, and common research programs.

Cooperation with doctors in private practice

We do not have a private practice system in child and adolescent psychiatry, but the experts on private panels also work in institutions.

Cooperation with non-medical institutions and professionals

A real collaboration between non-medical institutions and child and adolescent psychiatrists does not exist, because of its marginalization and sometimes it being ignored by the other institutions. Even in a 1971 report, the neuro-psychiatrists complained about the lack of an audience and cooperation with institutions such as special schools, help-schools, or phanages, etc. Usually, the relationships were begun upon diagnosis and scholarly orientation for children with psychic problems. The absence of psychologists and social assistants had, as result, strict cooperation only with services which included the few available experts. Rarely and only in some university centers there were better collaborations with centers for social assistance and scholar head departments more common after 1990, but even now there is poor cooperation with the Child Protection Department. Good work is possible with NGOs involved in child protection.

5. Graduate/postgraduate training and continuing medical education

Graduate training: The role of medical faculties

Between 1961 and 1989, at the medical universities which included a pediatric faculty (there were 6 such universities), child and adolescent psychiatry was taught as an independent discipline. Once the pediatric faculties were disabled, the students are still learning child and adolescent psychiatry in only three medical universities (Bucuresti, Cluj, and Timisoara). One of the major goals is to reintroduce the child and adolescent psychiatric departments in the university education.

Postgraduate training, a joint effort

Before 1995, postgraduate training to become a specialist in child and adolescent psychiatry consisted in gaining a place through competition and traversing a 3-year training in child neurology and psychiatry. Since 1995, the resident's postgraduate training consists also in gaining a place through competition, but the candidates have to spend four years in child and adolescent psychiatry and one year for complementary studies (pediatrics, neurology). To practice the specialty, a final examination (a written and a practical phase, with a case presentation) is necessary.

To practice psychotherapy, a two-year curriculum during the specialty training is needed and then another two years with supervision (this is the unofficial proposal of the Psychotherapeutical Association). The training curriculum is according to most countries from the EU, consisting of 720 h.

Continuing medical education

There is no obligation to fulfill a continuous medical education. The universities are organizing postgraduation courses with optional participation.

Training programs for other disciplines

In the university centers where the residents in other disciplines are trained, they can fulfill courses from 1–3 months (pediatrics, endocrinology, general practitioners). The residents in adult psychiatry have to fulfill a 6 month training. Also, the psychology and social assistance students are trained in this department.

6. Research

Research fields and strategies

Research activities are included in the universities as a complement to the teaching activity without an extra-remuneration, or it is an optional activity for physicians. There is a research plan of the Academy for Medical Sciences, but there is no place for research in child and adolescent psychiatry. The research is centered on the scientific interest area of the universities. After 1990, the interest for research was stimulated by participating at international congresses and exchanges between experts.

The centralized character which also affected the medical services allowed one to collect important scientific material, especially in the epidemiological psychiatric research, in the prospective and retrospective clinical studies, in the family studies, and more recently in the initiation of some multicentered researches with occidental partners.

Research training and career development

Since 1990 some initiation courses in research have been organized, especially for young residents and specialists, by important personalities, such as N. Sartorius, J. L. Terra, H. Remschmidt, F. Poustka, and P. Graham. Also, many young specialists have participated in international seminars or have benefited by training scholarships in research. In the future we hope that this cumulated experience and competence will materialize into important scientific research.

Funding

There is no funding for research in child and adolescent psychiatry, neither from the state budget, from the Health Department, nor private foundations. There were some attempts to participate in the Tempus programs, but these were not approved. The activity of some specialists in some NGOs allowed some research activities to sustain the research programs, with financial support from the European Community.

7. Future perspectives

The professional and scientific quality of the specialists in Romania gives us the right for high expectations about the evolution of child and adolescent psychiatry in the 21st century.

However, the economic and social environments are an objective obstacle in front of our optimism, especially about the practical realization possibilities of some initiatives of institutional and professional modernization.

Research

To achieve progress in the research area, some fundamental conditions are necessary and include:

- building an information net and a computerized infrastructure,
- assuring access to international literature and to specialty publications. Generally, this access is very limited compared to other countries.
- assuring further training for the younger generation applying special programs for scientific research,
- advocating child and adolescent mental health research among decision makers in politics and in the public, and
- securing some financial resources which should allow high quality scientific research.

The residents are further prepared – theoretical and practical – to know the research methodology and instruments for child and adolescent psychiatry and psychotherapy.

Training

One of the purposes is to generalize the child and adolescent psychiatry discipline in the university education system. The postgraduate training is possible in the recognized university centers in the country, according to the curricular program accepted by EFTA countries.

Improvement of services and care systems

Steps to improve the existing institutions and services by training and changing the present way of thinking of all personnel and the decision makers in management and health politics are being taken. The development of the psychological and social assistance education system is going to represent the guarantee of a better practical activity and of the community and family orientation. The specialist training in different directions of psychotherapy, such as systemic familial psychotherapy, cognitive and behavior therapy, Moreno psychodrama, existence analysis-axiological and anthropological, and Frankl's logotherapy, will provide more humanity and another dimension to the therapeutical act in child and adolescent psychiatry in Romania.

Selected references

Ghiran V (1998) Date privind structura si organizarea retelei de psihiatrie a copilului si adolescentului in zona Cluj. Cluj

Ionescu E (1971) Raport al comisiei de psihiatrie cu referire la schema de organizare a asistentei de neuropsihiatrie infantila in Romania. Timisoara

Lupu C (1995) 30 de ani in serviciul sanatatii mintale a copiilor si adolescentilor. Timisoara

Mircea T (1995) Proiect privind organizarea serviciilor de psihiatrie si a Centrului de Diagnostic Precoce si de Recuperare. Timisoara

Remschmidt H (1996) Changing views: New perspectives in child psychiatric research. European Child and Adolescent Psychiatry 5 (1): 2–10

UNICEF doc (1996) The situation of child and family in Romania 1992. Venice Working Group of IACAPAP – Mental Health Services and Systems for Children and Adolescents. In: Young JG, Ferrari P (Eds) Designing Mental Health Services and Systems for Children and Adolescents. A Shrewed Investment (pp 443–463). Brunner/Mazel: Philadelphia, PA

Urechia Ci (1929) Handbook for Neuro-Mental Pathology. Cluj: Lepage

Child and adolescent psychiatry in Russia

A. A. Severny, Y. S. Shevchenko, B. A. Kazakovtsev, and L. V. Kim

1. Definition, historical development, and current situation

Definition

Apparently, in Russia, "child and adolescent psychiatry" does not have a normative definition in official documents. As child/adolescent psychiatric care is a part of general psychiatric service, it is meant that child and adolescent psychiatry is psychiatry which applies to the appointed age – child (0–14) and adolescent (15–17) – according to official age framework. The point is that the Ministry of Health does not issue normative acts especially for child psychiatry, and nongovernmental professional organizations do not have the authority to establish these. To obtain the right to work as a child or adolescent psychiatrist, it is enough for any child physician to complete the 4-month course of appropriate specialization (see below). Since the Ministry of Health eliminated in 1995 the specialty of child and adolescent psychiatry from the official list of medical professions, it is not possible to reflect this specialization in labor documents.

Historical development

The first private hospital for children with severe mental retardation and epilepsy was opened in Russia in 1854. The first state schools for mentally retarded children appeared at the same time. Child psychiatry was founded in close connection with general psychiatry, pediatrics, child neurology, psychology, and other allied disciplines. The studies of European scientists greatly influenced the development of child psychiatry in Russia. The first scientific works in child psychiatry appeared in Russia at the end of the 19th and the beginning of the 20th century. A. S. Griboedov, child psychiatrist, founded a school for mentally retarded children in St. Petersburg's asylum in 1890 and a children's dispensary for neurological and psychiatric patients. In 1907 V. Bekhterev organized the Research Institute of Child Development in St. Petersburg, and G. I. Rossolimo founded the Institute of Child Neurology and Psychology in Moscow in 1914. A new stage of child psychiatry history in the former USSR began after the October Revolution in 1917 and was connected with the names of prominent psychiatrists, such as P. P. Kashchenko, V. A. Gilyarovsky, M. O. Gourevich, N. I. Ozeretsky, G. E. Sukhareva, T. P. Simson, S. S. Mnukhin, and others. In 1918 the Department of Child Psychopathology was founded in the Ministry of Health. A network of psychoneurological dispensaries all over the country was organized in the 1920s. Their tasks in particular were to detect for the first time and observe the mentally ill and intellectually retarded children and adolescents, provide outpatient care, sending them to hospitals and other outpatient institutions, providing preventive examinations of children in kindergartens and schools, as well as sanitary and hygienic education.

Recent advances

All types of psychiatric care in Russia are free of charge, but mental diseases including disorders in children and adolescents are not covered by the obligatory state insurance. Disabled children with severe mental retardation receive government welfare. The Russian Federal Law "On Psychiatric Care and Patient Rights as it is Rendered" of 1992 is very important for the modern state of psychiatric service. There were endorsed psychiatric examination norms for minors, rules for their hospitalization or admission to special educational institutions, as well as rules of discharge from psychiatric hospitals and other special institutions. The law founded the basis for legal and social regulations of psychiatric patients and gave public organizations the possibility to control the rights of mentally ill in psychiatric hospitals. At the same time the law excluded the possibility of preventive psychiatric examinations of children and adolescents. It has no regulations of children's mental health for the district outpatient psychiatrist, has no regulations for parents if they do not provide necessary psychiatric and psychotherapeutic care in time and do not consider children and adolescent's peculiarities of psychiatric disorders. In 1995 the federal program "Emergency Measures for the Improvement of Psychiatric Care" was approved by the government. This document devotes attention to the realization of a program to develop child and adolescent psychotherapeutic services, specialist's training, etc. But the majority of those programs still have not been realized in connection with the social-economic problems in Russia.

Current situation

At the beginning of 1997, the country's population was 147,000,000 with 37,000,000 (25.2 %) children and adolescents. The number of child and adolescent psychiatrists in 1994 was 1891. In the following 4 years, their number decreased by 30 %. Thus, at the present time, 1 child/adolescent psychiatrist serves 28,000 children and adolescents. Evidently, the majority of psychiatrists have more or less no large private practice. The number of child and adolescent psychiatrists practicing only privately (without working in any state medical system) is probably not very large, due to the economic situation (the negligible quantity of wealthy patients, the high tax system), negative public attitude towards psychiatry as a whole, and the low development both of psychotherapeutic service and of education of professionals. It is necessary to note that private practitioners work separately and out of any professional control.

There is only one non-governmental professional organization – Independent Association of Child Psychiatrists and Psychologists (IACPP), which was founded in 1992. The number of IACPP members currently is about 150 from 16 regions of

Russia. The IACPP unites child and adolescent psychiatrists, psychologists, and children's specialists of allied disciplines. IACPP together with other organizations hold almost every year conferences in actual social and mental health problems of children ("An Unusual Child and His Environment", 1993; "Orphans of Russia: Problems, Hopes, Future", 1993; "School Disadaptation: Emotional and Stress Disorders in Children and Adolescents", 1995; "Social Disadaptation: Behavior Disorders in Children and Adolescents", 1996 ; "Children of Russia: Abuse and Protection", 1997; "Social and Mental Health of Child and Family: Protection, Care, Rehabilitation", 1998). Materials of all conferences were published in abstract books.

There is also a Section of Child and Adolescent Psychiatry as a branch of the Russian Society of Psychiatrists. The real number of members in the Russian Society of Psychiatrists is unknown, because there is no registration nor membership fee.

The demographic situation and deteriorated state of children's mental health in Russia for the last years are closely connected with deep reorganizations in state and public life and continued social-economic crisis. Thus, from 1990–94 the number of newborns was 3.7 million less in Russia than in the previous five years; a normal course of pregnancy is observed only in 20 %, every fifth newborn is ill or became sick in the neonatal period; more than 1,000,000 children are practically disabled; in school the number of healthy children has decreased by five times and the adolescent's death rate has increased by 35 %. Only 14 % of public school graduates can be regarded as practically healthy. Prevalence of syphilis among adolescents for the five year increased by 20 times!

The data for children and adolescents "social health" are also very impressive. About 2 million school children (10 % of appropriate population) do not study anywhere and do not work (40 % of child/adolescent criminal activity is from this group); about 2 million children and adolescents are vagabonds; the number of orphaned children has reached 700,000; 40 % of children have undergone abuse in families; 16 % of school children have undergone physical abuse and 22 % psychological abuse by teachers at school. For the last ten years, the death rate from suicide attempts has increased by 100 %; in 1996, 2,756 children and adolescents committed suicide and suicide has been noted among children ages 5–9. There are 700,000 families with minors in Russia where one parent is unemployed, 60,000 families with children where both parents do not have financial resources. Criminal behavior of minors is growing twice as fast as in adults, especially in the field of severe crimes against persons. Children's criminal activity has grown 1.5 times in 5 years, while the number of crimes committed by girls is more than 57.1 %; the number of arrested minors has increased almost two times and exceeded 1 million in a year; 27 % of them are children under 14 years old. About 30,000 organized criminal groups of minors act in Russia. As a matter of fact, 60–80 % of minor's crimes are committed by minors with mental anomalies. About 35 % of school children have experience with the use of drugs and toxic agents. Compared with 1995, the number of children and adolescents in 1996 registered as drug addicts increased by 2.3 times, as toxic agents addicts by 2.7 times, alcohol dependence by 10 %, child/adolescent deaths caused by alcohol intoxication in 1990–1995 increased by 3 times.

How do the social and biological factors reflect on the mental health of children? 9.6 % of children 0–3 years old already have clear psychiatric abnormalities; only about 45 % of pre-school children do not have any morbid deviations in mental state, which are annually increasing by 8–12 %; among school children the prevalence has already reached 70–80 %. Only 14 % of school-aged adolescents can be regarded as completely mentally healthy. Among children with school disadaptations, 93–95 % have more or less mental disorders, and 80 % of those, who enter to special educational institutions for deviant children, need urgent corrective psychiatric care. Among homeless children vagabonds, mentally healthy children do not account for more than 6 %, the necessity of psychotherapeutic care for orphans living for extended periods of time in the homes for orphans reaches 100 %.

However, only 10 % of all children needing psychiatric service received it in the state system of psychiatric care!

There is no faculty of child and adolescent psychiatry in any of the Russian universities or medical institutes. There is a great lack of various specialists for child psychiatric service and a very large deficiency of scientific research in actual fields of child and adolescent psychiatry (borderline psychiatry, psychosomatic disorders, drug dependence, psychiatry of early childhood, social psychiatry, etc.).

2. Classification systems, diagnostic and therapeutic methods

Classification systems

ICD-9 is still used in Russia. The Russian version of ICD-10 was published in 1994, an adaptation of this classification is now in process, and in 1999 it will be installed. The universal form of report documentation for psychiatric institutions is in use throughout Russia.

Diagnostic methods

The majority of children's psychiatric hospitals use the modern set of technical diagnostic facilities including EEG examination, computer tomography, etc. The conditions for biochemical and genetic examination in laboratories are much worse, because of lack of equipment and reagents. In particular, the psychotropic medication concentration level in plasma is not tested. A large number of the psychological test battery used in Russia are adopted tests of foreign psychologists.

Therapeutic methods

Psychopharmacology has the most important role both in inpatient and outpatient clinics. Psychotropic medications could be indicated at any age, beginning at infancy. However, psychiatrists begin to cure children only after 4 years of age, so before this age psychotropic recommendations are usually made by other specialists (neurologists, etc.). It is difficult to estimate psychotherapeutic care in the child/adolescent because of its underdevelopment; family therapy is practically absent.

3. Structure and organization of services

Guidelines for services for children and adolescents with psychiatric disorders

There are no officially determined and adopted principles of psychiatric care for children and adolescents. The distribution of the psychiatric care is based on a principle of district service. There are no structures for specialized care for different forms of psychiatric disorders. Children with all types of mental pathologies are serviced by the same doctors in the same psychiatric institutions. Child psychiatrists service children ages 4–14 years old, adolescent psychiatrists service adolescents from 15–17 years old. Special psychiatric hospitals for adolescents exist only in some large cities.

Types of services

Care for children with mental abnormalities is divided into three departments: Public Health, Education, and Social Protection. Two main types of psychiatric care – outpatient (in psychiatric dispensaries and outpatient clinics) and inpatient (in the children's psychiatric departments of district psychiatric hospitals) – belong to the Public Health Department. All other forms of psychiatric service organization are not practically in use. Special kindergartens and schools for different categories of children (mentally retarded; with speech impediments; behavior disturbances) are under supervision of the Department of Education. Special invalid homes for the disabled as a result of mental illness, mainly invalid homes for the severely mentally retarded (more than 30,000 children, mostly orphans; about 200 children per invalid home), are under supervision of the social protection system.

Outpatient services

Outpatient care is rendered by child and adolescent psychiatrists of state district dispensaries. Child psychiatrists are usually located in the district outpatient departments and adolescent psychiatrists in psychiatric dispensaries. According to official norms, one child psychiatrist is allocated to every 15,000 children in cities and 25,000 in the country. One psychotherapist services 100,000 people (or 25,000 children on average). Because of staff reductions in some regions and towns, there are no child psychiatrists. Service for psychiatric care in early childhood is absent.

Private psychiatric practice is rendered by a few high-qualified specialists. But private care is mostly rendered by representatives of so-called nontraditional medicine (extrasences, parapsychologists, sorcerers, wizards, etc.). Parents with a child often visit medical doctors after several failed attempts of treatment by extrasences and sorcerers. The network of different centers (about 1500) providing specialized service for children has grown over the past few years. Obviously, the great part of those patients are in need of psychiatric and psychotherapeutic assistance, but as a rule there are no psychiatrists in the centers.

Daypatient services

Day psychiatric hospitals for children and adolescents are practically absent. There are only a few of them in some regions: day department in psychiatric hospitals (in Moscow) and selective day hospitals (in St. Petersburg).

Inpatient services

Almost all children's and adolescents' psychiatric departments are parts of regional or state psychiatric hospitals or dispensaries (there are 89 regions in Russia), as well as parts of city psychiatric hospitals in the larger cities. For every 100,000 people, there are 7 beds on average. Psychiatric clinics of universities do not have departments for children and use children's departments of district psychiatric hospitals. Only the Center of Mental Health of the Russian Academy of Medical Sciences has its own children's psychiatric department. Children are admitted to the psychiatric hospitals without mothers.

Complementary services and rehabilitation

Special rehabilitative institutions for mentally ill children and adolescents are also practically absent. Those institutions are now being establishing as a new form of child and adolescent psychiatric organization. Particularly, these forms are found in St. Petersburg. The foster family system is not developed.

Personnel

A system of special training for child and adolescent psychiatric personnel does not exist. Students of colleges for nurses study psychiatry together with other medical disciplines.

Funding of services

State psychiatric service on a whole is free of charge in Russia and is financed by state funding, but is not covered by obligatory state insurance. All patients of psychiatric hospitals, outpatients if their age is under 3 years old, and disabled children receive free psychotropic medications. But the list of free medications for outpatients (approved by Ministry of Health) is limited and is constantly being reduced. Nowadays it includes only the less expensive medications. Many patients do not have the possibility to use modern expensive medications. There is no other financing of psychiatric care for children and adolescents.

Evaluation

There is no research in comparative efficacy of different organizational forms for child and adolescent psychiatric care.

4. Cooperation with medical and non-medical disciplines

Cooperation with pediatrics

There are no pediatric hospitals in Russia with psychiatric or psychosomatic departments. Psycho-neurological departments in the pediatric hospitals invite as a rule psychiatrists when it is necessary to consult and do not include them on the staff. There are no child and adolescent psychiatrists in pediatric outpatient clinics. Children under 4 years are not examined by psychiatrists. Children from 4–14 years old are examined in a pediatric outpatient department by a psychiatrist from the district psychiatric dispensary. Children's psychiatric hospitals have a staff of all necessary specialists for diagnostic and therapeutic care.

Cooperation with psychiatry

Psychiatric care for children and adolescents is an important part of general psychiatric service. Child and adolescent psychiatrists are included on the staff of district psychiatric dispensaries; child/adolescent psychiatric hospitals are usually part of district general psychiatric hospitals. Case histories of patients older than 18 years transfer to a general ("adult") psychiatrist. There are no other special forms or fields of cooperation between child/adolescent and general psychiatry.

Cooperation with doctors in private practice

State child and adolescent psychiatric service predominates in Russia. Therefore, private practice is underdeveloped, and it is difficult to determine the forms of cooperation between them.

Cooperation with non-medical institutions and professionals

Cooperation between psychiatrists and non-medical institutions and professionals is hampered by their dependence to different departments. It is difficult for psychiatrists to start work in the non-medical institutions, because in this case they have lost their privileges, such as charge extra, vocation lengthening, etc. Psychiatrists of district dispensaries service special educational institutions (invalid homes for mentally retarded, schools for adolescents with deviant behavior, etc.).

5. Graduate/postgraduate training and continuing medical education

Specialists in child and adolescent psychiatry are trained in the institutes and faculties for postgraduate specialized education, as well as in the scientific institutes. There are no departments of child psychiatry in the medical institutes. The short-term training model in child psychiatry is the first specialization for primary care doctors (usually pediatricians) with medical experience of not less than 3 years. It is a four month training program in the department of postgraduate study. The second model is an internship – one year training program after graduating from the medical institute. This training takes place in the departments of psychiatry of children's psychiatric hospitals. The next model is "ordinatura" or clinical internship (two year program) for medical graduates, who have worked (usually as pediatricians) for not less than 3 years. Doctor "ordinators" study at the departments of the medical institutes, postgraduate institutes as well as at the research institutes of psychiatry. The period of study can be lengthened to 4–5 years. Routine study for raising the level of professionalism (2 month course of training) takes place in those institutes once every five years. Once in every five years psychiatrists must pass an exam which confirms their level of knowledge. After the exam, they receive a medical category of second, first or high level. Psychiatrists with psychiatric experience of not less than 3 years must pass a state license examination (in the form of computer tests) to receive a private practice license. Usually before the examination he should raise the level of professional experience for one month at one of the postgraduate institutions.

Three postgraduate departments of child and adolescent psychiatry are functioning in Russia: in Moscow, St. Petersburg, Chelyabinsk. The oldest of them is situated in Moscow in the Russian Medical Academy for Advanced Education and was founded in 1935. Prof. G. E. Sukhareva was the chief of the department before 1966, then Prof. V. V. Kovaliov. Since 1994, Prof. Yu. S. Shevchenko has been the chief. From that time, the department has enlarged the circle of functions and was named the Department of Child and Adolescent Psychiatry, Psychotherapy, and Medical Psychology. Besides specialization and raising the professional level, the department provides training of clinical (medical) and school psychologists, pediatricians, defectologists, logopeds, teachers of special educational and pedagogical institutions, and correctional classes, and social workers.

6. Research

Intensive scientific researches in child and adolescent psychiatry became possible in Russia from the end of the 1920s and beginning of the 1930s and conducted according with the conceptions of two leading scientific schools – Moscow and St. Petersburg (formerly named Leningrad). In the first one, the leading positions were occupied by V. A. Gilyarovsky, T. P. Simson, M. O. Gourevich, and G. E. Sukhareva. The second one was represented by N. I. Ozeretsky and S. S. Mnukhin. In 1929, the monograph of T. P. Simson "Neuropathy, personality disorders, and reactive states of infants" was published and has not lost importance up to now. The author wrote based on psychoanalytical positions. From the middle of the 1930s psychoanalysis was prohibited in Russia for more than half a century because of ideology. Then all efforts were strained to research schizophrenia in children. The first result was reflected in the monograph of G. E. Sukhareva "The symptoms of schizophrenia in children and adolescents" (1937). G. E. Sukhareva was the first who, while observing schizophrenia, differentiated three types of course (slow continuous, in the form of attacks, mixed). Further investigations of Sukhareva and her followers revealed a correlation between the type of course and of leading psychopathological syndrome, clarified the aged evolution of the disease, and showed the unity of main correlation of schizophrenia in adults and children besides of age peculiarities. T. P. Simson and her colleagues made an important contribution to understanding the nature of schizophrenia in early and middle childhood. In 1948 the monograph of Simson "Schizophrenia of early childhood", was published describing excessive catatonic forms of schizophrenia. At the same time in Leningrad, S. S. Mnukhin and his followers investigated peculiarities of circular psychosis in adolescents, psychosis in mentally retarded, residual-organic disorders after cerebral infections, brain trauma, and intoxication. Both psychiatric schools actively investigated problems of mental retardation, epilepsy, constitutional and organic personality disorders, and neurosis and neurosis-like states. The three volume manual of Sukhareva "Clinical Lectures of Child Psychiatry" was the result of clinical research from the first part of the 20th century, which completed the foundation of the independent Russian pediatric-psychiatric school. From the end of the 1960s the leaders of the so-called Moscow psychiatric school in child psychiatry were V. V. Kovaliov, G. K. Ushakov, M. S. Vrono, and V. M. Bashina and of the Leningrad school D. N. Isaev, A. E. Lichko, and V. E. Kagan. From that time the traditional clinic-dynamic approach in research of mental disorders of children and adolescents was completed by positions of mental disontogenesis. Generalized book of M. S. Vrono "Schizophrenia of Children and Adolescents" (1971) and later the monograph of V. M. Bashina "Early Children's Schizophrenia" (1980) were published. A. E. Lichko wrote books about problems of adolescent psychiatry (1977, 1985), D. N. Isaev about mental underdevelopment (1981), and V. E. Kagan about the syndrome of early autism.

In the 1990s the peculiar changes of generations are taking place in child psychiatry. Anyway, the main trends of scientific research have been preserved. New actual trends have developed: psychotherapy, psychiatry of early childhood, drug dependence of children and adolescents, PTSD, forensic aspects of child psychiatry, etc. Now Prof. I. A. Kozlova is the chief of the department for autism and schizophrenia in children (Research Center of Mental Health). The department of infant pathology is headed by Prof. G. V. Kozlovskaya. The chief of the department for deviant behavior and affective disorders in children of the Moscow Institute of Psychiatry is Dr. L. A. Ermolina. The chief of the department of child epilepsy in St. Petersburg Research Psychoneurological Institute is Prof. R. A. Kharitonov; the department of adolescent psychopathology of the same institute is headed by Prof. Yu. V. Popov. There is a department of psychotherapy in the St. Petersburg Medical Academy of Postgraduate Education. The department of child and adolescent psychiatry, psychotherapy, and medical psychology of the Russian Academy of Postgraduate Education investigated for many years the clinical and dynamic course of borderline disorders of children and adolescents. In recent years scientific interests of this department have widened and include the study of neurosis and neurosis-like disorders in early childhood, establishment of effective psychotherapeutic forms and psychocorrection as well as ontogenic oriented integrative methods, and art-therapy.

7. Future perspectives

Research

For further development and coordination of scientific research in the field of child psychiatry, it is necessary to organize state scientific and educational institutions in child and adolescent mental health and to publish special volumes of journals in child psychiatry, psychosomatic, and psychology. The fundamental directions of scientific investigations which required further development are psychiatry of early childhood, child and adolescent drug dependence, comparative estimation of efficacy of different organizational psychiatric forms of child and adolescent care for children and adolescents, borderline psychiatry, child/adolescent psychotherapy and family therapy, psychosomatic, and social and juridical problems in the protection of rights of mentally ill children and adolescents.

Training

The principal tasks of the training system of child psychiatrists consist of

- giving fundamental education and enough practical experience in general psychiatry/psychology before specialization in child/adolescent psychiatry;
- giving fundamental education and enough practice in general problems of child/adolescent psychiatry/psychology before specialization in the more narrow professional fields;
- giving the possibility to raise the level of knowledge in all aspects of child-adolescent psychiatry/psychology, as well as in methodological and practical aspects of cooperation with specialists of other disciplines connected with children for specialists in child and adolescent psychiatry;

- periodical confirmation of modern knowledge possession in allied professions for specialists.

A preventive program of child and adolescent mental health should be included to the training program for students of pediatrician and physician faculties aimed at increasing the preventive trend of medicine and orientation to consider the patient as a whole system.

Two-year training in "clinical ordinatura" is the first specialization in child and adolescent psychiatry for medical doctors after 1-year training in general psychiatry ("internatura" or internship) and a two year practice in psychiatric institutions; or with 3 years experience in general psychiatry. For pediatric faculty graduates, the length of clinical "ordinatura" is 3–5 years depending on the tasks. Improving professional skills further (if there is practical experience in child-adolescent psychiatry of more than 2 years) in general and special issues is possible in the departments of postgraduate study; duration may be from 2 weeks to 6 months. Every psychiatrist must be trained not less than once every five years. For postgraduate research, it is necessary to have 3 years experience in a child-adolescent psychiatric institution. Certification, attestation, and licensing examination for child-adolescent psychiatrists should be done by commissions which are independent from the institution where the student or doctor studies or works.

Child medical psychologist must have a fundamental high psychological education, diploma of medical psychologist, and training in psychopathology and clinical courses of mental disorders, patho- and neuropsychopathology, as well as child and adolescent psychotherapy. It is possible for general and school psychologists or teachers-defectologists or pediatricians (on the faculties of medical psychology in the medical institutes) to be enrolled for 2 year primary training in child and adolescent psychologists with different programs.

It is imperative to include courses on raising the professional level for allied professionals – general psychiatrists and narcologists, pediatricians, child neurologists, general and school psychologists, defectologists, logopeds, workers of penitentiary institutions for adolescents, social workers, etc.

The minimum list of specialists for child-adolescent psychiatric service includes:

- child-adolescent psychiatrist, psychiatrist of early childhood, child-adolescent narcologist, child psychotherapist, adolescent psychotherapist;
- psychologist of early childhood, child psychologist, adolescent psychologist, play-therapist, child-adolescent pathopsychologist, neuropsychologist;
- specialist in functional diagnostic methods in child psychiatry;
- manager of child-adolescent service, specialist in social-legal and social-psychological problems of childhood and family (social-patronage worker).

Improvement of services and care systems

Psychiatric service for children in the former USSR had some positive sides, i.e., free of charge, possibility to observe sick children very actively, receiving statistical data about child psychopathology, planning character. At the same time this system had many negative traits:

- it existed apart from the education system, social service, and other state institutions. Thus, children in psychiatric institutions could not receive multidisciplinary care and correction. On the contrary, mentally ill children in the boarding school and correctional institutions could not receive adequate psychiatric care;
- it was separated from general medicine (pediatrics), deprived from connection with important links such as psychosomatic care;
- absence of preventive and rehabilitative approaches. The whole system was oriented to the care of already severely mentally ill children with deep disadaptation, without any organizational principles for return to normal life after treatment;
- absence of psychiatric service for early age children;
- child-adolescent services for drug addicts was underdeveloped;
- the training system did not provide the necessary level of quality and set of specialists for child-adolescent psychiatric service;
- absence of social and juridical services for children with mental disorders and their families. Legislative protection of mentally ill children rights was absent;
- cooperation between state and independent organizations was weak; and
- there was no scientific-methodological center for coordination of psychosocial problems of childhood.

The Independent Association of Child Psychiatrists and Psychologists (IACPP) established the Project of Development Child-Adolescent Psychiatric Service in Russia. There are the following theses:

- Introduce the basic principles of children's mental health protection:
  - child-adolescent psychiatric service must receive independence as an organization and must closely be in contact with all departments and institutions dealing with the child population;
  - the multiple nature of mental diseases and profound disadaptation as a consequence urge a multidisciplinary approach for organization of child psychiatric care and their families in cooperation with specialists from different professions: psychiatrists, psychologists, social workers, etc.;
  - the child-adolescent psychiatric service must be as close to the population as required (for children, parents, allied professionals).
- Special laws must be approved for regulation of child psychiatric and psychological care. Those laws should give equal possibilities for receiving care and protection from any discrimination because of mental disorders for all children and their families.
- Limitation of age (as it is adopted all over the world) for the period of adolescence.
- Introduction of open program competition "Development of child psychiatric service".
- Taking part in organization and work of interdepartmental multidisciplinary social-psychological centers for children and adolescents.

The structure of child and adolescent service is organized as follows.

Child Psychiatric Service (CPS) as an independent structure uses the territorial principle of service for children aged 0–17 years old. Regional CPS is an institution with different units.

The central link of district CPS is a child psychiatric outpatient clinic with staff including all necessary specialists: child psychiatrist, adolescent psychiatrist, psychiatrist of early childhood, child-adolescent narcologist, child psychotherapist, adolescent psychotherapist, family therapist, psychologist of early childhood, child psychologist, adolescent psychologist, play-therapist, manager of child-adolescent service, etc. The outpatient clinic for mentally ill children is the center for consultations and methodology.

The head of the outpatient clinic is the chief child psychiatrist of the district and has all functions as an administrative and methodological director of district CPS.

The primary link of CPS is a psychotherapeutic office in the pediatric outpatient clinic. There is a minimum of three specialists – psychiatrist, psychotherapist and medical psychologist, as well as social worker. Besides correcting borderline mental disorders psychotherapists contact general pediatrics and cure psychosomatic disorders in outpatient clinics and in pediatric hospital (as a staff consultant). Together with medical psychologist he should provide child-adolescent and family psychotherapy. The medical psychologist, besides his professional functions, is an important link with non-medical institutions and cooperates with teachers, psychologists, police inspectors, and others.

District CPS besides having a psychotherapeutic office and an outpatient clinic also include a children's psychotherapeutic inpatient clinic in a pediatrics clinic, it also can be a psychosomatic department; children's psychiatric hospital; child-adolescent narcological outpatient clinic with an inpatient department; psychoneurological invalid home for mentally disabled children; psychotherapeutic sanatorium; and a school-sanatorium, psycho-corrective kindergarten for children with mild deviations in mental development and mental disorders at borderline level.

Specialists of district CPS take part in the foundation of interdepartmental institutions together with these interested in departments as well as with independent professional and charitable organizations (medical-psychological commission, commission on minor problems, center of social-psychological care, rehabilitative center, crisis center, crisis line, etc.).

Specialists of CPS take part in the accreditation of institutions that deal with psychiatric problems independent from the departmental and legal position of those institutions.

CPS works under the guidance of the Department CPS with the chief specialist in child-adolescent psychiatry in the Ministry of Health of the RF as a Head. A special information center was established for activity coordination of federal CPS and independent organizations in child psychiatry.

The principles of cooperation CPS with non-psychiatric institutions are as follows.

- Specialists of CPS provide consultant care in all state institutions of the allocated district.

- Specialists of CPS work in the non-medical and multidisciplinary institutions only if a license exists for medical care and medical psychological service with the chief in those institutions.
- Specialists of CPS work in the non-psychiatric institutions only if their professional rights and privileges (approved by Ministry of Health RF) are preserved.
- Specialists of CPS work in the non-governmental organizations on the basis of a contract and there is a license for medical care.

Realization of a CPS development plan is closely connected with the social-economical situation in Russia and overcoming out-dated organizational approaches, particularly with departmental separation of services for children with mental disorders. But those changes are necessary and inevitable because they follow the needs of the children's population and basic trends of child psychiatry all over the world.

Selected references

Bashina VM (1980) Early chlidren's Schizophrenia. Moscow: Meditsina

Governmental Report (1997) About the conditions of children in the Russian Federation (1996). Moscow, p 160

Gurovich IYa, Preis VB, Golland VB (1995) Psychiatric care for the population in Russia. Indices of activities from 1986-1993. Social and Clinical Psychiatry (Supp.) p 667

Iovchuk NM, Severny AA, Shevchenko YuS (1998) Current problems of mental health protection of children and adolescents. Independent Psychiatric Journal 2: 34–36

Isaev DN (1982) Child mental underdevelopment. Leningrad: Meditsina

Kagan VE (1981) Child Autism. Meditsina, Leningrad

Kazakovtsev BA (1996) The organization of psychiatric care (manual of lectures). Moscow 247

Kovaliov VV (1995) Psychiatry of childhood. Manual for doctors. Moscow 560

Lichko AE (1985) Adolescent Psychiatry 2nd edn Leningrad: Meditsina

Periodical report about the realization in Russian Federation of Convention on Child Rights in 1993–1997 (1997) Project. Family in Russia 4: 13–206

Severny AA, Smirnov AYu (1997) Current situation in mental health care for children in Russia. European Child & Adolescent Psychiatry 6: 50–52

Simson TP (1929) Neuropathy, personality disorders, and reactive states of infants. Moscow-Leningrad: Medgiz

Simson TP (1948) Schizophrenia of early childhood. Moscow: Medgiz

Sukhareva GE (1937) The symptoms of schizophrenia in children and adolescents. Moscow: Medgiz

Sukhareva GE (1955–1965) Clinical lectures on psychiatry of childhood. Vol 1–3. Moscow: Meditsina

Vrono MS (1971) Schizophrenia of children and adolescents. Moscow: Meditsina

Child and adolescent psychiatry in Serbia

V. Išpanović-Radojković, N. Tadic

1. Definition, historical development, and current situation

Definition

From the beginning of its development, around 1927, child and adolescent psychiatry in Yugoslavia has been given different names and definitions. At first, it encompassed the wide concept of "mental hygiene", and later "psychiatry of developmental age", "psychiatry of childhood and youth" and finally "child and adolescent psychiatry". Today the last term is in use. It is defined as a separate field of psychiatry covering diagnostics, treatment, prevention, rehabilitation, and scientific research of disorders in emotional, cognitive and social development, psychiatric disorders, and psychosomatic illnesses of children and young people. It is closely linked to pediatrics, and special branches of psychology, sociology, neuropsychology, general psychiatry, genetics, law, and other professional fields and sciences engaged in the care of children and adolescents.

Historical development

There are very scant medieval written documents and evidence about the care of mentally retarded, blind, and abandoned children and adolescents in monasteries, rare general hospitals, and foster families, as well about the treatments with folk medicine. At the end of the nineteenth and the beginning of the twentieth century, the organization of institutional education and the rendering of a certain amount of care to mentally retarded, blind, hard-of-hearing, and mute children and adolescents was started.

Organized prevention and treatment of children and adolescents with psychological disorders in present Yugoslavia (Serbia and Montenegro) was started after the Second World War. As children and young people found themselves in an adverse position (a large number of war orphans, stress-related disorders, poor economic situation), Dr. Vojin Matic, a psychiatrist and psychoanalyst, was asked by the Yugoslav Government in 1949 to organize courses on child psychiatry for special teachers and soon after that the lectures in child psychopathology for the students of Higher School for Special Teachers. Dr. V. Matic, together with a group of physicians, psychologists, special teachers, pedagogues, and social workers, founded in Belgrade (Serbia) in 1951 the first Medical Pedagogical Counseling Center for mental health care of children and adolescents with psychological disorders and disabilities. The Counseling Center was working on, at that time, advanced principles for mental health care. Diagnostics, psychoanalytic psychotherapy, pedagogic, and social work were carried out, emphasizing team work. At the same time systematic psychoanalytically-oriented education of personnel was started. In the same year, 1951, the Chair for Clinical Psychology and Psychopathology was established at the faculty of philosophy in Belgrade, and the subject "Psychopathology of childhood and adolescence" was introduced.

At the beginning, the child and adolescent psychiatry and its services (counseling centers, outpatient and hospital departments) developed predominantly within adult neuropsychiatry and more rarely within pediatrics, psychology or special education. The child and adolescent psychiatry gradually differentiated as a relatively separate branch with specialized counseling centers, outpatient and clinical departments, and even special institutes for child and adolescent neurology and psychiatry.

The first inpatient unit for child neuropsychiatry was opened in Belgrade in 1949, at the Neuropsychiatric Clinic for Adults at the School of Medicine, Belgrade University. Until then, the children with more serious psychiatric disorders, as well as mentally retarded children, were treated together with the adults. In 1978, this unit became an independent Department for Children and Adolescents and in 1982 the Institute for Neurology and Psychiatry for Children and Adolescents. Since 1986, it has been called the Clinic for Neurology and Psychiatry for Children and Adolescents. The first exclusively psychiatric department for children and adolescents was founded in 1963 within the Institute of Mental Health in Belgrade. In other larger cities (Novi Sad, Nis), the counseling centers, outpatient, and inpatient units of similar type began to be founded.

The founding of the first counseling centers, outpatient, clinical and hospital units for children and adolescents went closely in step with the education of physicians, neuropsychiatrists, psychologists, social workers, and other experts in the country and abroad, particularly in France and England.

From its beginning until the present, the theoretical orientation in child and adolescent psychiatry and psychotherapy has been psychodynamic and psychoanalytical, as well as biological, more rarely behavioral and gestalt oriented. A significant advance in the development of child psychiatry was made with the introduction of the subject of neuropsychology, based on the theories of Luria and Piaget.

The appearance of the first handbooks contributed to the faster development of psychiatric services and the psychiatry of childhood and adolescence, i.e. "The Psychopathology of Childhood and Adolescence" by V. Matic (1953); "Mental Hygiene" by V. Matic and M. Jojic-Milenkovic (1957); "Neuropsychology of Developmental Age and General Re-Educative Methods" by S. Bojanin (1979); "Childhood and Adolescence Psychiatry" by N. Tadic (1980); "Psychotherapy of Children and Adolescents" by N. Tadic (1984); "Social Psychiatry of Developmental Age" by S. Bojanin and K. Radulovic (1988); "Psychoanalytical Psychotherapy of Children and Adolescents" by N. Tadic and coworkers (1992).

There is no special journal for child psychiatry, but "Psychiatry Today" has been published (earlier Annals of the Institute of Mental Health) regularly since 1969, with topical issues devoted to child psychiatry.

Thanks to the development of services, increased interest and education of professionals, as well as publishing activities, the section for Child Neuropsychiatry of the Serbian Medical Association was established in 1970 and later the Yugoslav Association for Child and Adolescent Psychiatry and Related Fields (JUDEDAP) (1979) and the Association for Developmental Age Neurology and Psychiatry (1979).

In time, the sections and associations have become members of the European and international associations. In the work of the sections and associations, physicians (neuropsychiatrists, neurologists, psychiatrist, pediatricians) participate as regular members, and psychologists, special teachers, pedagogues, social workers, and other related professionals as associated members.

Recent advances

In the beginning, the development of child and adolescent psychiatry was initiated mostly by educated and highly motivated professionals and institutions. Later, the suggestions and recommendations for the organization and coordination of services, education, number of personnel and programs, were issued by the Sub-Commission for Child and Adolescent Psychiatry and Psychotherapy, established within the Commission for Psychiatry of the Ministry of Health of Serbia.

The division of neuropsychiatry into neurology and psychiatry (1989) was very significant for further development, as well as later separation of child and adolescent from adult psychiatry with the introduction of a separate four-year specialization in child and adolescent psychiatry (1992).

Current situation

According to the data of the Federal Bureau for Statistics, at the end of 1994 Yugoslavia had 10,536,183 inhabitants. Out of this number, there were 22.4% (2,346,446) children from 0–14 and 7.6 % (758,212) adolescents from 15–19 years of age. This means there are a total of 3,104,664 children and adolescents aged 0–19, i.e., 30.1 % of the total population.

The Subcommission for Child and Adolescent Psychiatry of the Ministry of Health recommended in 1985 that mental health care of children and adolescents in Yugoslavia should be organized on principles of comprehensive mental health care in the community. The proposed model emphasized the need for expansion of the network of Outpatient Mental Health Units for Children and Adolescents in Health Centers and their linking with the primary health care of women and children and the community.

Although the proposed model was accepted, its implementation was slow and partial and put into effect only in certain areas. The reasons are found in radical changes in social context and the fall in economic potential of the country, particularly during the last ten years.

The problem is that even the existing services are not uniformly distributed. There are parts without any service, mental health unit or even child development counseling service, thus, preventing rendering of mental health care to children and adolescents in areas far away from larger centers.

Another problem is the insufficient number of specialists for child and adolescent psychiatry and psychotherapy. Out of the total of 817 neuropsychiatrists and psychiatrists, the majority is engaged in psychiatry of adults in hospitals, and only 57 (7 %) are exclusively or predominantly engaged in neuropsychiatry of children and adolescents. This means that the ratio is one child neuropsychiatrist per 184,000 inhabitants, i.e., per 54,467 children and adolescents. The number of specialists engaged exclusively in psychiatry and psychotherapy or psychoanalysis of children and adolescents is even smaller. We expect that the situation will soon improve as the education of young professionals specializing in child and adolescent psychiatry, introduced six years ago, is in course. There remains the question, however, to what extent it will be possible to extend the services, i.e., to open new working posts for these young specialists in the present situation in the country.

Recent war and postwar events in the territory of the former Yugoslavia, economic sanctions, and the decrease in the number of professionals significantly affected overall mental health care of children and adolescents despite the aid provided by the humanitarian organizations in the country and from abroad (UNICEF, Save the Children, etc.).

There are about 700,000 refugees in the country, mostly from Croatia and Bosnia and Herzegovina. About 215,000 of them are children under 18 years of age (UNICEF data).

The number of children, adolescents, and their parents in need of help is increasing. According to some studies, 13,5 % of children in the general population and 62% of refugee children suffer from moderate or more serious psychological difficulties and disorders as a reaction to experienced traumas and chronic stress situations in which they live.

2. Classification systems, diagnostic and therapeutic methods

Classification systems

The classification system ICD-10 is officially adopted and obligatorily used in Yugoslavia. For scientific research, the system DSM-IV is also used.

Diagnostic methods

Classical methods like interviews, clinical-psychiatric observation, neurological, psychological, special education assessment methods, and EEG recordings are used in outpatient and inpatient services. More advanced methods like neuropsychological assessment, genetic, special laboratory and imaging technics are carried out by inpatient departments or services linked to university centers.

Therapeutic methods

The majority of services apply psychodynamic psychotherapy, Rogers' counseling, support psychotherapy, psychoanalytic psychotherapy (more rarely psychoanalysis), psychopharmacotherapy, sociotherapy, individual and group work with parents, and families, psychomotor re-education, speech therapy, and neuropsychological treatment and pedagogic re-education.

3. Structure and organization of services

Guidelines for services for children and adolescents with psychiatric disorders

The basic guidelines for the structure, organization, and development of services are issued by the Institute for Mental Health and the Clinic for Neurology and Psychiatry for Children and Adolescents in Belgrade. They were appointed by the Commission for Psychiatry of the Ministry of Health of Serbia as the republic methodological centers for development of child psychiatry. The Sub-Commission for Child and Adolescent Psychiatry consisting of prominent professionals has recommended the following:

- It is necessary to harmonize the basic conceptions about mental health care, programs of work, organization of services, and to synchronize the education, type, and number of personnel, equipment, and other significant components.
- Mental health care of children and adults should be organized according to principles of comprehensive psychiatric care. Each health center, responsible for basic primary care within a municipality with 150,000 to 200,000 inhabitants (i.e., 50,000–60,000 of children and adolescents from 0–18 years of age) should establish an outpatient mental health service with a special unit for children and adolescents. Each pediatric outpatient service should organize a child development counseling service (CDCS) for prevention of mental health disorders in at risk children. These services should be horizontally linked with other related medical, social, preschool, and school institutions, homes for placement of children and young people in their territories, and vertically with competent higher order services in the country.

These and other recommendations have been only partially implemented until the present.

Types of services

In Yugoslavia a three level system of services for mental health care of children and adolescents exists.

Level I

- Counseling Center for Pregnant Women
- Counseling Center for Preschool Children
- Counseling Center for School Children
- Child Development Counseling Service
- Psychological service in kindergartens and schools
- Center for Social Work

At the level of primary health care there are 399 Counseling Centers for Pregnant Women (one physician per 7,000 pregnant women), 452 Counseling Centers for Preschool Children (one physician/1,000 children), and 363 Counseling Centers for School Children (one physician/3,000 children). Nearly all schools and kindergartens have a psychological service (on average one psychologist per 1,500 children).

It is recommended that all pediatricians and home visiting and medical nurses in primary health care services should be trained for counseling.

Child Development Counseling Services (CDCS), as functional units within pediatric primary health care in health centers, have a special and important role in providing mental health care to at risk children and their parents. They are also responsible for treatment of children with mild psychological difficulties and disabilities and for referral of children with more serious disorders and disabilities to specialized psychiatric, social, and other institutions.

Child Development Counseling Service should follow the incidence and prevalence of at risk children and disabled children, as well as children with mild developmental disorders in its territory. The CDCS team consists of a pediatrician, a psychologist, special teachers, and eventually a social worker, employed on a full-time or part-time basis. The team undergoes a special one-year training in mental health care of at risk children and for psychodynamic and Rogers' type of counseling. At present, about 160 members of multidisciplinary CDCS teams and about 250 home visiting and medical nurses have passed the above training.

The CDCS network expanded rapidly during the last several years in response to a large number of refugees and traumatized children in need of psychosocial help. There were 16 CDCS in 1991, and now there are 40 CDCS. The training of personnel and the expansion of network have been significantly helped by UNICEF and the Swedish/Norwegian organization "Save the Children".

The Centers for Social Work (a total of 160) are entrusted, in addition to other functions, with adoption and placement of children without parental care and expertize in divorce and custody cases.

Level II

Outpatient mental health units for children and adolescents

There are 14 such units in health centers (an average of one unit per 220,000 children up to the age of 18). The problem is, however, the disproportionate territorial distribution of these services, so out of the total of 14 units 6 are in

Belgrade and there is only one in Montenegro. In regions without such services, the basic psychiatric care of children and young people is provided by adult mental health outpatient units.

The outpatient units diagnose and treat children and adolescents with more serious psychiatric disorders. They cooperate with the CDCS, psychological services in kindergartens and schools, centers for social work, and other related services and institutions. They also organize preventive measures and follow the incidence and prevalence of psychiatric disorders in their catchment area.

Professional teams in outpatient mental health care units consist of child psychiatrists, psychologists, psychotherapists, psychoanalysts, special teachers, social workers, and, if necessary, other professionals. Outpatient units, in cooperation with Child Development Counseling Services form Commissions for Categorization of Developmentally Disadvantaged Children and Adolescents.

Some outpatient mental health care units, particularly those within hospitals, clinics, and institutes, have specialized services for neuroses, psychoses, suicides, drugabuse, and psychotherapy and psychoanalysis of children and adolescents.

Level III

Level III services include:

- Inpatient services
- Daypatient services
- Institutions for placement of children without parental care
- Institutions for placement of mentally retarded and disabled children and adolescents
- Specialized institutions for treatment of children with social behavior disorders

There are 5 inpatient departments mostly at university centers. The total capacity is 80 beds, meaning 38,000 children per 1 bed. Some specialized units, for instance, for epilepsy, convulsions, and psychosomatic disorders, are situated in pediatric inpatient services. Inpatient services carry out more complex diagnostic procedures, treat, and rehabilitate children and adolescents with more serious psychiatric disorders (neuroses, psychoses, suicides, drugabuse, and others).

There are only two daypatient services (30 places). This is still an insufficiently represented form of mental health care despite its professional and economic justifications.

The accommodation and care of mentally retarded and disabled children and adolescents is provided by 26 specialized institutions with the total capacity of 2,400 places. They are funded by Ministries of Health, Education, and Social Welfare.

The rehabilitation of children and adolescents with the social behavioral disorders (pre-delinquent or anti-social behavior) is provided by six specialized institutions.

The institutions for adoption, family, and institutionalized placement, in cooperation with centers for social work, CDCS, and, if necessary, with mental health care units, place children without parental care in foster families and homes, and undertake their follow up. These institutions are only in small part funded by the Ministry of Health and in greater part by the Ministry for Social Welfare.

At present 2,000 children without parental care are in foster care and about 2,100 in institutions. About 300–350 children of younger age are adopted each year.

The trend is to treat and rehabilitate as many children and adolescents as possible under outpatient and non-institutionalized conditions, in families, and to reduce inpatient time of stay as much as possible.

Complementary services and rehabilitation

For the time being, there are no other forms of treatment and rehabilitation except the above mentioned ones.

Personnel

The relationship in number of personnel and patients in outpatient and inpatient services is partly regulated by the Ministries of Health and Social Welfare and partly by institutions, subject to specific activities and funds provided by health insurance.

Funding of services

After the Second World War, Yugoslavia introduced free health and social care of all children and adolescents up to 18 years of age for all types of health and social services. Health costs in GNP range from 4.6–6 %. However, due to enormous fall in the total social product after 1991, the funds allocated are insufficient to meet the previous levels of health care. The system of health care must undergo radical changes with a probable decrease in the level of services offered without payment.

Evaluation

Systematic or more comprehensive evaluation of mental health services for children and adolescents has not yet been made.

4. Cooperation with medical and non-medical disciplines

Cooperation with pediatrics

Theoretical and practical links between pediatrics and child psychiatry are the most obvious in the field of primary mental health care of children and adolescents, in the work of Child Development Counseling Services. In addition, children from 0–3 years of age with neuropsychiatric disorders (convulsions, epilepsy, encephalopathies, psychosomatic disorders, and mental retardation) are somewhat more frequently admitted to inpatient pediatric and neurological services, which are better equipped for their treatment.

Despite the observed and frequently emphasized need a psychologist is rarely included as a permanent team member in pediatric and other child services (endocrinological, nephrological, surgical, for malignant diseases). Most frequently the psychologist, psychiatrist, and eventually psychotherapists from inpatient psychiatric service are called as consultants.

Cooperation with psychiatry

The outpatient and inpatient psychiatric services for children and adolescents are frequently linked to general psychiatric services for adults. This facilitates the cooperation between the teams for children, adolescents, and adults (the parents). In addition to this, young people between 16 and 18 years of age are often treated in general psychiatric departments because child psychiatric units are inadequate for their treatment.

Cooperation with doctors in private practice

Private psychiatric and psychotherapeutic practice in Yugoslavia has only started to develop, and it is outside the health insurance system. There is no organized cooperation, except personal contacts.

Cooperation with non-medical institutions and professionals

The cooperation with related non-medical institutions, such as psychological services in kindergartens and schools, centers for social work, adoption commissions, family and home placement of children, as well as with other specialized institutions for children and adolescents, is generally good. In addition, occasionally, particularly under war conditions, good cooperation was established with mass media, humanitarian, religious and the Red Cross organizations.

5. Graduate/postgraduate training and continuing medical education

Graduate training: The role of medical faculties

There is no special subject in child and adolescent psychiatry in graduate curriculum at the four existing schools of medicine. Students are offered the basic knowledge in these fields within the subject of psychiatry. At the chairs of psychology at three faculties of philosophy, the subjects of psychopathology of childhood and youth are taught, and at the faculty for special education child psychiatry as a part of the subjects neurology, psychiatry, and neuropsychology.

Postgraduate training, a joint effort

Until 1989 the specialization in neuropsychiatry lasted only 3 years and later 4 years. A number of neuropsychiatrists have shown special interest in child and adolescent psychiatry. They received additional 2 years sub-specialistic training in developmental neurology and psychiatry. From 1982 until 1992, that is, before the introduction of child psychiatry as an independent specialization, 18 professionals completed this subspecialization.

In 1989 the specialization in neuropsychiatry was divided into neurology and psychiatry, and in 1992 two separate, basic 4-year specializations were added: child neurology and child psychiatry. The curriculum in child psychiatry includes theoretical and practical instruction in the following fields: child psychiatry (24 months), adolescent psychiatry (5 months), adult psychiatry (10 months), child neurology (6 months), pediatrics (2 months), otorhinolaryngology (15 days), ophtalmology (15 days). There are obligatory colloquia in the following fields: neuropsychology, psychological development theories, mental and behavior disorders in early childhood, school age, and adolescence, the treatment of psychiatric disorders in childhood and adolescence (psychodynamic, family, cognitive, behavioral psychotherapy and counseling), and psychopharmacotherapy. At the end of the specialist training, a final examination has to be passed before the commission of the School of Medicine.

A subspecialization "Psychodynamic psychotherapy of children and adolescents" was introduced in 1978 together with the subspecialization "Psychodynamic psychotherapy of adults" for specialists in neuropsychiatry, pediatricians, and clinical psychologists. In 1990, these two subspecialization were joined and transformed into the subspecialization "Psychoanalytical psychotherapy". It also provides knowledge and skills for psychoanalytical psychotherapy of children and adolescents. The psychotherapeutic curriculum includes about 200 hours of theoretical instruction, at least 300 hours of personal psychotherapy, 150 hours of individual, 100 hours of group supervision, and a specialist paper as a final examination.

We think that the International Psychoanalytic Association's recognition of the status of psychoanalysts and training analysts to six members of the Belgrade group for psychoanalysis will have very significant impact on further advance of the profession as they are predominantly working with children and adolescents.

Advanced education of professionals engaged in psychiatry of children and adolescents is also carried out in the form of master of science and doctoral studies in "neuropsychology", "social psychiatry", and a 3-year specialization in clinical psychology for bachelors in psychology.

Until the present, more than 30 psychiatrists and psychologists have obtained their M.Sc. and Ph.D. degrees in child and adolescent psychiatry, psychotherapy, and psychology. Educators from abroad (Great Britain, France) have also participated in the above forms of post-graduate studies.

Training programs for other disciplines

The institutes and university clinics organize the education for psychologists, social workers, pediatricians, special teachers, educators, psychiatric nurses, and other related professionals. The education is organized through special programs in mental hygiene, psychotherapy, neuropsychology, family therapy.

6. Research

Research fields and strategies

During the last twenty years, in addition to the research within individual master of sciences and doctoral theses, extensive research studies encompassing topics in child and adolescent psychiatry and psychotherapy were either completed or are still in progress, such as:

- Clinical, neuropsychological, and neurophysiological aspects of psychiatric disorders in childhood and adolescence (neuroses, depressions, suicides, schizophrenia, autism, hyperkinetic syndrome);
- Comparative investigation of classifications in child and adolescent psychiatry (ICD-10 and French Classification);
- Epidemiological and neuropsychological research of developmental disorders and possibilities for their prevention, treatment within the primary health care system and in schools;
- The promotion of psychosocial development of children through primary health care, WHO/EU Multicenter Study;
- Neuropsychological diagnostics and rehabilitation of children with focal and diffuse brain damage (joint project with Burden Neurological Institute, Bristol, U.K.);
- Children and adolescents in war and exile – reactions, consequences, possibilities of prevention and treatment;
- The evaluation of psychosocial help for children and adolescents living in adverse conditions.

It is obvious that the research in the field of epidemiology, evaluation of therapeutic methods, services and quality assurance are still insufficiently represented. In view of the significance of this research for the improvement of mental health care of children and adolescents, we consider they should be given priority in the future and be provided with necessary funds.

Research training and career development

The training for research is carried out within post-graduate master of sciences and doctoral studies. However, it is for general medical research. It will be essential to organize special courses for researchers in the field of psychiatry and psychology.

Funding

The majority of research projects have been funded by the Federal or Republic Ministry for Science and Technology. Joint programs with foreign partners enjoyed the support of the Federal Ministry, also in the form of the exchange of professionals, while all other costs were covered by the institutions responsible for projects. During the recent war years, the resources for funding of research were greatly decreased. It has been possible to continue with research, even in a reduced form, only thanks to the enthusiasm and devotion of the researchers. It is obvious that the question of funding will play a decisive role in the future development of research in child and adolescent psychiatry in Yugoslavia.

7. Future perspectives

The future work on mental health care and child and adolescent psychiatry in Yugoslavia should develop in several directions:

- The expansion and better organization and distribution of the network of comprehensive mental health care of children and adolescents, particularly of outpatient services. This also includes the development of psychiatric daypatient services and other alternative forms of mental health care (youth clubs, family placement of children without parental care, etc.).
- The education of medical and related non-medical personnel for prevention, psychotherapy, and sociotherapy both in the country and abroad.
- Stimulation of research, particularly evaluation of preventive and therapeutic methods and quality assurance.
- The admission of the Association for Child and Adolescent Psychiatry as a member in corresponding European and international associations.

There is no doubt that the fulfillment of these plans and future development of child and adolescent psychiatry in Yugoslavia will depend on the general development of the social and economic situation in the country.

Selected references

Bojanin S (1979) Neuropsychology of Developmental Age and General Re-Educative Methods (in Serbian: Neuropsihologija razvojnog doba i opsti reedukativni metod) Privredna stampa, Beograd

Bojanin S, Radulovic K (1988) Social Psychology of Developmental Age (in Serbian: Socijalna psihijatrija razvojnog doba) Naucna knjiga, Beograd
Matic V (1953) The Psychopathology of Childhood and Adolescence (in Serbian: Psihopatologija detinjstva i mladosti) Filozofski fakultet, Beograd
Matic V, Jojic-Milenkovic M (1957) Mental Hygiene (in Serbian: Mentalna higijena) Filozofski fakultet, Beograd
Tadic N (1980) Childhood and Adolescence Psychiatry (in Serbian: Psihijatrija detinjstva i mladosti) Naucna knjiga, Beograd
Tadic N (1984) Psychotherapy of Children and Adolescents (in Serbian: Psihoterapija dece i omladine) Naucna knjiga, Beograd
Tadic N (ed) (1992) Psychoanalytic Psychotherapy of Children and Adolescents (in Serbian: Psihoanaliticka psihoterapija dece i mladih) Naucna knjiga, Beograd

Child and adolescent psychiatry in Slovakia

J. Pečeňák

1. Definition, historical development, and current situation

Definition

Child and adolescent psychiatry is not an independent discipline in Slovakia. It is considered a special field of general psychiatry.

Historical development

The history of Slovak psychiatry can be dated back to 1919 when the Czechoslovak State University (nowadays Comenius University) was founded in Bratislava. The Clinic for Nervous and Mental Diseases existed as a part of the medical faculty from the beginning. It was transformed from the department for mentally ill people in the state hospital founded in the year 1864; this department had been a part of it ever since. It is quite clear from the name of the department that it was a neuro-psychiatric approach that dominated in psychiatry at that time. The division of it into independent psychiatry and neurology came in 1950.

The development of psychiatry in Slovakia was very insufficient until the end of the Second World War. The ratio of beds in the departments of psychiatry between the Czechia and Slovakia was 1:50. The first regional psychiatric departments were not founded before 1935. At that time the first psychiatric hospitals were also founded. In addition, a family care system for mentally ill people in agricultural regions in the south of Slovakia have been in existance since the beginning of the century.

Child and adolescent psychiatry separated as a field in general psychiatry after creating the first departments for children within the adult psychiatric departments and after the establishment of child psychiatry as a specialized field of psychiatry with the possibility of making an attestation (postgraduate examination) in the field. Previously, general psychiatrists, pediatricians, and neurologists with interest in child psychiatry provided care for children with mental disorders. There were no beds for mentally ill children, and those with mental retardation and probably other more severe mental disorders were placed in social institutions without a special therapy.

The first departments for children in psychiatric facilities were founded in 1941 and 1951 in the Psychiatric Hospital Pezinok. The departments were dedicated for children with epilepsy and reflected a neuro-psychiatric approach of the field. They both had only limited functions, i.e., were in existence for only a short time.

The first department for children, which is still in existence, is the Department for Children at the Department of Psychiatry affiliated with the University Hospital in Bratislava. It was founded in the first half of the 1950s. In this department worked the first psychiatrists who specialized in child and adolescent psychiatry. This department formed a basis for founding the Department of Child Psychiatry affiliated with the University Hospital for Children in Bratislava in 1982. The new department became the first and until now the only independent department of child psychiatry in Slovakia affiliated to a medical faculty.

The first physicians (pediatricians or general psychiatrists) passed their attestation (postgraduate examination) in Slovakia in child psychiatry in 1971. There has been the possibility to pass the attestation in child psychiatry as a specialized field of general psychiatry since 1962 in Prague. 51 child psychiatrists have passed the attestation in Slovakia since 1971; 12 of them passed their attestation since 1993 – in Slovakia as an independent state. In 1995 the subdepartment for Child Psychiatry in the Department of Psychiatry, Institute of Postgradual Studies in Medicine, was established. This department is a part of the Department of Child Psychiatry, University Hospital for Children, Bratislava. Three child psychiatrists passed their attestation at this subdepartment.

In 1971 the Pedopsychiatric Section of the Slovak Psychiatric Association was founded. It changed its name to the Section of Child and Adolescent Psychiatry in 1992.

In 1962 the first Child Guidance Clinics under the Ministry of Education were founded. These clinics are still existing in a transformed state. In 1964, the Institute for Study of Child psychology and Pathopsychology was founded. The institute started to publish the Journal of Child Psychology and Pathopsychology in 1966. The institute and its journal are orientated to a broad spectrum of psychological and pedagogical concerns. Many topics, which they are concerned with, are close to clinical child psychiatry.

Recent advances

The fundamental change during the recent years was the establishment of the subdepartment of child psychiatry as the base for postgraduate training in 1995. It is expected that this institutional basis will initiate further development in the field.

In 1997, the new Concept of Psychiatry was published by the Ministry of Health. Child psychiatry is defined as a special field of general psychiatry, not as an independent discipline.

Since the change of the political system in our country, an innumerable number of foundations have been established. Their activities are orientated toward helping children with various kinds of disorders or problems. The cooperation with child psychiatry in fulfilling these aims is insufficient.

One of the most important results of the political changes is a continuous changing of general approaches to people with mental retardation. There are positive changes in institutional care for children with mental retardation. Several new daycare centers or centers for week-staying were founded. Foundation of several centers for children with autism in healthcare and educational institutions is a very significant success. The activity of the SPOSA (Society for Help People with Autism) which is an organization for parents, professionals, and interested laymen has been an important stimulus. There are several other organizations which are very active, e.g., an organization to help people with Down's syndrome. In the health care system and in the non-state foundations, the activity for protection of maltreated and abused children is being developed continuously.

Since the split up of Czechoslovakia, the contacts and cooperation between Czech and Slovak psychiatry have been preserved. The journal "Czech and Slovak Psychiatry" is still the common journal for the both the Czech and Slovak Psychiatric Societies.

Since 1994 a new journal "Psychiatria" is published in Slovakia in which articles on child and adolescent psychiatry are also published.

The tendency of taking care of adolescents (up to 18 years) in all pediatric medical fields is important. Previously all pediatric fields only took care of the children up to 15 years. Considering the "child" as children up to 15 years and "adolescent" as people up to 18 years is a result of the rules of state statistics (up to 15 years there is a compulsory school attendance).

Current situation

At the end of 1996, the population of Slovakia was 5,373,810, among them 1,164,906 children up to 14 years and 468,872 adolescents between 15 and 19 years. This is 1.6 million children and adolescents, which is about 30 % of the total population. The tendency of the population trend is unfavorable. Since the 1980s the number of live births has been continuously falling. In 1992, there were 74,640 live births, in 1996 only 60,123.

At present there are eight inpatient psychiatric departments for children and adolescents in Slovakia with 318 beds. According to official statistics the ratio is 2.3 beds : 10,000 children. The number of children and adolescents hospitalized in 1996 divided by age and diagnosis is given in Table 1.

Table 1. Number of patients 0–17 years* hospitalized in psychiatric departments in 1996 according to age and ICD-10 diagnosis

ICD-10 diagnostic group	age (years)				
	4	5	6–9	10–14	15–17
F00 – 09			11	21	5
F10 – F19				33	274
F20 – 29		2	2	16	130
F30 – 39			1	6	30
F40 – 48		1	22	81	139
F50 – 59	1		4	8	26
F60 – 69			1	10	88
F70 – 79	12	10	71	154	137
F80 – 89	10	8	30	22	21
F90 – 98	34	46	320	602	113
F99			3	3	74
Total	57	67	465	956	1037

*No hospitalization up to 3 years

Three of eight departments for children and adolescents are affiliated with University Hospitals. The Child Psychiatry Clinic, which is an independent department, is part of the University Hospital for Children in Bratislava and is affiliated with the Faculty of Medicine. There is a subdepartment for Child Psychiatry (under the Department of Psychiatry) in the Institute for Postgraduate Studies in Medicine. The subdepartment is responsible for organization of postgraduate examination in child psychiatry as a specialized discipline within general psychiatry.

The departments of psychiatry (general) in Bratislava and Martin which are affiliated with the Faculties of Medicine, have units for children and adolescents. The University Department of Psychiatry in Košice has no beds for children.

Other departments for children and adolescents are within psychiatric hospitals; there is also only one specialized psychiatric hospital for children located in East Slovakia.

Some of the departments have specialized units or have specialized in some clinical problems. For example, the department for children at the Department of Psychiatry in Bratislava is orientated at treatment of eating disorders; the Psychiatric Hospital in Pezinok has a unit for treatment of drug-dependent adolescents. In the Department of Child Psychiatry in Bratislava there is a unit for preschool aged children.

There is not a sufficient regional distribution of inpatient departments for children. There are whole regions without any inpatient units. Adult departments also admit adolescents over 15 years, but it is not a very suitable solution.

In Bratislava there are two daycare clinics for children; one of them is orientated toward the care of preschool children.

Outpatient care is provided by 41 outpatient units. In a part of them, mostly in units which are affiliated to inpatient departments, child psychiatrists with only part-time duty are working. A part of the outpatient services are private. In 1996, 7,849 patients were examined for the first time with the diagnosis F 90 – F 98 (Institute for Health Information and Statistic 1996).

The Section of Child and Adolescent Psychiatry is a part of the Slovak Psychiatric Association. It has 113 members at this time. The section organizes two or three scientific conferences during the year, but the members of the section also take part in conferences organized by other societies within the Slovak Medical Association.

2. Classification systems, diagnostic and therapeutic methods

Classification systems

ICD-10 is the official classification system. It is obligatory and is used also for documentation and for the purpose of health statistics. In practice some other diagnostic categories, which are not components of ICD-10 are used, e.g., the diagnosis of minimal brain dysfunction or "neurotic development". In spite of using this kind of diagnosis, the psychiatrist is obliged to code the diagnosis according to ICD-10, using the most appropriate code. Formalized multiaxial diagnostic system is used occasionally.

At inpatient departments, the basic part of the patient's file is documentation of psychiatric assessment. It contains data about family and personal history given by the parents, data given by patient (if possible), objective findings, list of symptoms, psychopathological and differential diagnostic considerations, diagnosis and proposed therapeutic interventions, and recommended plan of other investigations. This structure of documentation is used generally, though not officially recommended. The documentation in outpatient units is usually not so detailed, but the documentation of the first assessment should contain similar components.

Diagnostic methods

A broad spectrum of diagnostic methods is used. The basis is psychiatric assessment and other diagnostic procedures indicated. Psychological testing is a common part of the complex investigation. The psychologist decides about the appropriate test for answering the questions given by the psychiatrist. Different tests for intelligence and projective performance tests are used. Drawing the person and other drawing tests or techniques are also broadly used by psychiatrists. Concerning the related disciplines, the pediatric, neurological, and genetic examination and consultation are required most often. EEG recording is possible in some of the departments. CT and very rarely MRI (because of little accessibility) are usually performed only after the recommendation by the neurologist.

Therapeutic methods

The spectrum of available therapeutic methods depends on personnel and technical equipment of departments and on the approach of the psychiatrist. The pharmacotherapy, psychotherapy (behavioral, psychodynamic, family therapy), methods of special pedagogy, and rehabilitation techniques are used.

In comparison to the data from Western Europe and the USA, a broader spectrum of psychopharmacotherapy is used for children, but not one psychostimulant clinically verified abroad (e.g., methylphenidat) is registered for clinical use in Slovakia. Neuroleptics are used for therapy of quite a broad spectrum of disorders. We have had a long clinical experience with clozapine, the first experience with risperidone in child psychiatry, and tiaprid is used for therapy of tic disorder. SSRI (citalopram) was used in clinical studies as a therapy for eating disorders. Recently, the process of new registration of drugs according to the standards in the European Union is running in our country. A restriction of the psychopharmacotherapy in childhood could be expected.

3. Structure and organization of services

Guidelines for services for children and adolescents with psychiatric disorders

According to the new Concept of Psychiatry published in the Bulletin of Ministry of Health in 1997, the basis for building up the net of psychiatric services should be the "standard region of psychiatric care". It is planned for a geographic area with a population of 100,000 – 150,000. Appropriate accessibility of psychiatric services is given either by the distance of 50 km or accessibility by public transportation lasting not more than one hour. Every region of standard care should have an outpatient unit for child psychiatry; the inpatient departments should serve more than one region.

No special standards for building up the net of psychiatric services for child and adolescent psychiatry exist. There are several reasons; one of the main ones has been a substantial change of regional organization of the country in 1996. Eight regions of state administration (four before 1996) and 79 districts (38 before 1996) were created. At the time when only 38 districts existed, every district should have its outpatient unit for child and adolescent psychiatry. The new organization of the country demands setting up of a new plan for regional development of psychiatric services. For example, in the region of Prešov with 770,000 inhabitants, there are three pedopsychiatric outpatient units and no inpatient departments; in the region of Bratislava (619,000 inhabitants), there are 12 outpatient units and more than 100 beds for children.

Types of services

Different types of child and adolescent psychiatric services in the health care system are given in Table 2, and complementary services which are outside the health care system in Table 3.

Outpatient, daypatient, and inpatient services

Table 2. Services of child and adolescent psychiatry in the health care system

Type of services	No of services/No of beds	Comment
Departments affiliated with university hospitals and faculties of medicine	3/56 beds	One of them an independent pedopsychiatric department
Departments for child and adolescent psychiatry which are parts of departments of psychiatry in general hospitals	2/33 beds	Both are separated from departments for adults. The Department of Child Psychiatry in Nitra is located in the Hospital for Children.
Departments of child and adolescent psychiatry in psychiatric hospitals	3/230 beds	One specialized psychiatric hospital for children (90 beds)

Studies in Medicine, the unit for early intervention for children with developmental disorders has been established. It is proposed to establish similar centers in other regions of Slovakia.

The capacity of inpatient pediatric departments has decreased (4,500 beds in 1992, 3,500 in 1996) because of the population trend and the privatization of pediatric outpatient units. Pediatricians in private practice recommend fewer patients for hospitalization.

In the process of transformation of the health care system, the number of specialized outpatient units for adolescents was rapidly decreased (177 physicians for adolescents in the state health care system in 1992, 22 in 1996).

Cooperation with psychiatry

The association with general psychiatry is essential for the existence and future development of the child and adolescent psychiatry at this time. The main support for the field comes from the side of general psychiatry – much more support than from, e.g., pediatrics.

Departments of child and adolescent psychiatry and some of the outpatient units belong to general psychiatry departments. The Section of Child and Adolescent Psychiatry is a section of the Slovak Psychiatric Association. The subdepartment of Child Psychiatry belongs to the Department of Psychiatry, Institute for Postgraduate Studies in Medicine.

Child psychiatry, similar as other pediatric disciplines, gradually starts to take care for adolescents (age from 15 to 18 years). Hospitalization of adolescents over 15 years is still more often realized at adult departments.

Cooperation with doctors in private practice

Privatization of health services brought new aspects. Funding of health services by insurance companies, which depends on the amount of diagnostic and therapeutic procedures, has changed some approaches compared with the past. The influence of privatization of services on the cooperation among physicians of different disciplines has not been evaluated. But physicians in private practice are supposed to try to manage more cases by themselves with fewer recommendations for hospitalization and for consultation with specialists.

Cooperation with non-medical institutions and professionals

Complex care for child psychiatric disorders requires coordination among several disciplines and institutions.

Pedagogical-Psychological Counseling Centers under the Ministry of Education have psychologists and pedagogues working in them. Some of them are orientated more to psychotherapy, some to diagnostic and therapy of learning disorders. The main objective is counseling in cases of behavioral or educational problems at school. They often manage children and families with problems, which would require psychiatric consultation. In some centers, child psychiatrists are working part-time.

Pedagogical-Psychological Counseling Centers also have the competency to recommend appropriate schools for children with some kinds of disorders. In some cases, hospitalization for diagnostic purposes of learning disorders in a child psychiatric department is recommended.

Children before being placed in foster homes undergo a diagnostic stay at the Diagnostic Center for Children which is a non-medical institution.

The Department of Care for Child and Family is affiliated with every district council. This institution can provide monitoring of families if there are some signs of abuse or neglect of children; social workers can also provide objective data about the family. Psychiatrists can initiate this monitoring. The council department is competent to decide (preliminary) about placing the child in institutional care. The definitive judgment on institutional care is in the control of the court.

The cooperation with psychologists and special therapeutists in private services is just starting to develop. There are two ways of running the private practice for clinical psychologists-psychotherapists. The first possibility is a contract with a health insurance company; the second is the independent service fully paid by clients. This kind of service is licensed by the Psychologist Chamber. Independent diagnostic and therapeutic activity of non-medical professionals is not fully legally covered; insurance companies usually require that recommendation for therapy should be done only after the assessment by a physician.

5. Graduate/postgraduate training and continuing medical education

Graduate training: The role of medical faculties

There are three faculties of medicine in Slovakia – in Bratislava, Martin, and Košice. Teaching and training of child and adolescent psychiatry is incorporated into teaching and training of general psychiatry and medical psychology. At the Faculty of Medicine in Bratislava, the teaching is organized in cooperation between two departments – Department of Psychiatry and the independent Department of Child Psychiatry. The exam questions on child and adolescent psychiatry represent 8 % of all the questions. In Bratislava the students have the possibility to select child psychiatry as one of the obligatory selected subjects of study. In Martin, the students have the possibility to receive some training in child psychiatry at their own decision, and in Košice, there is a lecture on adolescent psychiatry in the pediatrics course in the last year of study.

Postgraduate training, a joint effort

The system of postgraduate professional training in Slovakia is based on the categories according to the so-called basic disciplines and specialized disciplines.

As to the basic disciplines (psychiatry is among them together with internal medicine, surgery, pediatrics, etc.), so-called attestation (postgraduate examination) of the first and second degree can be passed. Child psychiatry is a specialized discipline. The training in specialized disciplines can officially start only after having passed the first or second attestation in the basic discipline. In the case of child psychiatry, the first attestation either in pediatrics or general psychiatry is obligatory.

This system of postgraduate attestation will probably be changed to the system of only one postgraduate attestation after six years of practice. This change is not fully prepared at this time.

Table 4. Training curriculum for attestation in child psychiatry

Theoretical knowledge:
(a) in the field of specialization • principles of prevention in child and adolescent psychiatry • normal development and basic theories of development • social influences involved in child development (environmental factors, family issues – communication within family, type of child rearing, etc.) • deprivation, separation, foster care, parents with severe somatic illness • nosology in child and adolescent psychiatry • drug dependency • suicidality • pharmacotherapy • psychotherapy, crisis intervention • daycare centers, cooperation with education system, cooperation with social and legal institutions • reeducation, rehabilitation, health resort care • long-term monitoring of children with mental disorders and children of parents with mental disorders • expert opinion for courts
(b) theoretical knowledge in related disciplines • human genetics and genetic disorders • emotional aspects of somatic disorders • physiology and pathophysiology of CNS, developmental neurology • basic knowledge in clinical psychology, effectiveness of psychological assessment
Practical knowledge, experience, and proficiency:
• complex clinical assessment of the child with an indication and interpretation of other examinations • setting up the plan for investigation and treatment • documentation of findings • gathering information about the child • ability to interact with the child in different manners • group interaction, therapeutic group • health education • preparing the parents for hospitalization of their child • organization and management of psychiatric care for children and adolescents
Principle of cooperation with other disciplines, expert opinion in the field:
• psychiatric emergency • liaison psychiatry • cooperation with district pediatrician • cooperation with educational system, assessment of ability for school attendance, recommendation for special education • occupational counseling

The candidate for specialization in child psychiatry with attestation in pediatrics has to spend 30 months at the pedopsychiatric inpatient department and 6 months at the department of general psychiatry. The candidate with the attestation in general psychiatry has to spend 30 months of training at the pedopsychiatric inpatient department and 6 months in the pediatric department. Three months of training in the department for drug dependence and three months in the department orientated on family therapy can be included in the curriculum.

There are no official criteria for the evaluation of postgraduate training before taking the examination, except the obligatory six week training in the Department of Psychiatry and subdepartment of Child Psychiatry of the Institute for Postgraduate Studies in Medicine. This Institute organizes courses, usually one week of lectures, that also include pedopsychiatric topics. But the structured training program for attestation in child psychiatry is not set up. The candidate has to write a thesis for the attestation. It can be a review of a special topic or one's own clinical study. The thesis should demonstrate the knowledge and/or scientific ability.

The components of the training curriculum are listed in Table 4.

Continuing medical education in child and adolescent psychiatry and psychotherapy

No formal requirements for continuing medical education exist. Participation at postgraduate courses organized by the Institute for Postgraduate Studies in Medicine is optional.

Training programs for other disciplines

Child psychiatrists give lectures in some faculties, e.g., at the Faculty of Pedagogy in Bratislava. Occasionally they are involved in courses or training programs in non-medical fields – especially for special pedagogues.

6. Research

Research is underdeveloped in the field of child and adolescent psychiatry. There are many reasons. Possibility to achieve a scientific degree for younger professionals is complicated by the fact that there is no associated professor or professor in the field. Three child psychiatrists have the Ph.D. title; no one is working directly in child and adolescent psychiatry at this time.

Funding of research, not only in child and adolescent psychiatry, is generally insufficient. Research can be funded to a small degree by institutional sources or by the state commission for grants.

Research orientation of child psychiatrists according to published studies are eating disorders and child autism (Department of Psychiatry, Bratislava), and electrophysiology, mental retardation, and psychopharmacotherapy (Department of Psychiatry, Martin). The Department of Child Psychiatry in Bratislava, which is the only independent psychiatric department for children affiliated with the Medical Faculty, devotes its research activities to drug dependency and abused children.

7. Future perspectives

The independent Slovak Republic has been in existence since 1993. This substantial change and previous change of the political system in 1989 brought up many consequences which have also influenced the health care system. The same is also true for state and regional administration. The system of funding health care by health insurance companies was introduced and works only with extreme problems. Mechanisms which would evaluate and monitor the process of privatization of the health care services are not sufficiently developed.

Child and adolescent psychiatry is not considered as a basic discipline and is much more influenced by changing social, economic, and cultural conditions than most of the other disciplines.

Research

It is very important to have basic epidemiological studies which would reflect the prevalence of mental disorders in our population of children and adolescents, and epidemiological data would serve as arguments for the future development of the discipline. Lack of sources devoted to research could be overcome by interdisciplinary designed projects and by involvement in international studies. Also, cooperation with adult psychiatry in projects covering both the child and adult psychiatry field would be helpful.

Training

It is unlikely to have child and adolescent psychiatry as an autonomous subject in pregraduate training at the Faculties of Medicine. The student's possibility to choose lectures or practical courses on child psychiatry as an optional subject at two of three faculties is an important achievement in comparison with the previous status. Cooperation with other disciplines (pediatrics, child neurology) should be improved.

In the field of postgraduate training, the main achievement is that the Subdepartment of Child Psychiatry of the Institute for Postgraduate Studies in Medicine was established in 1993. Preparing a new plan of postgraduate training which would be close to the new European curriculum is one of the most important aims of this new institution.

Improvement of services and care systems

There is a lack of adequate evaluation of the sufficiency of the psychiatric services net for children and adolescents. This evaluation is possible only in cooperation with the state authorities; however, child psychiatry should initiate this activity first. A new strategy for development of services should be prepared. The other important focus is to expand daypatient services and to create units with inter-regional character to treat children with severe mental disorders. Child and adolescent psychiatry also have to react to the increasing number of drug-dependent patients during recent years.

Future development in the field of child and adolescent psychiatry should make it more attractive for young professionals who want the branch to fulfill their professional and personal ambitions for the future.

Selected references

Dobrotka G, Fedor-Frybergh P (1995) Vyvoj pedopsychiatrie na Slovensku. (The development of pedopsychiatry in Slovakia). Psychiatria 2: 112–116

Koncepcia odboru psychiatrie. Vestník Ministerstva zdravotníctva Slovenskej rebubliky čiatka 9, ročník 45, 11. júna 1997. (Concept of Psychiatry (1997) Bulletin of Ministry of Health, Slovak Republic, part 9, vol. 45, June 9, 1997)

Psychiatria 1996. Ústav zdravotníckych informácií a štatstiky, 1997. (Psychiatry 1996 (1997) Institute for Information and Statistics in Medicine), Bratislava, Slovakia

Sedláčková E, Fleischer J, Kolibáš E, Žucha I (1996) Profesor MUDr. Zdeňek Mysliveček, DrSc. – zakladatel' slovenskej psychiatrie. (Professor Zdeňek Mysliveček, M.D. – the founder of Slovak psychiatry). Psychiatria 3 (3/4): 216–219

Statistical Yearbook of the Slovak Republic 1997. Bratislava, Slovak Academy of Sciences (1997)

Tichy M, Sedláčková E (1966) Prof. MUDr. K. Matulay. Bratislava, JUGA

Child and adolescent psychiatry in Slovenia

M. Tomori

1. Definition, historical development, and current situation

Definition

In Slovenia, the field of child and adolescent psychiatry joins all the professions and services dealing with children and adolescents with mental disorders or dysfunctional psycho-social development. The child and adolescent psychiatrist is a specialist who has completed his/her residency in psychiatry by a board exam and works in the field of child and adolescent psychiatry, comprising diagnostics, treatment, and prevention.

Historical development

Until the 1950s, the professional care of mentally disturbed children and adolescents in Slovenia was carried out rather unsystematically, dispersed among different specialties. Partly it was developed within the framework of general psychiatry and partly in the field of pediatrics where the main attention was paid to psychosomatic, developmental, and emotional disorders in children. The first outpatient clinic for child psychiatry was established at the Psychiatric Dispensary of the University Psychiatric Hospital in 1954 (B. Pregelj). The first professional team consisted of only a psychiatrist and a clinical psychologist, their activity being partly complemented by external co-workers, particularly social workers, nurses, and school pedagogues. In the same year, an institute for diagnosis and triage of adolescent delinquents was established, the socalled Transitory Home for Adolescents, which was run by a more comprehensive team of experts, including pedagogues and even a lawyer. In 1955, the first Child Guidance Clinic (H. Puhar) was established within the framework of the school system; its work was centered particularly on the problems of development, education, and school failure. The only child psychiatrist of many years (B. Pregelj) also took upon herself the responsibilities of educator by lecturing in the then schools for parents, thus, setting the foundations of prevention in the field of mental disorders of childhood and adolescence. In those social-realistic times, her report on the role of maternal care in early childhood had a dramatic impact on the attitude of government structures, which resulted in prolonging maternity leave from the previous 3 weeks to 3 months after childbirth. (Nowadays, mothers are entitled to one-year maternity leave, a part of which can be taken by the child's father.)

After 1960, more outpatient clinics for child psychiatry were set up in Slovenia, initially within the framework of the primary health care, in regional health centers – either as independent units at pediatric departments of those health centers or as part of general psychiatric outpatient clinics. Gradually, the number of child psychiatrists has increased as well; some of these emerged from among former pediatricians and school physicians (who added psychiatry to their basic specialty), but there were increasingly more of those who specialized in psychiatry of children and adolescents. After 1965, the outpatient clinics for child psychiatry were run by even larger and more comprehensive teams of professionals, which consisted of psychiatrists, clinical psychologists, consultants in different pediatrics-related specialties, phoniatrists, speech therapists, pedagogues, social workers, and nurses. A number of child guidance clinics were established within the framework of the schooling system throughout Slovenia; some of these, however, were later closed down when their responsibilities were taken over by school advisors and outpatient clinics for child psychiatry as part of the primary health service.

In 1970, a department for child psychiatry with 12 beds was established at the University Pediatric Hospital (A. Kos). The child psychiatrist and his/her team were in charge of the diagnostics and therapy of mentally disturbed children up to 14 years of age; they also performed counseling service for all of the University Pediatric Hospital. In 1975, a department for adolescents with 21 beds was established at the Mental Health Center of the University Psychiatric Hospital (M. Tomori). As there was no special psychiatric service for the adolescent population aged 14–20 years available in Slovenia at that time, this department developed a widespread outpatient psychiatric service with a daycare clinic for adolescents. The standard team of specialists was further supplemented by an art therapist, a psycho-drama therapist, a musical therapist, and other specialists.

Education for psychiatric work with children and adolescents reached beyond the scope of the general residency program in psychiatry available in Slovenia; therefore, child and adolescent psychiatrists had to upgrade their knowledge abroad, traditionally in Germany (Tübingen) and in Great Britain (London – Institute of Psychiatry, Tavistock Clinic). In 1976, the Faculty of Medicine of the University of Ljubljana, organized its first postgraduate study in childhood psychiatry (B. Pregelj). Since then, clinical psychologists and psychiatrists have been able to acquire additional knowledge needed for their work with mentally disturbed children and adolescents. The program covers two semesters and is completed with a board exam. Since 1992, an additional one semester postgraduate study in family dynamics (M. Tomori) has been organized by the Chair of Psychiatry of the Faculty of Medicine. An exam based on this study program is a prerequisite for further sub-specialist studies in family therapy.

In 1979, the Society for Child Psychiatry was established at the Slovenian Medical Association (B. Pregelj, S. Bertoncelj). This is an organizational-professional and professional-oriented association for child psychiatrists and clinical child psychologists in Slovenia.

Current situation

Slovenia is both a young and small European country. As one of the six Republics of the former Yugoslavia, i.e., its north-western most part, it gained its independence in 1991. The European Community recognized Slovenia as an independent country in January 1992. According to the census on 31 June 1996, of the two million population of Slovenia, there were 354,553 children up to 14 years of age and 151,199 adolescents, aged 15–19 years. The prevailing religion is Roman Catholic, and the language Slovenian.

Children start school at an age of 6–7 years; school is compulsory until the 15th years of age.

In Slovenia, the professional care of children and adolescents with mental disorders is carried out by a well-developed and adequately distributed network of institutions, all of which (with the exception of two hospital wards) are part of the community, i.e., run on an outpatient basis, and therefore readily available to users. In 1998, there were 12 outpatient clinics with child psychiatry as part of the primary health care service in Slovenia; these were joined by two private services for child psychiatry. Professional teams in these clinics are headed by child psychiatrists. There are four child guidance clinics, whose teams consist basically of psychologists and pedagogues. Their work is complemented by school counselors, who best know the situation in their community since they work directly at schools. Doctrinary and systematic counseling work is carried out by the Counseling Center in Ljubljana which emerged from the first child guidance clinic in Slovenia. This center is also connected with the Collaborative Center for Child Mental Health WHO.

Inpatient treatment is carried out at the Department of Child Psychiatry of the University Pediatric Hospital and at the Unit for Adolescents of the University Psychiatric Hospital in Ljubljana. The existing facilities of 30 beds available at these two departments (of the total 2,300 psychiatric beds for whole Slovenia) are basically sufficient, in view of the generally accepted doctrine that children and adolescents should remain as far as possible part of their families and natural social environment and indications for hospitalization should be restricted to the most severe conditions for the shortest possible period of time.

Presently, there are 24 child and adolescent psychiatrists active in Slovenia. The Society of Pedopsychiatry comprises 50 members – physicians (pediatricians, school and family doctors) and around a 100 other members of allied professions.

2. Classification systems, diagnostic and therapeutic methods

Classification systems

Since 1996, all medical institutions and private clinics treating children and adolescents with psychiatric disorders have been exclusively using the classification of psychiatric disorders according to ICD-10 system. This enables cooperation of several institutions in the diagnosis of psychiatric disorders, comparability of clinical experience, as well as research work and the evaluation of the epidemiological situation in this field.

In 1995, the 10th revision of the International Statistical Classification of Diseases and Related Health Problems was translated (under the supervision of experts in the different fields) for the needs of the Slovenian health service. It was the very uniform approach to the classification of all diseases and health disorders – be it somatic or mental – that contributed to psychiatry being better recognized and acknowledged as one of the branches of medicine by other medical specialties. The psychiatric section of the WHO's ICD-10 classification was prepared in collaboration with Slovenian experts in the field of psychiatry (J. Lokar, M. Tomori). Particularly in the field of child psychiatry, our relevant specialists (A. Kos) contributed considerably toward education and establisment of the multiaxial framework.

Diagnostic methods

In Slovenia, we use a complex and comprehensive approach for the diagnosis of psychiatric disorders of children and adolescents, which considers somatic – particularly neurological – as well as psychological, developmental, family and social factors associated with the onset and development of disease.

The choice and combination of different diagnostic approaches depend on the type of disorder or disease, as well as on the type of institution where the diagnostic procedure is being carried out and on its staffing. If the diagnostic process is not feasible in, e.g., a child guidance clinic, the procedures can be complemented in a university affiliated health institution where a comprehensive diagnostic team is available, thus, enabling more differential investigations to be carried out.

Neurological diagnostics include EEG and other neurophysiological diagnostic methods; the findings are interpreted by child neurologists, most of whom possess adequate knowledge and understanding of the problems of children's mental health, which qualifies them for performing this task. Also the somatic diagnostics can be carried out by adequate counseling services of all medical branches.

Psychodiagnostics are carried out by clinical psychologists using standard psychodiagnostic procedures as well as other tests and instruments (inventories, scales, questionnaires) needed in the diagnosis of individual cases.

The child and adolescent psychiatrist not only performs psychiatric exploration of the child but also carries out interviews with the child's relatives. When necessary and approved by the child's relatives (or the adolescent himself), the psychiatrist also collects relevant heteroanamnestic data from other sources, e.g., from the child's teacher or responsible social worker. Diagnostics also include basic psychodynamic factors and evaluation of family function together with the properties of the child's closer social environment.

University affiliated institutions also implement their diagnostics by including special questionnaires which enable systematic collection of data needed for clinical work and scientific research purposes.

Therapeutic methods

The choice of the therapeutic method to be used as help in the treatment of an individual child or adolescent depends on the type and nature of the problem and also partly on the professional orientation and objective facilities of the institution where the treatment is carried out. Slovenia being small, the professional education at the specialist level is uniform, which ensures that therapeutic doctrine in the whole country has been practically synchronized. The prevailing professional ideology is based on the respect of bio-psycho-social integrity of the child; comprehension of mental disorders is generally psychodynamicaly oriented without ignoring biological factors. But, certain individual differences and specific therapeutic preferences are, nevertheless, present among the child psychiatrists. The range of therapeutic techniques is wide, including everything from professional counseling, psychodynamically oriented individual or group psychotherapy, to family counseling, systemic familial therapy, and the eclectic approach in outpatient clinics and university departments. Indications for the use of psychoactive medication in children are very restricted, while in adolescents such medications are used mostly in the case of severe depression or psychoses. Particular care is also taken that the patients maintained on drugs are not deprived of psychotherapy and that their families are intensively involved in the therapeutic process. The most integrated therapy is available at hospital wards, where an adolescent is offered individual psychotherapy while he/she also takes part in psychotherapy-oriented treatment group, psychodrama, art therapy, music therapy and kinesiotherapy, and attends individual sessions. His/her parents or other relatives take part in the family groups. Nevertheless, despite the general psychodynamic orientation, psychoanalysis is used only in older adolescents, who are highly motivated for therapy and have already reached a certain level of personal autonomy.

3. Structure and organization of services

Guidelines for services for children and adolescents with psychiatric disorders

Although the majority of services taking care of children and adolescents with mental disorders are affiliated with the national health care service, a part of the treatment is carried out within the framework of education and social care programs. Those activities are financed from the government budget, the main share being contributed by the Ministry of Health, and minor shares by the Ministry of Education and Sports and the Ministry of Labor, Family, and Social Affairs.

Schools counseling services are the domain of the education program. Most primary and secondary schools in Slovenia have one or more school counselors, who are either psychologists or pedagogues by their basic profession. A minority of these have specialized in clinical psychology, while a few have completed postgraduate study in child psychiatry. Those experts are the first in line when it comes to recognition of children and adolescents at risk, their counseling being able to solve some less complicated psycho-social problems of pupils and high school students. More complex cases are referred to specialists for psychiatric treatment, while a school counselor will resume the role of their advocate in the school.

Such psychologists and pedagogues also collaborate with social workers at regional centers for social care. There they are responsible particularly for children with conduct disorders and for adolescents from dysfunctional families (frequently burdened with alcohol abuse problems). They also carry out preparatory procedures when a child is to join a foster family or is being adopted or a delinquent adolescent is to be sent to a correction institution. Apart from that, they are responsible for socio-therapeutic management of adolescent delinquents. Centers for social care supervise and run dwelling communities for adolescents from dysfunctional families.

Child guidance clinics function partly within the framework of the national health service and partly within the educational system. Their professional teams are responsible for counseling in developmental disorders, school problems, and conduct disorders. Their therapeutic activity is carried out at different levels; it uses individual approach rather than a group one, involving the families of mentally disturbed children as well. The central institution of national importance is the Counseling Center in Ljubljana, which – apart from dealing with study and development related problems – also carries out psychotherapeutic work. It takes care of the education of teachers and other pedagogues by organizing regular seminars in children's mental health and by preparing text books and other publications dedicated to the pedagogic work with children at risk.

Further, different services functioning in the field of child and adolescent psychiatry within the framework of health system offer a wide range of different forms of help to the population at risk and to children and adolescents with mental disorders.

Outpatient services

The regional network of outpatient psychiatric services in Slovenia is relatively consistent.

Most of the outpatient services are performed by clinics of child psychiatry as part of the primary health care service within the framework of regional health centers. These clinics are run by therapeutic teams consisting of a psychiatrist, psychologist, pedagogue, and social worker. Other specialists, such as neurologists, phoniatrists, and speech therapists, are also available at health centers.

Some of these clinics are a constituent part of outpatient clinics of psychiatry comprising also a psychiatric service for adults. The work of experts in such clinics is easier, because they have ample opportunity for peer-revision, supervision, and consultations in psychotherapy. All outpatient child psychiatrists work in close collaboration with pediatricians and school physicians in health centers, the latter often referring children for diagnosis and treatment to those specialists.

Outpatient clinics are also maintained at both psychiatric hospital departments, (Department of Child Psychiatry and Department of Adolescent Psychiatry). While many children and adolescents are treated there on an outpatient basis, others are referred from outpatient departments to hospital wards and/or continue treatment as outpatients after discharge from the hospital.

The university hospital of psychiatry also runs an independent clinic of psychiatry, which carries out the most complex and demanding outpatient treatments, and at the same time serves as a teaching basis (likewise at both hospital departments) for undergraduate and postgraduate studies in psychiatry.

Since 1992, private psychiatric practice has been legally approved in Slovenia. Presently, there are only two private clinics for child psychiatry available in the country; there, a restricted team of professionals is supervised by a child psychiatrist.

Daypatient services

A daypatient department is run only at the hospital ward for adolescents at the University Psychiatric Hospital. This department is intended for children and adolescents who can and should stay in close contact with their families, or the daycare treatment represents an introduction to their hospitalization. Many patients from hospital wards are transferred to the daypatient facility in the intermediate phase of treatment, before their discharge from the hospital.

Inpatient services

There are only two specialized hospital wards for the treatment of children and adolescents with mental disorders available in Slovenia. Both wards are part of the university hospitals and represent a teaching basis for undergraduate as well as postgraduate studies in different psychiatry-related specialties. The ward of child psychiatry functions within the framework of the University Pediatric Hospital; it comprises 12 beds. Its complete team of professionals carries out complex diagnostic and therapeutic treatment of children up to 14 years of age, and also functions as a psychiatric consultation service for the needs of the University Pediatric Hospital. The team has established bilateral collaboration with other pediatrics-oriented specialists, particularly neurologists and endocrinologists. Apart from other mental disorders, it pays special attention to the treatment of somatoform disorders in children. Great therapeutic importance is also attributed to working with the patient's family and family therapy.

The ward for adolescents is run by the University Psychiatric Hospital; it has a capacity of 19 beds and is intended for the treatment of adolescents older than 14 years of age. The upper age-limit is determined by the type of psychiatric disorder; therefore, patients at an age of 20 or 21 years are not an exception, when their specific problems are associated with dysfunctional individuation and separation.

In the diagnostic work, a team approach is used, and communication with schools and social centers is bilateral. The available therapeutic activities are versatile and adjusted to the adolescent's stage of development. Adolescents with all types of mental disorders are admitted to the ward. However, this being an open type ward (which means that some patients attend school during the course of therapy and all of them spend weekends at home), severely suicidal patients and those in acute psychotic episodes are for the shortest possible period transferred to a safe-guarded hospital ward for adults at the University Psychiatric Hospital. The diagnosis at this department is complex and the treatment eclectic. The patients receive medication when necessary; all of them are subjected to psychotherapy (either individual or group) and join art therapy, psychodrama, or training of social skills and assertiveness while their relatives participate in the therapeutic group for parents or/and in family therapy.

The ward for adolescents is also a teaching basis providing education in the treatment of mentally disturbed adolescents not only to physicians but also to experts of other areas (school physicians, pediatricians, clinical psychologists, pedagogues).

The problem of lacking facilities for psychiatric inpatient treatment of children and adolescents in the northeastern part of Slovenia was partly solved by the Children's Hospital in Maribor, which admits children and adolescents (with mental disorders) to their general pediatric department. The professional team led by a pediatrician with a postgraduate degree in child psychiatry also includes other adequately qualified professionals, such as clinical psychologists and pedagogues.

Complementary services and rehabilitation

Children and adolescents with long-lasting and chronic mental disorders receive support of social services and all the above mentioned psychiatric services.

Youth centers

Children with conduct disorders, whose families are unable to ensure conditions for their healthy development and adequate schooling, and delinquent adolescents are placed in institutions which provide educational programs, sociotherapy, schooling, and vocational training. In these institutions, the help of a consultant psychiatrist is available, when needed. The institution personnel maintain active contacts with boarders' relatives and the social services which will continue the rehabilitation process after discharge from the center. There are six such centers in Slovenia.

Residential communities

These facilities are intended for adolescents who cannot live with their families, but are attending regular school or are already working. While the educational work is the domain of pedagogues, possible psychiatric help is provided by the regional psychiatric outpatient clinic for adolescents.

Foster care

Children and adolescents with mental disorders, whose development and personality formation still require a family shelter, which for various reasons cannot be provided by their own families, are placed in foster homes by social services. Placement in a foster family is suitable for psychotic adolescents who do not need inpatient treatment. Regularity of medication treatment and nursing care is the responsibility of a field nurse who pays regular visits to the foster family.

Civil, non-institutional organizations

Groups of children and their parents are joined in special associations on the basis of their mutual problems. Thus, the associations of parents with handicapped and mentally retarded children and children with cerebral palsy, as well as of adolescent drug-addicts already have a tradition for decades in Slovenia. In recent years, quite a few associations for psychotic patient rehabilitation have been established (ŠENT, Ozara, Altra). Some of these associations have developed good systematic rehabilitation programs and offer possibilities for socialization of psychiatric patients. They maintain good bilateral communication with psychiatric services. On the other hand, some associations are anti-psychiatry-oriented and, therefore, a relatively poor support to the psychiatric patient.

Personnel

The mental health services for children and adolescents in Slovenia is carried out by 24 specialists in child and adolescent psychiatry. Their professional teams consist of 35 clinical psychologists, 25 pedagogues, 42 social workers and a number of other professionals who work on a full-time or part-time basis.

Funding of services

Slovenia has a compulsory health insurance system. Children during their obligatory schooling and adolescents until their education is completed are entitled to free health care, including psychiatric help. The Health Insurance Institute pays the cost of health care services directly to the responsible institutions. The payment of treatment in private psychiatric clinics is made possible through concession contracts signed between the private psychiatric practitioners and the Health Insurance Institute. Rehabilitation services are financed partly by the health care and partly by the social care systems.

Evaluation

In Slovenia, we do not have a uniform or systematic approach for the evaluation of child psychiatric service functioning. When introducing new programs or evaluating the requirements for personnel and new equipment investments, certain institutions may be occasionally interested in the evaluation of individual therapeutic programs and in the assessment of rationality and effectiveness of diagnostic procedures.

Partial evaluation programs make constituent parts of some research studies (e.g., comparison of the effectiveness of two therapeutic methods).

The whole system of child and adolescent psychiatric service lacks the facilities for part-time institutional treatment, i.e., daycare departments. In addition, the care available to children and adolescents with mixed emotional and conduct disorders is also insufficient. On the one hand, child psychiatric institutions are reluctant to admit patients whose disturbing behavior may jeopardize the treatment of, e.g., depressed children, while on the other, reformatories with their relatively rigid systems represent too much of a strain and a source of permanent frustration to such children. We also need a special psychiatric department intended for adolescents with eating disorders, which should develop its own specific regimen of work, as well as a hospital ward for acutely psychotic adolescents, so that these need not be admitted to wards intended for adult patients.

4. Cooperation with medical and non-medical services

Cooperation with pediatricians and school physicians

Bilateral and close cooperation of pediatricians and school physicians with child psychiatrists is traditional. Specialists/consultants and supervisors in psychotherapy are always consulted when mental disorders in children and adolescents with primary physical ailments are to be assessed and treated. Children and adolescents in whom psychiatric problems have been suspected on routine and other physical examinations are referred to child psychiatric services for comprehensive diagnostic and therapeutic treatment. Cooperation of a child psychiatrist is also sought whenever there is the need for an isolated and focused psychiatric intervention (e.g., preparation of the child and his/her relatives for a demanding and risky surgical procedure, or treatment of a child whose reaction to somatic disease or its treatment entails an acute psychoreactive disorder).

On the other hand, pediatricians and school physicians also participate in the somatic part of the diagnostic process undergone by children treated for psychiatric disorders. They too offer their consulting services to psychiatrists, with respect to their specialty (neurology, endocrinology, orthopedics, ophthalmology, etc.). This cooperation applies to outpatient as well as inpatient services. While at the level of primary health care (health centers), it is part of the regular routine work; at the level of university affiliated institutions (the University Pediatric Hospital and the University Psychiatric Hospital) this cooperation is carried out on the highest academic level. This cooperation is easier and more functional since pediatricians and school physicians already learn the basics of child psychiatry within their regular residency programs, while some of them will also attend a postgraduate course in child psychiatry. Thus, they become more aware of the psycho-social problems of childhood and adolescence, and they also learn the basics of professional terminology specific to this branch of medicine.

Cooperation with psychiatry

General psychiatry is more closely connected with that part of psychiatric services that concerns adolescents. Also, the hospital ward for adolescents with mental disorders and a part of outpatient services intended for those patients are organized within the framework of the University Psychiatric Hospital. The most direct form of cooperation is inpatient treatment of acutely psychotic or severely suicidal adolescents who require temporary hospitalization in a special, safe-guarded ward for adults of the psychiatric hospital.

Certain cooperation is also needed in the treatment of children and adolescents whose parents are mentally ill. Steady communication is also maintained between child psychiatrists and family psychotherapists.

Cooperation with doctors in private practice

The cooperation of child and adolescent psychiatrists and the members of their professional teams with the doctors in private practice (psychiatrists as well as family doctors and general practitioners) is bilateral and flexible. There are no formal or financial problems regarding this cooperation as all mental health care for children is payed by the Health Insurance Institute.

Cooperation with non-medical institutions and professionals

The psychiatric services for children and adolescents in Slovenia maintain permanent and active contacts with non-medical services that play a special role in the care of children.

Wide-spread connections have been established with social services dealing with families at risk and dysfunctional families, and children from socially deprived environments; social services also direct delinquent adolescents into schooling and employment and arrange placement with foster families or youth centers. When necessary, centers for social work provide information on social conditions of children receiving psychiatric treatment. On the request of psychiatric services, they arrange financial, accommodations, and other help to the families of children at risk.

Cooperation with schools and other pedagogic institutions is also good. The degree of understanding and their readiness to pay special attention to children and adolescents with mental disorders is generally satisfactory; in individual cases, however, it is necessary to alert psychologists to those children and motivate them to work with them. Furthermore, the role and possibilities of school counselors may differ from one school to another. While at some schools, these professionals perform generally administrative and triage work; at others they have the possibility of comprehensive counseling and supportive psychotherapeutic work – even under the supervision of a child psychiatrist affiliated with a health institution.

Cooperation of child and adolescent psychiatry experts with the judicial and legal system is mainly in the field of expertise activity. This is most frequently required when dealing with delinquent adolescents, drug and alcohol abuse, and in cases of child abuse.

5. Graduate/postgraduate training, and continuing medical education

Graduate training

Faculty of medicine

There is one Medical faculty in Slovenia, which is affiliated with the University of Ljubljana. The study of psychiatry is organized and carried out by the Chair of Psychiatry; the teaching staff consists of 9 full professors and 6 members with academic titles.

The total number of enrolled students and undergraduates is 1,500; about 160 of them graduate every year. The study of psychiatry consists of lectures, practice with patients, and optional seminars in the 4th year. Unfortunately, the number of hours dedicated to child psychiatry is insufficient. This drawback is partly compensated by additional practical training (bedside teaching) which is conducted in both University Hospitals, i.e., of Pediatrics and Psychiatry.

Pedagogic Faculty

With respect to the number of hours dedicated to child psychiatry, the situation is somewhat better at the Pedagogic Faculty. In the 3rd year, the independent subject "Psychiatry in childhood and adolescent period" is attended by approximately 90 students of defectology and social pedagogics. The topics included in the program are further upgraded by seminar work.

Other faculties

At the Department of Psychology, child psychiatry is included in the curriculum of the 2nd year, within the subject "Clinical psychopathology". At the faculty of law, selected topics of child psychology are covered by the subject "Forensic psychopathology" in the 3rd year of study.

Postgraduate training, a joint effort

Residency program

For the time being, there is no special residency program in child and adolescent psychiatry available in Slovenia. The future child psychiatrists train in general psychiatry for three years. Students can attend this residency program after having completed two years of internship during which the graduate from the Medical Faculty acquires knowledge needed for practical work in all branches of medicine (during this two year internship, the student can already choose psychiatry as a 4 or 6 month option). The internship is completed by a board exam which officially qualifies the candidate for the independent physician's work.

Residency in psychiatry takes three years. During that period, the candidate rotates through all the main departments of psychiatric services and is actively involved in both inpatient and outpatient work with patients. The residency is completed by a practical and theoretical state board exam.

It is planned that in the near future the concept and duration of psychiatric residency program in Slovenia will be changed in accordance with the European criteria (Chair of Psychiatry – M. Tomori, S. Ziherl, B. Kores). There will be two residency programs available, i.e., in general as well as in child and adolescent psychiatry, each lasting 5 years. After a three-year period of common studies, there will be two more years of study, which will differ with respect to the selected line (either child or general psychiatry). For the difference from general psychiatry, the program for child psychiatry has more time dedicated to practical training in pediatrics, developmental neurophysiology, and neurology, as well as to direct work in child and adolescent psychiatry under supervision, and to consulting work in the community and social system.

Postgraduate study

There is a two-term study in child and adolescent psychiatry organized at the Faculty of Medicine every other year, while the alternate years are reserved for the study of psychotherapy. Both study programs are compulsory for all the residents in child psychiatry. Candidates and non-residents in medicine (i.e., psychologists, clinical psychologists, pedagogues, sociologists) can also enroll into these two studies.

The study lasts two terms; besides lectures in subject-related topics, a considerable proportion of hours is dedicated to practical work with the patient, under supervision. It is completed by a written seminar work (presentation of psychotherapeutic treatment for the child or adolescent) and a board exam.

Future child psychiatrists studying at the Faculty of Medicine in Ljubljana can also enroll in the one-term study in systemic family dynamics.

Continuing medical education in child and adolescent psychiatry and psychotherapy

In Slovenia, physicians have to undergo a regular continuous education process in order to reconfirm their medical practice license. The conditions of this education are determined by the Chamber of the Medical Profession of Slovenia.

Such programs for child psychiatrists consist of various forms of medical education, including regular professional meetings of the Society of Child Psychiatry, case conferences at the university psychiatric departments, and professional conferences, which can be either dedicated to a single topic or aimed to give an overview of the state of the art.

Training programs for other disciplines

Professionals with no preceding medical or psychological education can extend their knowledge in child and adolescent psychiatry at specially organized courses, professional meetings or under individual tuition and supervision of child and adolescent psychiatrists. Regular seminars on various child psychiatry related issues organized by the Chair of Psychiatry at the Faculty of medicine are traditional and well attended meetings for professionals of all allied disciplines.

6. Research

Research fields and strategies

In Slovenia, scientific research in the field of child psychiatry, likewise in general psychiatry, has certain advantages as well as drawbacks. Among the advantages, Slovenia's accessibility and its convenient geographic position should be pointed out: its small size renders Slovenia very suitable for various systematic studies. This facilitates the coordination of research, as well as data collection and communication. The country's position in Central Europe, at the crossroads of East-West and North-South communication pathways, give ample opportunity for the study of heterogeneous factors on an area of interest.

The drawback lies in the methodology of research: thus, investigations carried out in Slovenia using the methods of humanities and social sciences are not very interesting for the world and are difficult to publish, while studies based on the methods of neurobiology are too expensive for a country as small as ours. In addition, we lack multidisciplinary research teams. Prospects are anticipated in international cooperation and trans-cultural comparative studies. All studies in psychiatry should be approved by the Ethical Committee at the Ministry of Health, which is a prerequisite for their performance.

All research fields are at the same time among the priorities of the Slovenian health care program and are in one way or the other dealing with problems specific to Slovenia: epidemiology of mental disorders, depression, suicidal behavior, drug and alcohol addiction, and eating disorders are studied most frequently. Studies for the evaluation of treatment success and those comparing the effectiveness of individual treatment programs are interesting because of their clinical value and possible applicability in daily practice.

Research training and career development

In Slovenia, knowledge and skills required for medical research can be obtained through corresponding postgraduate studies at the Faculty of Medicine, as well as through work in research teams.

Funding

Like other research in medicine, studies in the field of child and adolescent psychiatry are also financed from the government's budget. The funds are generally provided by the Ministry of Science and Technology and the Ministry of Health. Every year, the former invites research teams to cooperate by a public announcement. After having submitted their project proposals, which should be well-grounded, the teams are evaluated for their research competence. This is evaluated according to several criteria, the most relevant of these being the number of points collected by number of publications in professional journals with an impact factor (SCI). In view of the well-known fact that it is much easier to publish reports in basic medical sciences and in somatic medicine than those in psychiatry, the researchers/child psychiatrists are in a disadvantaged position in comparison with others, which poses an additional rather realistic obstacle to research in this field.

7. Future perspectives

Research

Research in the field of child and adolescent psychiatry is directed toward studies, whose findings should help diminish the most pressing problems that jeopardize the mental health of children in Slovenia. Studies of depression, psychosocial disorders in children from dysfunctional families, self-destructive and suicidal behavior in adolescents, alcohol and substance abuse, and nutrition-related disorders are all challenges that call for response. The existing research teams, which presently still lack investigators skilled in the use of modern research methodology, should be expanded and educated accordingly. The results of these studies are needed not only for a more effective clinical work, but also for further development of efficient prevention programs.

Training

The relative rigidity of the undergraduate study program at the Faculty of Medicine cannot ensure a significant increase in the child and adolescent psychiatry curriculum for physicians. Therefore, we plan to introduce an optional subject dedicated to this topic.

Introduction of a new, longer residency program, which will provide more knowledge on child psychiatry, is the priority of postgraduate studies. It will be necessary to ensure better possibilities for mentorship and supervision work in the practical part of the educational program.

The relatively large publishing activity at the national level, including everything from lay texts intended for parents and pedagogues to professional monographs, should be enhanced with publications at the international level. This could form a sound basis for better communication of Slovenian experts with their colleagues worldwide, which would further promote and implement their research and education activities.

Improvement of services and care systems

In the past few years, a lot has been done to ensure that children's rights be considered and respected. Nevertheless, in order to improve mental health of children, much more could be achieved by the development of non-governmental services. Better communication and coordinated cooperation of different factors promoting general health of the population and humanization of (interpersonal) relations will be necessary. Focusing on the field of child psychiatry, we should strive to:

- develop better communication between professionals in the social, educational, and health care systems (with special emphasis on personal data protection as including more non-medical institutions may render this issue questionable);
- promote further development of outpatient and day-treatment psychiatric facilities evenly throughout the country;
- improve personnel and equipment facilities of professional teams by offering pediatricians and school physicians the possibility for additional education and training in child psychiatry;
- enhance education at all levels, including parents and teachers/pedagogues as well as experts; and
- develop prevention programs at primary, secondary, and tertiary levels; these should be logically adjusted with respect to specific risk factors which jeopardize the mental health of Slovenian children and adolescents.

Self-evidently, all these endeavors are largely dependent on general socio-economic conditions, the degree of awareness of the structures making decisions about the distribution of funds, as well as the development of an up-to-date health care system in general. Of course, there is no reason why child and adolescent psychiatrists should not take an active approach to all these issues.

Selected references

Kobal M, Tomori M (1979) Organizacija psihiatrijskog tretmana adolescenata. Aktualni psychiatricke problemi mladezi, Praha: 365–373
Pregelj L (1965) Odvisnost duševnega zdravja od materine nege. Zdr Varstvo 3: 41–43
Tomori M (1982) Skupinsko delo z mladostniki. Pedopsihiatrija 4: 15–24
Tomori M (1992) Grupna psihoterapija dece i omladine. In: Tadić N (ed) Psihoanalitička psihoterapija dece i mladih. Beograd: Naučna knjiga, pp 181–187
Tomori M (1992) Psihoterapija toksikomanija. In: Tadić N (ed) Psihoanalitička psihoterapija dece i mladih. Beograd: Naučan knjiga, pp 376–379
Tomori M (1992) Psihoterapija mladih od 15 to 18 godina: In: Tadić N (ed) Psihoanalitička psihoterapija dece i mladih. Beograd: Naučna knjiga, pp 282–287
Tomori M (1994) Mental health care in Slovenia. Ljubljana: Psihiatrična klinika, pp 1–11
Tomori M (1995) Challenges facing psychiatry in Slovenia. World Psychiatry 3: 27–28

Child and adolescent psychiatry in Spain

J. L. Pedreira-Massa, J. L. Alcázar, J. T. i Vilaltella

1. Definition, historical development, and current situation

Definition

The specialty of Child and Adolescent Psychiatry and Psychotherapy in Spain does not have a precise definition and is generally not officially recognized as an autonomous specialty. Nevertheless, the Spanish Association of Child and Adolescent Psychiatry (AEPIJ) has defined the specialty in a recent document (Pedreira et al., 1996) in the following way: "Child and Adolescent Psychiatry and Psychotherapy includes the promotion of the psychosocial development in children and adolescents, the prevention of possible mental dysfunctions in children and adolescents, the diagnosis, the therapeutic intervention, the treatment in its social group of the disorders detected – in pharmacologic, as well as psychotherapy, family support and the psychosocial intervention – and the rehabilitation and social integration of the children and adolescents with mental disorders, psychosomatic conditions, developmental disorders, sensorial dysfunctions and other psychological and behavioral problems and disorders and social adaptation that occur in children and adolescents, considering that this stage includes from the moment of birth to 18 years". Nevertheless, it is necessary to wait until the National Council of Medical Specialties (CNEM) approves in a definitive way the Area of Specific Training and Accreditation (ACE) in child and adolescent psychiatry to be able to formulate as much the definition as the professional competitions and the program of the Spanish professionals' training in this scientific and professional field.

Historical development

Child and adolescent psychiatry in Spain has its historical roots as much in pediatrics as in psychiatry, but it has also received contributions from other related sciences such as psychology, pedagogy, and social sciences (including the judicial field). Occasionally, the relationships have not been very flowing, because of the great heterogeneity of the sources and of those sciences, the different levels of scientific development, and social interaction of all of them. However, in the current state of our professional field these and other influences can be considered, without a doubt, of great value and with an important capacity, both theoretical and practical.

In the 19th century, Hospital Asilo of the Niño Jesús, the first pediatric hospital, was opened in Madrid in 1879 two years after the Hôspital des Enfants Malades in Paris, which was the first pediatric hospital of Europe. Still health attention given to children was not differentiated and only the perseverance of some medical doctors obtained this advance (Aguilar, Tolosa Latour).

In the first third of the present century in Spain, the study of child and adolescent psychopathology was indeed developed: in 1908 Dr. Augusto Vidal Perera published the first book titled "Summary of Child Psychiatry", a copy of which is in the Royal National Academy of Medicine. Some years later the first class of child psychopathology is believed to have been held at the University of Barcelona, but it was located in the Department of Pedagogy with Prof. Mira-López as its first chairperson.

The Spanish Civil War reduced later developments, and the scientific and intellectual marasmus at the time of the dictatorship also affected this specialty. Since 1950, the first scientific organization is believed to have studied the mental disorders in children and adolescents: the Spanish Association of Child Neuropsychiatry which later became the current Spanish Association of Child and Adolescent Psychiatry (AEPIJ). The founders were pediatricians and psychiatrists worried by these topics; Vázquez Velasco, Córdoba, Moragas, Folch i Camarasa, Sarrate, Mendiguchía, and Prieto Huesca are the first professionals of child psychiatry in Spain. During those years, the Catalan Society of Child Psychiatry was founded and continues its activities at the present time.

These pioneers did not obtain, in spite of their efforts, the specialty in an autonomous way. Nevertheless, they carried out annual scientific meetings and congresses every three years which initially encompassed neuropsychiatrics, but went on to include pychiatric topics and psychopathology with the theoretical perspectives that were dominant in Europe. They also contributed to the creation of the European Union of Child Psychiatry, predecessor of the current ESCAP. Prof. Sarrate became the president of the European Union of Child Psychiatry and in 1979 AEPIJ organized the European Congress in Madrid, with Prof. Mendiguchía as president of the organizing committee.

Also starting in the 1950s in Spain, the National Patronage of Psychiatric Attendance (PANAP) started Orientation and Diagnosis Centers for children, having built four child and adolescent psychiatric hospitals: Ciudad Real, Madrid, Teruel, and Zamora. Their operation has been a point of great debate; beyond the efforts carried out by the professionals who carried out work in them, they represented to a certain degree the exclusion of the children who entered and an objective demonstration of the marginalization of this profession in our country. In other words: the situation was criticized without giving real alternatives or proposing real solutions for children with severe mental disorders except for their condemnation to institutionalization for life, which is something that then has obvious repercussions in the operation of the psychiatric hospitals of adults.

From 1978 to 1984 other scientific societies were established with different perspectives: the Section of Child Psychiatry of the Spanish Association of Pediatrics was the first one started (1978), because during the 1960s the only child psychiatric services were bound to the pediatric hospitals (La Paz in Madrid, Vall d'Hebron in Barcelona), since by law those younger than 18 years could not be admitted into the psychiatric hospitals. The Spanish Society of Child and Adolescent Psychiatry and Psychotherapy (SEPYPNA; 1981) is focussed at professionals who had emigrated to Switzerland and returned to Spain after the dictator's death, their roots with the original Spanish sources are scarce and their orientation is a psychoanalytical perspective, being a society open to other types of professionals (psychologists) and not only to doctors. Finally, the Section of Child Mental Health of the Spanish Association of Neuropsychiatry (1983-84) is concerned with assistance policy, and it integrates medical professionals and non-doctors (psychologists, social workers, psychiatric nurses) in their constitution.

Thus, it is paradoxical that in a country that does not have a specialty of Child and Adolescent Psychiatry, five scientific societies with different objectives and perspectives exist, including theoretical and assistance. Nevertheless, since 1992 AEPIJ has facilitated the convergence of the scientific associations, including the Catalan Society of Child Psychiatry, the Section of Child Psychiatry of the Spanish Association of Pediatrics, and the Section of Child Mental Health of the Spanish Association of Neuropsychiatry (in 1995 it opted to abandon this integration when modifying the objectives and their advisory board).

In the early part of the 1980s, AEPIJ published the Journal of Child and Adolescent Psychiatry quarterly, which was the only periodic scientific publication on the market that was simultaneously in the Spanish language and specifically dedicated to child and adolescent psychiatry, psychopathology, and psychotherapy.

Recent advances

AEPIJ has continued carrying out its annual scientific meetings and its journal continues to be the only one that is published regularly in Spanish about child and adolescent psychiatry and psychotherapy topics. It has the Spanish representation in the European Union of Specialist Doctors (UEMS), but in a generous way it has shared the delegation with the delegate proposed by SEPYPNA.

The fruitful collaboration of the group of the scientific associations, contained around AEPIJ, has been possible to elaborate an accreditation proposal in child and adolescent psychiatry and psychotherapy, following two parameters: that of professionals and services accreditation according to the approaches of the joint commission and that of the training programs from the UEMS. This document was submitted to the official organizations, the National Council of Medical Specialties, and the UEMS. We are certain that it has been a very appreciated document for its content and the bringing up to date the treated topics, which has facilitated an open dialogue with other Spanish scientific associations (Spanish Society of Psychiatry), the National Commission of Specialty of Psychiatry, and some Spanish professors of psychiatry.

Simultaneously, scientific publications written by Spanish professionals of child and adolescent psychiatry have appeared: "Psychopathology of the Children and the Adolescents" (1995) is an important text directed by Prof. Rodríguez-Sacristán, in which nearly fifty authors (thirty from Spain and twenty from other European countries) collaborate. Other authors who have contributed to our specialty include: Dr. Mardomingo (1994 and 1996), Dr. Pedreira (1995), Prof. Toro (1998), and Dr. Tomás (1995–1998).

The results of the perseverance of child and adolescent psychiatry professionals in Spain are the verification that the societies of pediatrics and psychiatry, as well as other professional groups, include in their scientific activities psychopathological aspects, clinic and treatment of the mental disorders in children and adolescents, inviting SEPIJ or the associations so that they participate in these topics.

Current situation

Spain has 10,589,961 children under the age of 18 years, of those 5,434,232 are male and 5,155,729 are female (Ministry of Social Matters, 1991).

Several perspectives that are of interest to us in the consolidation of child psychiatry in Spain are real alternatives for professionals:

- The National Commission of Psychiatry has written a document granting the Specific Accreditation in Child and Adolescent Psychiatry and Psychotherapy, which is highly valued and which basically coincides with the document produced by AEPIJ (see postgraduate training, p. 343).
- The normalization of the Spanish representation in the ESCAP should be by means of AEPIJ, since legitimately and historically it corresponds to it and because it represents a place of open debate without prominence of any theoretical perspective in an explicit way nor to any other ownership and, finally, because it facilitates the convergence of other scientific societies with the active presence of those that are represented in their association carrying out training activities, scientific meetings, publications, and members on the AEPIJ advisory board.
- AEPIJ has organized a permanent research work group that has funded the following lines of research: elaboration of a model of clinical assessment in child and adolescent psychiatry (Coordinator: Dr. Ballesteros); epidemiologic research, in which there have been integrated several communities (Director: Prof. Rodríguez-Sacristán and Coordinator: Dr. Pedreira-Massa); attention deficit disorders and behavior disorders (Coordinator: Prof. Benjumea); eating disorders (Coordinators: Prof. Toro and Dr. Velilla); psychosis and pervasive developmental disorders (Coordinator: Prof. Agüero); psychopharmacology in children (Coordinators: Drs. Gutiérrez and Ballesteros).

2. Classification systems, diagnostic and therapeutic methods

Classification systems

Spain has collaborated in an active way in the work of ICD-10, from the WHO Spanish Collaborating Center under the direction of Prof. López-Ibor (Jr.). The Spanish version dates to 1992, and gradually they have published the glossary, the equivalence between ICD-9 and ICD-10, the classification for research projects, the multiaxial system and the manual to the primary care services. In all of them child psychiatrists have collaborated in the field work. Nevertheless, the DSM-IV is of greater importance, as it is more commonly used for research and its use is propelled by certain groups of university professors and professionals with a stronger American than European influence.

We hope that the ICD-10 will have more possibilities in child and adolescent psychiatry if there were multiaxial developments, similar to the Rutter's system, mainly because the current code Z facilitates a better description of the family and social axis.

We want to verify the criticism of the categorial classification systems although we accept and use them. We would like to defend a more dimensional concept of mental disorders in children and adolescents, mainly because of the impact of the developmental process. In this sense we value the New Classification of the Mental Disorders in Children carried out by the French school, although it may still be in need of improvement and its value needs to be checked from different child and adolescent psychiatric perspectives, for different work systems, and for more countries.

Diagnostic methods

The complete spectrum of current diagnostic procedures is available for use. The use of various techniques (CAT, MNR, SPECT, and PET) facilitates the cooperation among several medical disciplines. Studies ranging from the simplest to those of structural and molecular interest are possible and are carried out in laboratories of different hospitals and research institutions of our country.

Recently translation, adaptation, and validation of diverse psychological and clinical evaluation scales for children, structured interviews, and semi-structured interviews have begun. Thus, a certain neuropsychologic and neuropsychiatric tradition is returning. It is necessary to single out in this field the work developed by the teams of Drs. Rodríguez-Sacristán in Sevilla, Domenech and Tomás in Barcelona, Polaino in Madrid, and Pedreira in Asturias among others.

The evaluation of family dynamics and early mother-child interaction (inherited from child psychoanalysis and the attachment theories) is also practiced in some groups of professionals and researchers. It is necessary to point out the work of C. Costa, Sánchez, and Domenech in Barcelona, Bayo in Madrid, and Pedreira in Asturias.

Therapeutic methods

A wide range exists in the therapeutic procedures from the use of the new psychopharmacology to various psychotherapeutic perspectives. In fact, in the Official Bulletin of the State (BOE, February, 15, 1995), the Royal Law published that there are adequate "Therapeutic Procedures of the National Health System", two excellent sections were included: in the maternal-infantile section, they ensured the prevention, promotion, and therapeutic care from birth until adulthood, integrating the bio-psycho-social perspective. The presence of a mental health condition guaranteed the treatment of acute exacerbations of chronic conditions in appropriate units of general hospitals, it also guaranteed psychopharmacological treatment, and psychotherapeutic treatment which was defined as individual, family or group psychotherapies. The psychotherapeutic concept, the requirements to be a psychotherapist, and the accreditation of the services to provide these treatments were not defined.

Of the different theories, the systemic perspective is obtaining a large audience among the professionals of the public services, mainly in certain regions of Spain. The cognitive and behavioral perspective has been developed, mainly, in the university services. The psychoanalytical and psychodynamic perspectives remain in the minority, at the moment, after a period in favour among hospital services. The existing assistance services carry out more eclectic and operationalized interventions in order to address crisis intervention and the resolution of problems.

3. Structure and organization of services

Guidelines for services for children and adolescents with psychiatric disorders

The General Law of Health (1986) discusses the appropriate care with regard to child mental health (Chapter three, Art. 20, Para. 1); however, it has still not been developed or even approached in a serious and rigorous way.

The report of the National Commission for Psychiatric Care Reformation (NCPCR) (p. 34) recognizes the specificity of mental disorders in children and adolescents, but neither appropriate and balanced development of the care nor human resources have existed to assist this stage of human development, despite the recognition that child mental health should be "a high priority and permanent program".

On January 15, 1990, the Royal Law 1.691/89 of December 29, 1989 was published in the BOE; the recognition of accreditation, certificates and doctor's titles, and specialist doctors of each member country of the European Union (EU) was regulated: in this ordinance in Appendix IV it was established that four years of training for child psychiatry are necessary.

In 1987 the European Parliament approved the Hospitalized Child's Rights, one year later they were debated in Oviedo (Asturias) and the Ministry of Health and Consumption published the works. Unfortunately, this has not been taken further. Hospitals still have inadequate physical conditions or resources for the hospitalization of children. They continue to be a copy of adult hospital centers.

In 1988 a national commission was constituted to study child abuse and neglect. The next step was the creation of a study group by the Ministry of Health and Consumption which included: Andalucía, Asturias, Baleares, Cataluña, Madrid, and Valencia; their studies are not yet completed. The General Office of Protection of the Minor assumed responsibility. It began specific professional training programs and financed alternative forms of intervention for children and families at social risk, but an administration change was made that eliminated this office, thus paralyzing its programs and eliminating (without warning of any type) the publication of documents related to child psychosocial topics.

It is important to point out the good intentions of the laws and successive commissions of experts (Castilla-León, Madrid, Galicia, and Cataluña), which have campaigned for attention to the mental problems of children and adolescents:

- Territory and community attention.
- Formulation of the demand by the family, except in the cases who have relapsed into social institutions.
- Coordination with other institutions and services that assist children.
- To avoid duplicities in the attention of the child mental problems (i.e., in the case of mental retardation, child abuse and neglect).
- Gradual functional integration in the area of different services.
- Multidisciplinary teams in order to develop integrated attention that includes: prevention and promotion of the psychosocial development, diagnosis of child mental disorders, early treatment, social rehabilitation.
- Teamwork
- Postgraduate and continuous medical education in a specific way.

Unfortunately, 13 years after the beginning of the reformation process the situation is much as it was. The realization of these objectives has not been fulfilled in a meaningful way.

In 1989 the UN approved the International Declaration on the Rights of Children. Some aspects remain debatable, but there are two significant rights: children should be assisted in their physical, psychic, and social requirements by professionals especially qualified for this developmental stage. The second right is that children should be helped in appropriately set up institutions. These premises are unfulfilled in Spain: specific training does not exist, and children (even new borns) are often mixed with drug addicts and elderly people, demonstrating the scant regard toward the necessities of childhood. However, these rights are not in Art. 39 Para. 4 of our Spanish Constitution of 1978.

Types of services

AEPIJ has defined the types of services. Their roles and the type of therapeutic interventions that they would offer are listed in Tables 1 and 2. Clear delimitation between the three complementary institutions is attempted, but they to some extent overlap or duplicate interventions, because of the differences between the health system (child and adolescent psychiatry), educational system (psychopedagogic services and special education), and social services.

Table 1. Therapeutic interventions in child and adolescent psychiatry

Healthy ministry	Education & science ministry	Social affairs ministry
– Psychopharmacology – Psychotherapies: • Individual • Group • Family – Therapeutic consultations (counseling) – Liaison-consultation – Promotion of psychosocial development	– Psychopedagogy – Rehabilitation: • Speaking disorders • Writing disorders • Calculation disorders • Psychomotr – Orthophonist – Psychopedagogy in mental retardation – Others	– Economic support – Early stimulation – Detecting and follow-up in cases of child abuse and neglect – Social support: • Parents' separation • Divorce • Adoption • Family support – Institution for children – Behavior disorders connecting with justice – Social rehabilitation

Table 2. Therapeutic interventions in child and adolescent psychiatry: tasks and devices

	Healthy ministry	Education & science ministry	Social affairs ministry
Tasks	– Clinical diagnoses – Detection and early intervention of developmental risks – Follow-up – Treatments – Support to the institutions of territory – Social rehabilitation supports	– Cognitive diagnoses – Pedagogic diagnoses – Follow-up – Psychopedagogy – Pedagogic supports	– Assessment of social risk – Detection of risk factors – Follow-up – Social supports – Social rehabilitation
Devices	– Child and adolescent mental health centers – Hospitalization, in contact with pediatric services – Day hospital	– Special teaching – Units of special education – Others	– Homes – Day centers – Specific unit for child and adolescent social services – Others

Outpatient services

The outpatient services are located in the child mental units of community mental health centers, which have a psychiatrist with experience in child and adolescent mental disorders, a clinical child psychologist, a social worker or psychiatric nurse, and an administrative assistant. In these services the service offers a clinical diagnosis, advice to families, and treatment. They have been developed in some areas of Spain, with a very irregular distribution, due to the changes in the composition of the members of the work teams and have received only little recognition.

A consultation service of some NHS hospitals also exists. Their operation is more clearly limited to diagnosis and treatment of the affective disorders. Some pediatric hospitals – such as La Paz, 12th October and Niño Jesús in Madrid, Vall d'Hebron and San Joan de Deu in Barcelona, La Fe in Valencia, University Hospital of Sevilla – have already been open for several decades, but remain isolated not integrated in any assistance net.

Daypatient services

In Spain this type of service is lacking. Except for a day hospital in the Consorcio Uribe Costa in Bilbao (directed by Prof. Lasa), another in Alcazar de San Juan in Ciudad Real (directed by Dr. Jiménez), and a few in Barcelona and Madrid, no others exist. This service type does not also figure, at present, in the assistance planning, and it is not well accepted or understood by the responsible administrators.

It is curious that without existing day services for child and adolescent mental disorders specific day hospitals have been developed for eating disorders. It represents an absurd situation that these should have been set up prior to provision for more general or common problems.

Inpatient services

The existing child psychiatric hospitals described in the preceding section, have been transformed into other types of institutions and no longer function as child psychiatric hospitals.

Hospital units do not exist for child and adolescent mental disorders; one has to choose between inpatient beds in the pediatric hospital services or inpatient beds in the units of adult psychiatry hospitals. Both options are, in our opinion, inadequate and they present numerous deficiencies and difficulties.

Recently, under pressure from the judicial system, a hospital unit is to open in Madrid for child mental disorders, mainly behavior disorders. This situation is complicated by two things: the Law of Rights of the Minor refers to the hospitalization for the child mental disorders and this is recognized by the Catalog of Therapeutic Benefits, but where this should be established or who should be responsible is addressed. Paradoxically, the anarchical and disordered development of specific units for eating disorders was approved.

Complementary services and rehabilitation

Issues relating to rehabilitation continue to be considered; rehabilitation is associated with physiotherapy in the health system and language delays with the ortophonist. The degree of integration of these services remains poor.

Psychopedagogic support is part of the Ministry of Education and Science. Its intervention is pedagogic in many mental disorders that alone in the face of the failure of psychopedagogy are admitted in precarious situations to the child psychiatry services, where present.

In the case of social services, the operation has some peculiar characteristics. Their operation processes are antiquated, and its theoretical perspective and the training of professionals is very heterogeneous (i.e., besides services formed such as those in Catalonia and Navarra, the great majority of Spain does not have agencies for resource information or administration). The degree of development of the services also reflects territorial inequalities.

Personnel

The previous discussions demonstrate that child psychiatry is not a field or a specific task of another specialty of medicine (Ramos-Gorostiza & Casas-Losada, 1991). Nobody in Spain seeks to debate the clear psychiatric origin of the specialty of child psychiatry, but rather it is necessary to recognize the contributions of other disciplines to understand the complex situation, including the Spanish historical perspective and the specific peculiarities.

With this background it is clearly necessary to have a specific training in child and adolescent psychiatry and psychotherapy. In Spain the situation is precarious; the human resources for treating child and adolescent mental disorders are not exactly known, neither those who work at the moment nor the projected number necessary. Diverse committees of experts have suggested the following requirements:

- Child and adolescent psychiatrist: one properly accredited for each 20,000 inhabitants younger than 18 years, as a minimum, more appropriately 1/15,000, and even better 1/12,500. In Spain there are 10,589,961 children younger than 18 years; 5,434,232 are male and 5,155,729 are female (Ministry of Social Matters, 1991).
- It is necessary to have a more homogeneous reference to be able to calculate the number of necessary professionals (Flirtz, 1991). For the clinical evaluation of adults, an average of 1–1.5 h is used; for the same type of professional intervention in children, 4.5–6 h are necessary. With these values, the number of professionals currently needed in Spain is estimated to be between 700 and 800 child psychiatrists. At present, the scientific societies have around 300, after removing double memberships.
- Clinical child psychologists, properly accredited: in a relationship of one to one with the child psychiatrist.
- Nurse: specialized in psychiatry, at least one per child psychiatrist.
- Social worker: to be based in the social centers in the community, a professional who is specifically dedicated to childhood and adolescence requests. One social worker per center in child and adolescent mental health is required.
- Administrative assistant: One per unit.

Funding of services

Funding is public by means of the NHS, meaning that the NHS is both, the agent and supplier of the health services, as well as the coordinator of some types of assistance. Nevertheless in the case of child and adolescent mental disorders the situation is much more varied.

The public attention to child mental disorders is precarious; generally, families look for the private care, at least initially, and for acute services and hospitalization. Some institutions that give assistance for sensorial deficiencies exist. Some centers also exist to assist mental retardation. But the treatment of chronic cases is not covered by existing insurance. This is in spite of the promulgation of the Royal Law of the Catalog of health benefits of the NHS that includes health services as a public service.

Evaluation

As assistance resources are scarce, evaluation studies are an exception. An Accumulative Psychiatric Case Register (APCR) in Asturias began in 1986; its theoretical foundations are similar to those expressed by the Department of Social Psychiatry of the University of Groningen directed by Prof. Giel. Some other autonomous communities have begun partial registration systems (activity registration), but they have not published their results.

Several published works of the APCR data of Asturias exist (Pedreira & Serrano, 1990; Pedreira & Eguiagaray, 1996). They include data of singular relevance, bearing in mind that the APCR does not solve the problems but rather attempts to demonstrate them. The APCR discusses the analysis of two longitudinal studies: the evolution of diagnoses, treatment, and their effectiveness in child and adolescent mental disorders: The first looks at the longitudinal evolution of the persons in contact with assistance services (pattern of use of services) and the second at the evolution of the interventions of the professionals involved in the services.

4. Cooperation with medical and non-medical disciplines

Table 3 shows a summary of the areas of intervention in child and adolescent mental disorders in several disciplines, pointing out the impact that each one of the different services has on the child's life. It is evident that in many cases the impact can be similar, but it is useful to emphasize the importance of coordinated and complementary work.

Table 3. Impact from the assigned tasks to different services and levels of attention in the mental dysfunctions of child and adolescent psychiatry

	Social services	School	Psycho-pedagogy	Primary health care	Adult mental health	Child mental health
Promotion	+	++	+	+++	±	++
Prevention	+	++	+	++	+	++
Detecting	++	+++	++	+++	+	±
Referring	++	++	+	+++	±	–
Assessment	±	±	+	+	±	+++
Diagnosis	–	–	±	–	+	+++
Treatment	–	–	–	±	±	+++
Social support	+++	++	+	±	–	±
Follow-up	+	+	+	++	–	+++
Rehabilitation	+	++	+++	+	–	++
Relapse programs	++	++	+	–	–	+

(–) = It doesn't have reason to develop the function or task; (±) = It develops partial and limited aspects of that task; (+) = It develops active collaboration (i.e. specific programs); (++) = It carries out impact activities; (+++) = Excellent task.

Cooperation with pediatrics

The pediatrician is a professional who enjoys great social prestige in children's care, prestige granted by the families (they have a great trust in the pediatrician) which contributes to their easy accessibility. Their position in primary health care allows them to be very close to the families' demands in child health care. The tradition of psychosocial concern, which Spanish pediatrics has historically had, has been paralyzed by the appearance of North American influenced pediatrics with technological demands that have moved away from the theory of child care in pediatric teaching.

We know that the pediatricians are not very sensitive but very specific in detecting child and adolescent mental disorders (Garralda & Bayley, 1990; Pedreira & Sardinero, 1996) (Table 4). Liaison-consultation and child liaison-psychiatry is fundamental, and aims to increase pediatrician sensibility. The use of liaison-

Table 4. Prevalence of child mental disorders in primary health care

Author and country	Year	Sample	Age	Prevalence rate (%)	Refer rate (%)	Risk factors
Costello et al. USA	1988	789	7–11	22 %	3.8 %	Behaviour disorders: boy + repeat class Anxiety disorders: girls + parental stressor life events
Garralda & Bailey United Kingdom	1990	137	7–12	47 %	–	Somatization vulnerability: 1) Children: demanding and sensitive personality + depresive symptoms + stressor life events + general anxiety 2) Family: mother without work + family stress and/or family health problems
Giel et al. India, Sudan, Philipine	1988	1.294	5–15	10–29 %	–	–
Goldberg et al. New York (USA)	1984	18.351	0–19	5.21 % (1.4–11.9)	2.5 %	Sex: male, poverty Monoparental family
Jellinek et al. USA	1988	206	7–12	39 %	–	–
Starfield et al. USA	1980	166.398	0–17	a) 15.5 % b) 5.4 % c) 15.0 % d) 5.7 % e) 14.2 %	–	Increased age Adolescent black race Poverty
Pedreira & Sardinero Asturias (Spain)	1996	235	6–11	30.2 %	8 %	–

consultation and child liaison-psychiatry, in the hospital environment as well as in primary health care, has encouraged the development of protocols and health programs for intervention in child mental disorders. Periodic health exams observe psychosocial risks and developmental issues are common until the child's chronic condition improves (including support in the usual activities for this age).

Spanish pediatricians are accustomed to providing assistance for families, who have problems. They are experts of their own limitations and they request cooperation of other institutions. If they observe however that the other institutions are not competent, then the cases will no longer be referred to these services.

Collaboration does exist, recently at the Congress of the Spanish Pediatrics Association, contributing information on certain common child disorders in pediatric care, i.e., depressive disorders (Pedreira & Tomás i Vilaltella, 1995), suicidal behaviors in adolescence (Mardomingo, 1996), sleep disorders (Bielsa, Martín-Alvarez, Pedreira, Rodríguez-Sacristán and Tomás i Vilaltella, 1998). A session on psychosomatic disorders is planned for next year.

Cooperation with psychiatry

Although a mental health plan was contemplated by the NCPCR, except for a few exceptions, it has not been developed. Spanish psychiatry is a specialty focussed on serious pathologies with particular attention given to the chronic ones. A second area is centered around drug abuse and a third focusses on elderly psychiatry. Their current orientation is very descriptive and categorical, with a limited psychopathological perspective and an almost absent developmental perspective.

The general use of the new mental disorders classification systems has improved the capacity of understanding in the use of scientific language. To these achievements, it should be added that a disadvantage has been the impoverishment of developmental psychopathology and of clinical observation. Child and adolescent psychiatry continues however to contribute to this forgotten aspect of current psychiatric practice in Spain. Our specialty continues to carry out case analysis, the integration of biological with developmental issues, dynamic, family and social issues, as well as understanding child mental disorders and planning and developing therapeutic intervention.

The relationship with adult psychiatry has not been easy in Spain. Very recently a new approach has been tried and results are awaited. Indeed, the publication of the Document of Accreditation from AEPIJ has been a forming point with the positive and receptive attitude of some important Spanish university professors, among these it is necessary to name in particular Profs. Conde and López-Ibor (Jr).

It is important to point out that recent topics in child and adolescent psychiatry have also been presented at the meetings of general psychiatry, e.g., eating disorders (Toro et al.), setting up a research group in child psychiatry (Rodríguez-Sacristán et al., 1995), continuity versus discontinuity of mental disorders in children and the adult (Agüero, Conde, Ballesteros, Rodríguez-Sacristán, 1997), assessment and treatment in child and adolescent psychiatry (Alcázar et al., 1998).

Cooperation with doctors in private practice

In Spain, private and public care are clearly separated; in many occasions they are in clear contradiction, sometimes having confrontations. Although the GHL contemplates cooperation between both types of care, this is unfortunately only a declaration of intentions (Table 4, p. 340).

Two exceptions exist: Cataluña and the Basque Country. In Cataluña the development of the private care sector or scarce development of the public sector, according to one view, has resulted in the ICS being integrated in the private sector in a complementary way. In the Basque and Navarre Country, the special economic policy allows the public financing of some care benefits to private services, when these benefits are appropriate and they are not available in public services. The creation of a cooperative of professionals in Catalonia and Unions in the Basque Country has been selected.

In our opinion this field will develop in Spain, but will have to overcome sterile confrontations over a rather ideological content. Nevertheless, we favor legislating public financing of services, which should have accreditation for a period of time, allowing professionals and services to be updated.

Convergence fields could include: the psychotherapies (individual, family, and group) that could not be undertaken by the public services because of pressure on services; intermediate services (day center and hospital, rehabilitation services), because these are not present in the public service and, finally, services of social care to chronically ill patients. The collaboration with family associations, the constitution of professional cooperatives, and the creation of foundations will be fields to develop in the immediate future.

Cooperation with non-medical institutions and professionals

The uncontrolled growth of some university degrees and the serious unemployment situation that exists in Spain are two factors that have hindered cooperation with other institutions and professions.

In recent years in Spain a reluctancy has existed in identifying child mental disorders; attempts have been made to diffuse the idea that identified disorders needed to be treated by psychiatrists, but this stops psychologists. On the other hand, the nonexistence of services and professionals in child and adolescent psychiatry has resulted in the services being manned by two types of professionals: the psychologist (who found in these programs an entrance door to the health system), and the nonexpert professional, who used these programs as a springboard to carry out professional progress to another type of more grateful and more prestigious sevices.

Clinical psychology, having the same accreditation as our specialty, is still to be recognized officially. It is evident that a cooperative effort is needed to establish meeting points in fields like child development, assessment, clinical instruments for the assessment, psychotherapeutic interventions and advice to families and community institutions. On the other hand, the social work professionals in Spain possess, in general terms, more enthusiasm than solid training.

Pedagogy and psychopedagogy are well established fields. The importance of these institutions in the child's life demands a joint effort; the differentiation of the pedagogic from the psychotherapeutic, combined pursuit of cases at risk and those with detected mental disorders, assessment instruments, aspects of learning and of the relationship with parents and in groups are some of the fields they share in common.

With the judicial system the importance is growing, not only for the increment of behavior disorders or for child and adolescent institutionalization, but also because the field of the rights in these stages of life is a new field needing harmonic and permanent development.

5. Graduate/postgraduate training and continuing medical education

Graduate training: The role of medical faculties

Rodríguez-Sacristán (1989) carried out a study where the time dedicated to the topics of child and adolescent psychological and psychopathological aspects in the medical undergraduate was evaluated; the results were not very encouraging (Table 5).

The total number of programs shows that pediatrics has as much time as medical psychology and psychiatry. However, little time is dedicated to the topics of child psychology and child psychiatry in the three areas.

The new plans for university studies are being currently approved and allow two types of subjects: optional ones and obligatory ones (they can be imparted in some specialities but not in all universities). The undergraduate teaching of child psychiatry does not have an appropriate place, i.e., in the University of Sevilla the subject of child psychiatry is considered as obligatory for the specialty in the study of medicine. The medical faculty at the University of Barcelona has declared it an optional subject and it already works with an educational program from the present academic course.

Table 5. Teaching of developmental psychology and infantile psychiatry in those specialities of medicine

Subjects (*)	Topic's numbers	% Child psychology	% Child psychiatry
Medical psychology	46	3	0.1
Psychiatry	45	0	4
Pediatrics	92	0.1	0.2

(*) It mediates of topics and percentage of the group of the specialities of medicine.

Postgraduate training, a joint effort

In 1990, the full General Council of Medical Specialties approved the proposal from the National Commission of Specialty of Pediatrics to recognize a specialization named pedopsychiatry, whose access would be mixed (from psychiatry and pediatrics), the same as in other specialties for the infanto-juvenile stage, such as intensive care, oncology, allergy, cardiology, and neurology. Psychiatry and other medical specialties were compared with respect to training in the draft of Real Ordinance about Medical Specialties (Guimon, 1990, p. 56). It was stated, "The most important novelty that the project introduces to the area of psychiatry is the inclusion of a new specific area named child psychiatry, which is a combination of psychiatry and pediatrics". Nevertheless, it should not be forgotten that all these organizations alone are of an advisory character, whereby their capacity is seriously limited and the linking of administration with their reports is usually applied in a very non-homogeneous way and without objective approaches.

The B.O.E. of January 15, 1990, included a Royal Law for recognition of training in the countries of the EU starting January, 1, 1993. In the transitory phase the minimum time required for recognition in child psychiatry, for example, is four years. With this real situation and with legal mark that supports it, the Spaniards have a double comparative offense with other professionals of the rest of the EU countries: if in our own country blocks of child psychiatry are summoned (assistance, educational or research), the Spanish professionals could not choose them or they would prefer those of other EU countries and that they would have the title; on the other hand, if another EU country summoned a block of child psychiatry (assistance, educational or research), the only professionals of the EU would be chosen or the Spaniards would have a disadvantage.

The previously exposed dilemma has some clear consequences: training programs do not exist in child psychiatry because an expressed recognition of this field of psychiatric knowledge and of the assistance practice does not exist. This non-existence results in a shortage (if not absence) of accredited services, as much for training as for care and research in this field. The two previous factors help us understand the shortage of professionals in the field of child and adolescent psychiatry.

Continuing medical education in child and adolescent psychiatry and psychotherapy

The continuous medical education in Spain constitutes a pending subject of the health system, since it is left up to the individual professional. Nevertheless AEPIJ is promoting that its scientific activities obtain the corresponding official accreditation.

On January 22, 1998, the National Commission of Continuous Medical Education of the NHS was constituted in Spain. They coordinate the health ministries of the various communities, the Ministry of Health and Consumption, and the Ministry of Education and Science. According to the specificity of the topics, the advice of the National Council of Medical Specialties, of the commissions of each specialty and of the representative scientific societies will be requested. AEPIJ has requested to be an adviser for the topics of its professional environment.

AEPIJ agrees on accepting the document from the UEMS, which has more than enough continuous medical education, for the scientific activities of our scientific society. The formative areas recommended in this document include: psychotherapeutic tendencies for the treatment of the child and adolescent mental disorders, child and adolescent psychopharmacology, child and adolescent psychopathology (classification systems of the mental disorders – both categorical and dimensional – and clinical expression of the disorders), mental retardation, research methodology, community mental health prevention in childhood and adolescence, management of the assistance services for the child mental disorders, law perspectives (international, national, autonomous with special reference to the International Declaration of the Rights of the Children), and improved quality of care and ethics as applied to our professional field.

In addition we are aware of having to establish a minimum of credits to execute on the part of the specialists for continuous medical education. These topics are a good incentive to promote professionals. A 4–5 year term to complete 40 credits seems reasonable.

Training programs for other disciplines

In Spain child psychiatrists have classically collaborated with other disciplines (psychology, psychopedagogy, pedagogy, professors, social workers, nurses, occupational therapists, phoniatrist, law professionals), but an atmosphere full of difficulties is detected for multidisciplinary teaching, which has increased certain cooperation, thus making it difficult to contribute this to a type of training program. Maybe the economic crisis and the increasing unemployment rate (also among professionals) has made this difficulty worse.

In spite of these difficulties, some professionals of child psychiatry and AEPIJ are renewing this activity in a slow and continuous way with combined day-work, participation in scientific activities, and increasing the presence of these topics in the daily activities.

6. Research

Research fields and strategies

The estimated prevalence in the child population, according to diverse international works of emotional or behavioral disorders, is calculated to be 10–25 % of children 0–18 years of age, who need specific help. In our country direct data do not exist; for this reason, AEPIJ favors a research denominated National Epidemic Plan (PEN) that includes 11 autonomous communities of Spain, with epidemiological methodology in double phase over three years (directed by Prof. Rodríguez-Sacristán and coordinated by Dr. Pedreira). This research will allow the completion of several important objectives, among those we highlight: creation of an atmosphere for discussion and training in research methodology, increasing collaboration and team work among diverse teams of several geographical locations and collecting data with the purpose of evaluating the assistance needed.

We have research on the estimated prevalence rates in the pediatric primary care setting stating that 30 % of children who consult the pediatrician with somatic complaints suffer emotional disorders that influence the origin, evolution and eventual cure of the processes. Of these, half are identified by the pediatrician and less than half are referred to a specific service of a child mental health center (Pedreira & Sardinero, 1996). These results are similar to those contributed by other groups of investigators at the international level.

These data have several implications:

- Of the 30 % of the children with mental disorders who consult a pediatrician for reasons of somatic complaints, only half are detected and half of them are referred to specific services.
- The possibility to receive psychopharmacotherapy for a child who presents a problematic behavior depends on the professional: GP 34 %; pediatrician 30 %; general or adult psychiatrist 26 % and child psychiatrist 3.5–5 % (with tendency to increase to 15–20 %, for the growing use of new psychopharmacological products).
- According to the expert groups from WHO Europe, most child psychiatric disorders do not receive appropriate care, which results in increasing social costs, increasing psychiatric morbidity rates in the adult age, and increasing delinquency rates.
- Therefore, the preventive component and promotion of psychosocial development are the basis of the practice in child and adolescent psychiatry.

Research groups are developing some lines of special relevance: the attention deficit disorder with hyperactivity, collaborating with the European group on the matter (Prof. Benjumea, from Sevilla); the work promotes psychosocial development from primary care services, WHO Europe program with Prof. Tsiantis as coordinator (Dr. Pedreira, from Asturias); the interesting works on child depression and suicidal ideation (Profs. Domenech from Barcelona and Polaino from Madrid); the use of the new psychopharmacology in child and adolescent mental disorders (Drs. Ballesteross from Valladolid, Gutiérrez from Badajoz and Rey from Salamanca); eating disorders, collaborating with European investigations (Drs. Morandé from Madrid, Velilla from Zaragoza, and Prof. Toro from Barcelona); the field of chronic conditions, pediatric oncology and transplantation in childhood and adolescence (Prof. Tomás, from Barcelona); psychosomatic disorders and child liaison-consultation (Prof. Pedreira from Asturias); continuity versus discontinuity of mental disorders (Prof. Agüero from Valencia); attachment and early psychopathology (Profs. Polaino from Madrid, Domenech from Barcelona, and Pedreira from Asturias) which represent some fields of interest developed by different teams in Spain.

Therefore, in spite of the administrative precariousness, the Spanish professionals develop strategies of investigation of excellent importance in some fields of interest:

- Clinical and applied epidemiology.
- Developmental psychopathology.
- Clinical assessment.

- Pharmacological and psychotherapeutic treatments.
- Longitudinal follow-up (continuity versus discontinuity).
- Research and ethics: informed consent in child psychiatry.
- New imaging techniques, genetic studies.

Research training and career development

Research training is obtained in Spain in university departments and by means of working in international research departments, fundamentally of North American influence.

AEPIJ has published during the last two years in its journal a complete course on research methodology, in order to contribute to this training and to sensitize professionals about the need for further development.

Funding

The funding in Spain for these topics is scarce and difficult to obtain. In their official organizations, high priority lines of financing for this research does not exist; it is necessary to look for the "cracks" in the official funding for research assistance.

The most important financial source is the Investigations Fund of the Social Security (FISS), but it does not have a category of mental disorders and it is necessary to apply for research funds in child psychiatry from another area: epidemiology, child health, services evaluation. Psychiatry is always of secondary importance and in childhood it becomes third. Thus, to find specific financing from a select group is hindered.

University R&D funds are also limited in each university department and, at the present time, there are not enough university professors with an educational and investigator profile in child psychiatry.

Funding from private foundations are not being pursued with enough persistence in this field, because priorities of the foundations are changing according to the opportunities and private interests. Therefore, the financing for research is in a precarious situation. However, Spanish groups search for it with tenacity and persistence and with a lot of work and dedication, they have been able to carry out projects.

7. Future perspectives

Research

Research is basic for the progress of any scientific branch; the stimulus for research in child and adolescent psychiatry should come from several environments:

- A concrete source of funding should be clarified as to where research funding can be requested to study various areas, mainly projects of multicenter and collaborative research of several services and autonomous communities.
- To support training in research methodology in child and adolescent mental disorders, in, for example, basic sciences (genetics, neurophysiology, diagnosis for image) and clinical sciences (psychopathological processes, clinical pictures, clinical assessment, psychopharmacology, psychotherapies), management of services (longitudinal evaluation, organization and services administration, process-cost), and in clinical epidemiology (population studies, computer science, statistics, evaluation instruments).
- To include research in postgraduate training, such as in continuous medical education, as contemplated in the diverse proposals carried out by CAPP-UEMS.
- To participate in international projects, promoted by official organizations (i.e., WHO Europe) or in multicentric research headed by university departments or research groups from scientific societies.

We believe that to promote and develop the Research-Shop proposed by AEPIJ is a step with future perspectives. This Research-Shop should continue to publish periodic updates in the journal of SEPIJ, organize scientific meetings and, above all, publish quality results.

Training

The aim in the future will be to develop training, according to the guidelines from the National Commission of the Specialty of Psychiatry, which will be approved by CNEM. The proposal is to be an ACE at least two years after completing the

Table 6. Priorities in training of child and adolescent psychiatry and psychotherapy

• International classification of mental disorders in children and adolescents: assessment and management	
• New diagnostic possibilities:	NMR
	PET
	EEG
	Biochemistry
• Developmental and psychopathological approach	
• Therapeutic interventions:	Psychopharmacology
	Psychotherapy
	Psychopharmacology + psychotherapy
	Community developments
	Liaison-consultation & liaison-psychiatry
• Family and social changes:	Monoparental families
	Divorce
	Family behavior
	Suicide behavior
	Eating disorders
• The impact and/or interaction between biological, emotional and social factors in mental disorders of children	
• Behavioral genetics	
• Longitudinal follow-up	
• Ethical issues	
• New technologies: informatic, internet, statistical approach	

specialty of psychiatry or three after that of pediatrics, which facilitates the historical duality of the child psychiatrists' origin in Spain.

The contents and objectives of the training would clearly complete the standards of the CAPPS-UEMS if they were based on the proposal of AEPIJ:

- Study of normal development.
- Factors that influence development and risks.
- The theoretical bases of child and adolescent psychiatry.
- Child and adolescent psychopathology and clinical approach.
- Psychopathological and clinical assessment in children and adolescents.
- Therapeutic interventions in childhood and adolescence.
- Research in child and adolescent psychiatry.

We emphasize the necessity of including these teachings in pre-graduate studies of the specialities of medicine (Table 6).

Improvement of services and care systems

The professional and services accreditation dates from 1917 when the American School of Surgeons set up minimum standards covering surgical services; it was summarized in the "Joint Commission Report" in 1951.

The accreditation process for a professional or health service is voluntary with an external audit, in order to evaluate the quality and standard approaches previously proposed by an independent committee, which published a report for obtaining professional accreditation.

For the previously exposed concept, the accreditation is dynamic and specifies continuous evaluation and accreditation. The AEPIJ's proposal includes a document of audit services with some minimum standards; therefore, this document closely mirrors the process of continuous improvement in quality of health services. This audit document is based on evaluating the minimum standards in the following areas: the library (a minimum list of journals, books, and handbooks is recommended), assistance quality, organization of the assistance services, access to a diagnostic service for imaging, access to clinical laboratory services, clinical child psychology, pharmacy, clinical documentation, hospitalization and agreements with complementary services.

Final considerations

We believe that child and adolescent psychiatry in Spain is already accepted by the population and many professionals. First, it was necessary to pass the General Law of Health and later the Reformation of the Psychiatric Care. Now, capacity of acceptance should not be confused with subjection; for this reason it is necessary to recognize minimum of professional requirements in the training of these professionals (Espino, 1992).

Finally, in Spain enough reports and proposals already exist for child and adolescent psychiatry training. None, however, has the degree of detail of the AEPIJ proposal. It is now necessary to develop this proposal into reality.

References

Available upon request from the author

Child and adolescent psychiatry in Sweden

K. Schleimer

1. Definition, historical development, and current situation

Definition

In "Child and Adolescent Psychiatry in Sweden during the 1990s" (Swedish Association for Child and Adolescent Psychiatry, 1993) it was stated that the discipline is a resource on specialist level within the national health service system. The goals to be fulfilled are to recognize, cure, relieve, and prevent any psychiatric disease or disorder that could be an obstacle to a child's personal development and maturity. The discipline should also take responsibility that the interests of children be covered in society through their parents and the school, social welfare, and health care systems. Characteristic of child and adolescent psychiatry is its field of knowledge to be of multidisciplinary nature. Medical, psychological, and social knowledge are integrated into a central focus on psychopathology and how to release resources in the child and its family.

Historical development

In Sweden, child and adolescent psychiatry has its roots more in pediatrics than in general psychiatry. However, since the first decades of this century, a common interest in children's mental development and health and in the prevention of deviant behavior has also existed among general psychiatrists, psychologists, pedagogues, and social workers. In 1932, the first child guidance clinics were opened. In 1934 the Erica Stiftelse, a foundation, was established to train teachers, psychologists, physicians, and social workers in diagnosing and treating children with mental health and school problems. This foundation still exists and today educates professionals in psychotherapy. It is also open to patients in need of psychotherapy. The first physicians to work with mental health problems in children were appointed in 1941, and during the 1940s some inpatient wards for these children were opened, linked to either pediatric or psychiatric clinics. The need for knowledge of children's normal and deviant behavior and development came from many sides and resulted in the multidisciplinary cooperation and planning for Swedish child psychiatric clinical work. In the middle of the 1940s it was decided that child and adolescent psychiatry was a new discipline in medicine, and in 1951 it was introduced as such officially in the Swedish Medical Association. In 1956 it was introduced as an autonomous section of the Swedish Society of Medicine. Since 1969 its official designation is child and adolescent psychiatry. Professorships were established in Stockholm in 1954, in Uppsala in 1963, in Umeå in 1966, in Lund 1983, and in Gothenburg 1984.

In the 1960s, Swedish child psychiatry was built up. In 1960 there were 10 independent clinics; 1965 there were 21! In 1971 all county councils had an organization with in- and outpatient services for child and adolescent psychiatry. Today, there is a nationwide child and adolescent psychiatric health care organization. Treatment homes, often necessary after a session in inpatient care, are today the responsibility of communities. After years of discussion whether child psychiatry should belong to the medical disciplines, to child social welfare or to behavioral science, it was confirmed in 1985 in an official report of the Swedish Government (BFU-81) that child and adolescent psychiatry is a medical discipline. However, in Stockholm county, the Child Guidance Clinics Organization (PBU), based on its historical development belongs to another non-health service organization, dealing more with psychotherapy compared to outpatient care in clinics and departments.

Daily clinical work today is based on clinics and departments with inpatient and outpatient services, the latter mostly sectorized and decentralized to be closer to their patients. Many clinics have organized daycare wards, especially since budget cuts have been common in the 1990s, and the number of beds had to be reduced, while at the same time the demand for child psychiatric services has increased by almost 100 % over the last 5 years throughout the country.

Recent advances

All treatment for child and adolescent mental disorders is funded by the county councils and, thus, has to compete with other medical disciplines. The social welfare system is responsible for social welfare of children and their families, which often intervenes with their mental problems and is a never-ending source for discussion between the two organizations. Considering the general development of our society with violence, drug abuse, unemployment, and reduction in school services, child and adolescent psychiatry received this year (1998) extra governmental resources not to expand but to cope with the increased demand for our services, depending on the budget cuts in other fields of society. The university hospitals with their child and adolescent departments are basically funded in the same way as the community clinics. However, since training of medical students is depending on clinical work, some of the university budget is transferred to the department equivalent to the number of students and scientific work produced.

Current situation

On January 1, 1998, the population of Sweden was 8,847,625, among them 1,956,826 children and adolescents aged 0–18 years, which is 22 % of the total population. On average about 2 % of the population 0-18 years are in contact with child psychiatry. There are 30 clinics and departments for child and adolescent psychiatry, among them 6 university departments, two of them without a chair but with associate professors responsible for teaching and training. There are 282 specialists in our discipline; 58 % of them are women. Most of them are publicly employed; only a handful work in private practice. In 1994, the UEMS/CAPP section showed that Sweden had 12.5 specialists for 100,000 inhabitants under the age of 20 years (Switzerland and Finland came next). The Swedish Association for Child and Adolescent Psychiatry has about 250 members, only child psychiatrists. We have no association for all mental health professionals compared to our international association (International Association for Child and Adolescent Psychiatry and Allied Professions), which also holds allied professions like psychologists, social workers, pedagogues, etc.

2. Classification systems, diagnostic and therapeutic methods

Classification systems

In Sweden, the ICD-9 classification system was used from 1987–1996 in child psychiatry but only in inpatient services, where we had to use it for statistical reasons. For many years in outpatient services nearly every clinic or department had its own way of documentation with data from the history, a list of symptoms, and therapeutic measures, for their own purpose. According to that, quite different data were noted. In 1997, we changed to the ICD-10 system, which now has to be used in all services. At the same time, in accordance with general psychiatry, child psychiatry also used and still uses the DSM classification system, from 1994 the DSM-IV. This system is mostly used for scientific purposes and also as a reference system, being more detailed and descriptive.

Diagnostic methods

In Swedish child and adolescent psychiatry, diagnostic methods of all kinds are used depending on the patient's problems. To start with a thorough history is taken, a physical examination including a neurological one is performed, and once again, depending on the results of these together, examinations like EEG and special brain imaging techniques are used. According to the raising interest for neuropsychiatry, specific examinations can be performed, often in teams specializing in this field. Even in the field of neuropsychology new diagnostic methods have been developed and are used if appropriate. Today in almost every special field of child psychiatry, special psychological instruments are available. Cooperation with pediatrics, the laboratory disciplines, and general psychiatry is well developed. All child psychiatric clinics have a hospital school and pedagogues may take part in the diagnosing process.

Therapeutic methods

Family therapy has for several decades now held the front position as a therapeutic method, normally using a psychodynamic orientated approach. This has to do with the fact that within the organization clinical psychologists and social workers outnumber child psychiatrists and, thus, the approach to a child and his family from the start has often been family focused. Psychoanalysis is rare. However, today with a growing interest in child neuropsychiatry and better understanding of the individual child with respect to biology and genetics, there is greater interest in using other more individually orientated methods, including behavioral techniques and cognitive therapy besides medication.

3. Structure and organization of services

Guidelines for services for children and adolescents with psychiatric disorders

The medical discipline child and adolescent psychiatry is organized within the county council's health service on the specialist level. The primary activity is to diagnose and treat psychiatric diseases and mental disorders. A clinic should be headed by a senior specialist in child and adolescent psychiatry, especially if patients will be treated under the law of compulsory psychiatric care. Otherwise today, any other mental health professional within the discipline can be the administrative head of a clinic. However, the child and adolescent psychiatrist is always responsible for medical issues. In the region of every county council, the discipline should be organized into outpatient teams, where child psychiatrists, clinical child psychologists, and social workers as well as trained nurses, occupational therapists, and social pedagogues work together. Even if almost 90 % of our activities are handled in outpatient services, inpatient wards, day units for infants and mothers and for children, family units, therapeutic schools, and treatment homes will still be necessary for emergency cases, e.g., more severe problems needing difficult investigations and longer treatment periods. In Sweden, a patient is free to ask for consultation throughout the whole country on an outpatient basis. However, most children and adolescents are seen within their home region, since school and social welfare systems and other organizations are normally integrated in evaluation and treatment. Every county council is expected to be self-supporting as to care for special disorders or diseases, but nevertheless there will always be departments and clinics with special interests and special services which might be open to patients from other regions.

Types of services

Practically all child and adolescent psychiatric services are organized publicly and localized to general, mostly regional, hospitals and university hospitals. Just a handful of child psychiatrists are working in private practice. Around larger cities there are enough services but in the countryside and the sparsely populated, northern part of the country, there is a shortage of child psychiatric services, although people in the north are used to overcome the inconvenience of long distances. To bridge this difficulty, child psychiatric teams in these regions travel from their center out to smaller locations, closer to the patients. Because of ongoing budget cuts in recent years there is a shortage of inpatient beds and even severely mentally ill children and adolescents may have to be treated at home with complementary, frequent consultations as outpatients. A shortage of treatment homes and other facilities for rehabilitation of young people with long-lasting and chronic psychiatric illnesses is dependent on the difficult financial situation of the communities, which are responsible for these complementary services. Thus, many patients will have to stay much too long in hospital inpatient units. As a consequence, quite a few private treatment homes were started during the 1990s with varying quality. Their problem is to make a financial agreement with the county council to keep the charges down.

There are 30 clinics and departments for child and adolescent psychiatry in Sweden. All of them are responsible for their region's outpatient services. Outside these services there are just a few private practices, all of them in larger cities. In pediatrics, child welfare centers and in general medicine parents can receive mental counseling, but as said before child and adolescent psychiatry is practised on the specialist level. The Swedish Association for Child and Adolescent Psychiatry has suggested there should be 10 specialists for 250,000 inhabitants, which is about equivalent to one county council region. Twenty years ago the need of child psychiatrists was estimated to 320 positions for specialists all over the country – this has not been achieved yet. However, in 1978 we had 18 positions for postgraduate students in our discipline; in 1998 we have about 80! The 30 clinics and departments also have inpatient units; some have several units for better differentiation, and others just one for all purposes. Some inpatient units have been transformed into daypatient services, mostly associated with outpatient units, as a bridge between out- and inpatient services. Inpatient wards seldom exceed 10 beds, 6–8 beds being the normal situation. Quite often a parent is admitted together with the child up to the age of about 12 years. There is no national proposal as to the number of beds per inhabitant, since the counties are self-determined concerning the extent of their health care.

Complementary services and rehabilitation

Children and adolescents with long-lasting and chronic psychiatric disorders should after assessment and treatment in a clinic come to more home-like services, if it is not possible for them to return to their families. These services belong to either the social welfare system in a community or are private initiatives, selling their activities to the communities whenever requested. Services belonging to complementary ones are treatment homes either for children or for adolescents, often specialized for different groups of chronic disorders and foster homes in private but well-trained families. There still are, but probably to a reduced number, group homes/big foster homes for young people who for some reason cannot stay in their families and need certain guidance before becoming independent.

Personnel

Different vocational groups work within child and adolescent psychiatry such as doctors, psychologists, social workers, trained nurses, practical nurses, occupational therapists, social pedagogues, and preschool teachers. The traditional outpatient team is manned by child psychiatrists, clinical psychologists, and social workers. In day- and inpatient units, the number of personnel is calculated in relation to the number of patients, taking into special account the mental and behavioral problems these patients show.

Funding of services

All child psychiatric facilities are paid for by the county councils as is all other health service according to the Health and Medical Services Act. Sweden has a compulsory national health insurance system, financed by the state and employer contributions, where all children and young people are insured in the name of their parents up to the age of 16, after that in their own name. This health insurance system in connection with the county council is responsible for physical and mental health for all patients. For treatment over years outside their families, chronically ill psychiatric children may be subsidized also by the social welfare system, especially with regard to their general dysfunction and insufficiency in society. For deviant youngsters with antisocial behavior or drug abuse there are training centers, paid by the state.

4. Cooperation with medical and non-medical disciplines

Cooperation with pediatrics

Liaison and consulting services from child psychiatry exist in most pediatric hospitals, though many of them also have their own social workers and clinical psychologists, especially in neuropediatric units. This work is carried out by senior specialists in child and adolscent psychiatry or by child psychiatric teams, who for part of their working time are situated within the pediatric department. Thus, psychosomatic patients may be cared for either by the pediatrician or by the child psychiatrist, depending on the patient's situation. Special psychosomatic wards are today rare if they still exist at all. However, chronic somatic disorders including oncologic diseases, crisis intervention, and intensive care are examples where child psychiatry should assist. Handicapped children are normally seen in special habilitation centers belonging to pediatric clinics, where support or direct cooperation from child psychiatry is the rule. This includes mental retardation, motor handicaps, metabolic disorders, and other diseases of the central nervous system and DAMP/ADHD disorders. Autistic spectrum disorders are therapeutically normally taken care of by child psychiatry. However, sometimes pediatric staff is involved in the evaluation.

Cooperation with psychiatry

In practical work, cooperation is much more intensive with pediatrics, but administratively CAP normally belongs to the block of psychiatry. CAP shares its age groups of patients with pediatrics but a diagnostic approach with general psychiatry, with special regard to older youngsters and adolescents. For older adolescents, we would wish to have special services, since this agegroup mostly does not feel at home either in child psychiatry or in general psychiatry. Other important groups where cooperation between the disciplines should increase are children of mentally ill parents, of abusing and neglecting parents, and of parents with drug and alcohol abuse. Also, cooperation is especially necessary when transferring an adolescent of age to general psychiatry.

Cooperation with general medicine

General medicine is practised on a basic level. They have a primary responsibility for children, adolescents, and their families both regarding physical and mental health. Doctors and trained nurses within this organization are in charge of baby and child welfare centers, school health care, and special treatment homes outside larger municipalities, where consultants from child psychiatry would be in charge. They should be able to intervene early and refer to child psychiatry cases they could not deal with. A condition of their intervention is they know something about child psychiatry, which in turn is our responsibility to give to them by teaching, training, and supervision.

Cooperation with non-medical institutions and professionals

Cooperation is divided into work with individual cases, education and training of non-medical staff, consultation, and supervision. The most important non-medical institution to cooperate with is, first the social welfare system, where social secretaries are responsible for children's and adolescents' welfare according to our legislation. Every professional working with children and adolescents under age is compelled to announce to them any suspicion he may have that a child or an adolescent is not living in the best conditions with regard to physical abuse, protection from sexual abuse, insufficient care, antisocial behavior or abuse of drugs or alcohol, etc. Also, children of divorced parents may be object to evaluation because of custodial disputes. Second, cooperation with the school system including both elementary comprehensive school and high school as well as the special school for mentally retarded children is important in daily practice. Children of normal intellect but with learning disabilities, speech and language disorders, behavioral and conduct disorders belong to the normal school and will receive special support and help there, for which consultation and supervision may be necessary from child psychiatry. Third, the police and court systems may need consultation as well. In Sweden we have no special juvenile court. Therefore, special knowledge of the situation of children in custodial disputes and in cases of sexual abuse is scarce and depends very much on who is in charge of the juridical case.

Fourth, consulting services are offered and delivered to different types of treatment homes especially for adolescents.

5. Graduate/postgraduate training and continuing medical education

Graduate training: The role of medical faculties

Not every medical faculty in Sweden has a chair for child and adolescent psychiatry. At four medical faculties (in Stockholm, Uppsala, Lund and Gothenburg), there is a professor. In Umeå the chair is temporarily not in use and in Linköping the professor of pediatrics is responsible for the child psychiatric department. In all six university departments of child and adolescent psychiatry graduate students are trained, normally for one full week, integrated into pediatrics. In 1944 a decision had already been made that child psychiatry should be taught in the medical curriculum but on an optional basis. When in 1951 child and adolescent psychiatry became an independent speciality, the course for graduates from 1953 onwards was obligatory. A compulsory basic clinical training program (internship) after medical school (for 5 1/2 years) was introduced in 1972, today comprising 18 months of clinical work including an internship for 3 months in either general or child and adolescent psychiatry. This has been an excellent way to recruit new physicians for our discipline.

Postgraduate training, a joint effort

After the university degree and the license to practise (after internship), specialist training for 5–7 years will start. This means that it is more important to fulfill the official objectives of the training program than to work for a certain period of time, as it was until 1992. An official description of required knowledge, skills, and attitudes was made by the Swedish Association for Child and Adolescent Psychiatry and was authorized by the National Board of Health and Welfare (Socialstyrelsen). The postgraduate student is entitled to have an individual training program with goal orientation, specifying the required practical training in various departments together with needed theoretical education in order to acquire the described knowledge, skills, and attitudes (see supplement). He is also entitled to have a personal tutor or supervisor (a senior specialist) who will give him professional guidance throughout his training for 5 years at a minimum. The specialist training will have to be fulfilled for 3 years in child and adolescent psychiatry, for about 1 year in pediatrics and general psychiatry, respectively. In addition, the student will have to attend about 6 national or regional specialist courses in various main subjects, including one course in basic psychotherapy, that is compulsory since 1986. This, however, does not allow him to announce himself as a psychotherapist – for that competence he will need more training to come after specialization. Every postgraduate student will have a training logbook with all instructions and demands for achieving the specialization license. The head psychiatrist of the department/clinic has the ultimate responsibility for the specialist training and has to decide when the student has reached the goals set up for the specialist training and thus can be recognized as a specialist. The head psychiatrist has to state this by issuing an official certificate. The National Board of Health and Welfare will then grant the doctor the formal competence as a specialist. There is no compulsory final examination as of yet before being granted a licence as a specialist. Other medical disciplines have accomplished optional examinations for many years. Child and adolescent psychiatry will at end of 1998 start with its first examination.

Continuing medical education

Continuing medical education (CME) is not yet formalized. The various specialist associations are responsible to organize this – in child psychiatry with the help of directors of studies.

In Sweden there are 6 directors of studies, each of them covering a geographic area of the country in order to supervise the postgraduate training given in this region by staying in regular contact with the postgraduate students, their tutors, and their heads of the departments/clinics and by arranging special symposia or workshops for them as a complement to national specialist courses. They are elected for a certain period of time by the Swedish Association for Child and Adolescent Psychiatry. The directors of studies also have taken on the responsibility of inspecting departments/clinics, where postgraduate students are trained. These inspections are aimed at assessing the structure of the training center (size, qualification of medical staff, premises, equipment, library, etc.) and the process (educational environment, tutoring, variety of assigned duties, etc.). Re-inspections take place about every 3 years. The directors of studies also have the responsibility of organizing CME according to the UEMS/CAPP regulations.

Training programs for other disciplines

Other medical and non-medical professionals also need training in child psychiatry. For instance, regularly students of psychology and social work have to serve for some time in CAP during their curriculum. Trained nurses specializing in our discipline have to serve for several weeks in inpatient units for practice, so will students of social pedagogy. Special teachers receive training when specializing.

6. Research

Research fields and strategies

The history of how child and adolescent psychiatry developed in Sweden also held important consequences for the establishment of research in the discipline. Current knowledge in Swedish and international child and adolescent psychiatry has mainly been achieved by two different methods. These are the retrospective "anamnestic" method in psychiatry and psychoanalysis with a retrospective view on deviant behavior and psychiatric disease – and the prospective "descriptive" method in pediatrics and behavioral sciences with prospective approaches for the study of development and maturation from birth to adulthood. To promote research even in our discipline the Swedish Medical Research Council has created a "planning group for child and adolescent psychiatric and social-psychiatric research", which in recent years has effectively stimulated new research programs, covering most fields within our discipline. Since the beginning of child and adolescent psychiatry in Sweden, 43 dissertations have been defended.

Research training and career development

Some positions for postgraduate students are linked to research training for future high quality research. These positions may be extended to make a dissertation possible within the training program. Many graduate students start their research career in preclinical fields, thus, postponing their medical degree. Clinical research is more difficult to fulfill with respect to the time it takes, especially when research is of a prospective, longitudinal character. A position as specialist at a department or clinic requires so much time and energy in practical work that research can hardly be fulfilled at the same time without a leave of absence. Postdoctoral training programs hardly exist.

Funding

Research in child and adolescent psychiatry is mainly performed at the universities, mostly in our departments but sometimes also in the departments of psychology and behavioral sciences. Since the universities also have had serious budget cuts, research can hardly be funded by institutional resources. The Swedish Medical Research Council has shown special interest in furthering research in our field by allocating special positions to postdoc students or funding special research programs. Otherwise organizations and foundations may sponsor research in their own field of interest. A normal child psychiatric clinic will hardly have the possibility to participate in research programs.

7. Future perspectives

The Swedish Association for Child and Adolescent Psychiatry has in the program "Child and Adolescent Psychiatry in the 1990s" (1993) presented goals covering four different areas, all aiming at better treatment for our patients:

- improve quality in clinical daily work both for patients and professionals,
- develop methods for measuring quality in treatment,
- improve education both for students and for specialists,
- promote both basic and clinical research and development,
- improve research methods, and
- have more interdisciplinary cooperation in research in order to develop research in the border area between the medical disciplines and the behavioral sciences.

Some of these goals have been achieved, some remain to be fulfilled.

Positions for postgraduate training should be increased to achieve a situation with about 320 active child and adolescent psychiatrists, according to programs both in the end of the 1970s and now the one from 1993. With respect to the extension of child neuropsychiatry and better understanding of biological and genetical factors influencing development and maturation, more doctors are needed in our discipline. As of today practically all other vocational groups in our discipline are outnumbering them. Services and care systems can be improved and focused on outpatient and daycare services with lesser budgeting without loosing effectiveness. More specified services are needed in step with modern knowledge and better techniques. Society and politicians have started to realize that child and adolescent psychiatry is an important discipline and have shown this with promises of lesser or no budgets cuts in the future.

Selected references

Den barn- och ungdomspsykiatriska verksamheten. Slutbetänkande från BFU-81. Official report of the Swedish Government, 1985: 14

Löfqvist A (1983) Child and adolescent psychiatry. In: The Swedish Society of Medicine 175 years – the establishment and development of its sections. Acta Societatis Medicorum Suecanae, Svenska Läkaresällskapets Handlingar Hygiea. 92 (6): 28–30

Rydelius P-A (1993) Child and adolescent psychiatry in Sweden – from yesterday until today. Nord J Psychiatry 47: 395–404

Swedish Association for Child and Adolescent Psychiatry (ed.) (1993) Barn- och ungdomspsykiatri under 90-talet. Kristianstad Boktryckeri AB, Kristianstad, 1993

Training logbook for postgraduate students of medicine. Child and adolescent psychiatry, chapter 14: 3. Edited by The Swedish Medical Association and The Swedish Society of Medicine, 1997

Child and adolescent psychiatry in Switzerland

D. Bürgin, W. Bettschart

1. Definition, historical development, and current position

Definition

It is remarkable that the definition of child and adolescent psychiatry, as given by M. Tramer at the launching of the Zeitschrift für Kinderpsychiatrie in 1934, has remained essentially unchanged. He wrote, "Child psychiatry or pediatric psychiatry is that part of medicine which is concerned with psychologically abnormal children and adolescents". He noted that the field of interest of child psychiatry overlaps with neurology, adult psychiatry and pediatrics, but that it occupies a special position for the following reasons: 1. the special research methods used; 2. the structure of the different forms of psychopathology, i.e., since time has a different significance in the development of psychopathology in childhood and adolescence (in psychological structure, the child is not simply an adult in smaller format); 3. the demands of therapy; and 4. the differing prognosis.

Historical development

D. J. Duché (1990) describes the long road our discipline has travelled from its early history in the eighteenth century. Because of German, French, and Italian linguistic groups Swiss child and adolescent psychiatry has been closely connected with these various European countries, but there have also been personal and scientific contacts with colleagues in England, America and Russia. There has been access both to the German (H. Emminghaus 1887) and to French (J. E. D. Esquirol 1818, P. Moreau de Tours 1888) traditions. On the Italian side there is, above all, Sancte de Sanctis.

In the 1930s came a new development, introducing modern child and adolescent psychiatry. There has been increasing collaboration between our discipline and related ones, such as psychology, educational theory (especially remedial education), pediatrics, and psychiatry, which have given and continue to give impulses to its further development. Deepening professional awareness and familiarity with the different areas of knowledge have improved the exchange between child psychiatry and these other disciplines. Nevertheless, there have been areas of tension, sometimes paralysing and sometimes enriching.

In Switzerland health and education are organized on a cantonal basis, giving plenty of scope for both personal and regional development. The founding of new cantonal child and adolescent psychiatric services in different parts of the country, regular exchange of clinical experience and scientific findings, institutionalized meetings to clarify administrative and organizational matters, and the development of a common program for further education under the auspices of the Swiss Society for Child and Adolescent Psychiatry have gradually built up a strong national identity in the speciality. The Swiss National Foundation was particularly important in the encouragement of research.

Development of the speciality

In 1921 Prof. H. W. Maier founded a psychiatric children's institution on the Stephansburg in Zürich "as a children's home that was under medical direction but with pedagogic staff and its own school" (J. Lutz & R. J. Corboz, 1992). The first outpatient clinic was started by A. R. Repond in canton Wallis in 1930. This was based on psychohygienic (represented in Switzerland predominantly by H. Meng in Basel) and psychoanalytic principles. On November 19, 1938, the Swiss Commission for Child Psychiatry, with J. Lutz as president, was founded in Lausanne within the framework of adult psychiatry, but there was still considerable resistance to be overcome before the independence of child psychiatry was accepted by colleagues in the adult field. In the same year L. Bovet established a private clinic for psychiatric treatment of children (Le Bercail) and within the framework of pediatrics. The "Office Médico-Pédagogique", which he set up in 1945, was within the Department of Justice and was at first intended primarily for juvenile delinquents. In Basel the Child and Adolescent Psychiatric Service, founded and directed by C. Haffter in 1960, evolved out of an adult psychiatric unit and a psychosomatic department of pediatrics, while in Bern child psychiatry was closely connected to the Child Guidance and School Psychology services. The observation and treatment unit for epileptic children in Tschugg (Bern) was also led by a psychiatrist for children and adolescents. Educational institutes for difficult, neglected, retarded, and mentally defective children, and those with impairments of hearing or vision, or with epilepsy, were increasingly led by child and adolescent psychiatrists. In both residential and day units psychologists were valued for their work in diagnosis, counseling, therapy, and research.

In terms of scientific research, the "Zeitschrift für Kinderpsychiatrie", later the "Acta Pedopsychiatrica", started by M. Tramer, has appeared since 1934. His book on general child psychiatry, "Allgemeine Kinderpsychiatrie", appeared in 1938. J. Lutz made an important contribution to clinical understanding and research with his work on childhood schizophrenia (1937). In 1951 L. Bovet published a monograph on adolescent delinquency, commissioned by WHO. In the realm of developmental psychology, creative impulses were provided by E. Claparède, a medical doctor and psychologist, and the pioneering ideas of J. Piaget (both from Geneva). Many of the child psychiatrists of that time had personal, clinical, and scientific connections to L. Kanner. The work of Sigmund and Anna Freud, and also that of Melanie Klein and August Aichhorn, opened up new perspectives for many colleagues in terms of prevention, diagnosis and treatment. The Rorschach test (1921) was soon introduced into the psychological diagnosis of children, as was the Z-test developed on the same basis by H. Zulliger (1954), a teacher and psychoanalyst. He became known through his publications on interpretation-free child analysis.

During the second world war, many European and international connections were ruptured. After the war Professor A. Friedemann (Biel) organized the "European Symposium for Child and Adolescent Psychiatry" in Magglingen, where not only old contacts were renewed and new ones made, but scientific collaboration revived. On May 4, 1957, the Swiss Specialist Group for Child and Adolescent Psychiatry was formed, introducing the specialist title for our discipline. The first president was Professor J. Lutz. In 1960 Friedemann's European Symposium gave birth to the "European Union for Paedopsychiatry" in Paris, which in 1970 became the "European Association for Child and Adolescent Psychiatry".

The post-war period was an extremely fruitful one for scientific activity. Textbooks were published by Lutz (1961), Züblin (1967), Ajuriaguerra (1970), and Herzka (1981). All five Swiss Universities (Basel, Zürich, Bern, Lausanne, and Geneva) had a professorial chair after the 1970s. In Geneva, the psychiatry of small children (B. Cramer), questions about the persistence of symptoms from childhood into adult Life (J. Manzano), and adolescent psychiatry were studied. In Lausanne, there was psychodynamic (R. Henny) and later epidemiological research, as well as research into the pathology of migration (W. Bettschart). Psychoanalytic psychotherapy, psychosomatics and relationship crises were the focus in Basel (D. Bürgin), while in Bern sects, rites of puberty (G. Klosinski), aspects of family therapy and the problems of children of divorced parents (W. Felder) were investigated. In Zürich there was research on disturbances in cerebral functioning (R. J. Corboz), child psychiatry in connection with remedial teaching (H. St. Herzka), and in epidemiology and classification (H. Ch. Steinhausen).

Recent advances

Swiss medicine is based on cantonal law. Qualification as a specialist is given by the FMH (Foederatio Medicorum Helveticorum, a private grouping of Swiss doctors). An important change occured in 1960 with the introduction of disability insurance, which took over responsibility for psychiatric treatment, special schooling, and educational measures (e.g., speech therapy) for children with mental and physical defects or birth injuries (e.g., autism or psychoorganic syndromes in early childhood). The disability insurance not only paid for individual treatment, but also made generous subventions toward the building and running of institutions and special schools. However, the contributions were only available to day hospitals and child psychiatric institutions, that included a special school under a qualified remedial teacher. A major question was, therefore, whether and how such a school (and the teacher in charge of it) could be incorporated into a psychiatric-psychotherapeutic concept. Each child and adolescent psychiatric service had to find its own way to fruitful cooperation with special school teachers, remedial educationalists, workers in children's homes, psychiatrists, and psychotherapists.

Current situation

On December 31, 1997, Switzerland had roughly 7.1 million inhabitants, of whom about 1.5 million (21 %) were children and adolescents under 18. There were 315 child and adolescent psychiatrists (157 = 50 % f, 158 = 50 % m); 256 of these had some form of private practice (130 = 48 % f, 126 = 49 % m). In the same year, 22 colleagues received the specialist qualification from the FMH (14 f, 8 m).

In relation to the population, there is one child psychiatrist for 22,500 or 27,700 inhabitants. If only children and adolescents under 18 are considered, the figure is 1 for 4,760 or 1 for 5,560. This may seem high, but there are four reasons why these figures need to be looked at carefully. First, the term "private practice" includes specialists in child psychiatric services, who can only devote a small part of their time to private work. Second, a large number of child and adolescent psychiatrists work part-time. In addition, many are employed part-time in institutions, children's hospitals, and school psychiatric services on a consultative basis or as clinicians or therapists. Finally, the greater part have a "mixed practice", i.e., they also treat adults. When these factors are taken into account we can count one child psychiatrist per 10,000 to 13,000 for the under 18 year olds.

Most cantons now have an outpatient psychiatric service, many with psychiatric day hospitals, inpatient observation and treatment units for children and/or adolescents, and liaison services. In the institutional field there is a lack of consultants, as a result of differentiation of services and creation of new ones (e.g., liaison services, day and night hospitals, emergency services), research posts, the incorporation of new forms of pathology and areas of work (e.g., drug dependency, post-natal depression, neonatology, or oncology), the expansion of preventive work (especially suicide prevention), caring for refugee children and their families, and pathology related to migration and to child abuse. There are still not enough child and adolescent psychiatrists in small towns and rural areas.

2. Classification systems, diagnostic and therapeutic methods

Classification systems

Throughout Switzerland the ICD-10 is used for clinical and comparative epidemiological purposes, in the German-speaking areas usually in the form of the "Multiaxial Classification Scheme (MAS)", which Remschmidt and Schmidt reproduced in 1994 based on Rutter. In the French-speaking areas, the French system of classification by Mises et al. (1988) is used. Basing their work on the "Operational Psychodynamic Diagnosis (OPD)" and as a supplement to MAS, an international German-speaking group is working on a "Child and Adolescent Psychiatric OPD" to systemize psychodynamic aspects. For research purposes the DSM-IV is more often used.

Diagnostic methods

Many psychodiagnostic procedures are used on an ambulant basis – individual-interactional, psychological testing (intelligence and projective tests, questionnaires, computer tests, neuropsychological methods), as well as psychodynamic and family-oriented methods – and are intended to give a complete picture of the patient as a biosocial individual and in the context of the family, school, social, ethnic, and community settings. These form the basis for the recommended therapeutic measures and the prognosis. In an inpatient setting the therapeutic milieu is foremost, whereby remedial education, psychotherapy and psychopharmacological treatment mutually enhance each other's effects. Switzerland is densely populated and well supplied with pediatric care; the majority of physical, neurological, and psychosomatic ailments in children are therefore recognized, and detailed somatic investigation is seldom necessary within child psychiatry. Nevertheless, such somatic investigation by appropriate specialists is often needed in marginal situations or for psychosomatic problems in adolescents.

Therapeutic methods

The different forms of therapy used not only depend on the age, diagnosis, setting, patient acceptance, and the situation, but are also influenced by the preferences and basic orientation of the service concerned. This produces a wide palette of psychoanalytic-psychodynamic, family-dynamic, cognitive-behavioral and psychopharmacological forms of treatment. Most services base their psychotherapy on one clear theoretical system and avoid unnecessary mixtures providing "a little bit of everything". This means that although particular forms of therapy are often chosen for official psychiatric services (mostly psychoanalytic in Basel, Geneva, Jura, Lugano, Luzern, Schaffhausen, St. Gallen, and Thurgau, in Aarau, Bern, and Neuenburg more systemic, and Zürich has a predominantly epimediological-biological system of reference), others are used as complements and it is rare that only a single form of therapy is used. The regulations covering further training as a specialist require that, on the completion of the qualifying examinations, the psychiatrist for children and adolescents should not only be able personally to provide a particular form of therapy but must also have a good understanding of the indications for other forms and of their therapeutic process.

3. Structure and organization of services

Guidelines for services for children and adolescents with psychiatric disorders

In Switzerland there are no national, official guidelines for the running of psychiatric services for children and adolescents. Each canton organizes this as they choose. At least eighteen cantons have their own services, which submit bills to the health and disability insurance, but whose deficit is then covered by the canton. In addition, there are about eight charitable services, whose deficits are also covered by local government. Five of the eighteen cantonal services are connected to the universities (Basel, Bern, Geneva, Waadt, and Zürich).

Unfortunately, not all cantons have a psychiatric service for children and adolescents. These cantonal services are usually run by the Department of Environmental Health, less often by the Department of Health or Social Services, rarely by the Department of Education or by several different departments.

The responsible professional societies and FMH together have divided the available psychiatric services into the categories A, B, C, D. In the A services, for example, it is possible to complete the whole professional training, whereas employment in a D category is only recognized as providing one year of professional training (see also p. 376).

Types of services

An overview of this is given in Table 1. The organization of the services differs from canton to canton for historical reasons. Outpatient services are given more importance than inpatient provision. In the larger cantons (e.g., Zurich, Bern, St. Gallen), the service is usually divided between a main center and various outposts. Units for inpatient treatment are usually small, with only 10–15 beds. There are twice as

Table 1. Facilities for caring for children and adolescents with psychological disorders

Outpatient care
Psychiatrists for children and adolescents in private practice Non-medical psychotherapists for children and adolescents Psychiatric outpatient facilities for children and adolescents State-run psychiatric outpatient clinics for children and adolescents Family counseling and child guidance centers Centers for early intervention Social-psychiatric institutions
Day or night care
Day hospitals, independent or integrated into other institutions Institutions offering night care Psychiatric-therapeutic kindergartens
Full-time care
Hospital units attached to university psychiatric clinics for children and adolescents (including, for example, specialized adolescent units) Hospital units attached to cantonal child and adolescent psychiatry services Psychiatric units for children and adolescents in pediatric of psychiatric hospitals
Other possibilities for care
Children's homes and crèches with child and adolescent psychiatry liaison services Communal living groups for adolescents Rehabilitation institutions for special groups of patients (e.g., epileptic patients)

many institutions which are fully inpatient as are partially so. Seen as a whole, the number of daycenters and rehabilitation units for mentally disturbed children and adolescents is still too small.

Unfortunately, the majority of pedagogic institutions (reception centers, children's homes) do not yet have organized interdisciplinary liaison and cooperation with child and adolescent psychiatry.

Outpatient services

The type of treatment is dependent on the pathology, the patient's age, and the family structure. In all cases, the most basic element is the therapeutic relationship. This is why our professional society has retained the double name "specialist (FMH) in Child and Adolescent Psychiatry and Psychotherapy".

Outpatient treatment is the central element of training. The child and adolescent psychiatrists in private practice, who are well represented in towns, care for the majority of patients, and to some extent also treat adults. Child guidance centers, school psychological services, and child and adolescent psychologists also carry out assessments (Bürgin 1980; Bürgin & Dudé 1986; Bürgin 1990).

By far the largest number of child and adolescent psychiatric patients are treated on an outpatient basis either with psychotherapeutically orientated interviews or with specific forms of psychotherapy. They range from occasional control or supportive interviews (once per month) to very intensive psychotherapy (several times per week). The parents are always encouraged to take an active part in treatment.

This type of cooperation is formative for the treatment setting and also influences the therapist's training. Most disorders can be defined as specific forms of pathological interaction. The pathological etiology, therefore, seems to belong to the field of social relationships. This implicit concept of a pathological interaction directly affects the way treatment is established. Nevertheless, even in cases of serious, largely internalized pathology in the child or adolescent, the parent-child relationship has also to be taken into account and attention paid to its changing course. At the same time the functional elements of the relationship have to be extracted from the pathological area, since they form the major resource for any type of therapeutic process. In addition to their theoretical learning, those in training in the various services have practical hands-on instruction in interview techniques, psychotherapy, and other forms of treatment. Outpatient treatment is carried out by an interdisciplinary team (e.g., including child and adolescent psychiatrists, child and adolescent psychologists, social workers and speech therapists). Particularly seriously disturbed children and adolescents require coordinated intervention by representatives of various specialities.

The first assessment of small children with psychological difficulties usually takes place in a pediatric practice or clinic, where many patients with functional disturbances are seen, and child and adolescent psychiatrists are often called in for consultation.

Special classes can be therapeutic instruments where children with marked personality or learning difficulties can be supported emotionally and given remedial education during their time at school.

Adolescence is a time of enhanced risk to psychological health. Between the 13th and 25th year of life, severe psychological disturbances appear with greater frequency (in about 5 % of adolescents). Access to treatment is often problematic, since traditional institutions tend not to meet the specific needs of young people. Nevertheless, there are increasing possibilities for informal basic contacts: surgeries for young people, special resources for drug dependency or those at risk of suicide, etc.

Everything which can motivate adolescents, give them a sense of purpose, and appeal to their potential is actively included in the care offered. Treatment is a question of creating a framework where the therapeutic alliance can grow and provide a space conducive to building up relationships. Supplying a treatment network has the great advantage of enabling many individual but interrelated approaches to be used. Dual control (for example, by a psychiatrist and psychotherapist at the same time) may be indicated for adolescents with severe psychotic or borderline disorders. Psychiatric emergencies are frequent in adolescence and often require hospitalization. On the one hand, it is important not to underestimate the severity of the disturbance, but on the other hand escalation of acting-out must be avoided.

Daypatient services

The need to offer daycare may arise from the severity of pathology in the child or from the degree of disturbance in the family. In earliest childhood a crèche or a "day mother" may take over this function, especially when there is very marked pathology in the parents or the immediate surroundings. For children at risk, those with severe early developmental problems or with serious physical illness and accompanying psychological symptoms, a therapeutic kindergarten is appropriate from the age of about 2 ½ years. The immediate care will usually be taken over by a professionally qualified nursery nurse. The psychiatrist, psychotherapist, speech therapist and psychomotor physiotherapist only intervene at special points. The major part of the treatment is, thus, carried out during daily contact in the institution and supported by specialists. The therapeutic care offered by such an institution works on a similar principle as the classic psychotherapeutic day hospital. These kindergartens or nursery schools are specifically intended for children up to 4 years and facilitate care on a daily basis which is appropriate to severe pathological disorders in early development or can be used to deal with a risk situation, where development may become pathological in the absence of intensive treatment. Such a therapeutic procedure makes it possible for the child to remain in the family and still receive the same intensive therapy as an inpatient – on the basis of a therapeutic milieu – which dialectically complements the therapeutic activity with parents and child in the institution.

Day hospitals offer patients with severe psychological disturbances a place for middle-term to long periods. In general, such units provide both ongoing daily care and psychotherapy. They aim for the young people's social and family integration, and work with them to avoid, as far as possible, any later social difficulties. Their role is to offer a temporary space with various forms of intervention, helping to establish the ability to cope with conflict, changes within relationships, and alteration of symptoms. Various forms of therapy are offered in a coherent manner. This form of treatment is appropriate for those patients who have psychological problems which cannot be adequately met by outpatient treatment, with severe personality disorders, or whose social situation is so unfavorable that it puts their further development in question. Day hospitals for psychotic, autistic or deprived small children are highly specialized units, with a high ratio of carers to children. Sadly, there are only a few such institutions in Switzerland.

The psychotherapeutically-orientated day hospital offers a constant therapeutic milieu to children of school and pre-school age (usually between 4 and 12 years) with severe psychological disorders. Although the day is spent in the unit, the child remains within the family, who can be drawn into the treatment process. There is, thus, global planning for the children and their families, by a multidisciplinary team (child psychiatrists, psychologists, painting-, music-, psychomotor- and occupational-therapists, speech therapists, social workers, remedial teachers and educators, and other carers). They aim to treat the psychological disorder and to offer help for a new start in school and social life. These children are usually accepted for longer periods. The basic understanding of this treatment is a milieu therapy in which the daily activities can be used for therapeutic purposes to assist the patient's psychological re-integration. In addition to child psychiatric care, there are pedagogic and educational activities which are all aimed at the same goal in the total therapy plan.

Liaison psychiatry covers a variety of specialized interventions, which have been developed for use in somatic hospitals, on the one hand, and social-pedagogic institutions, on the other. In hospitals, we are considering here organized consultations with the child and adolescent psychiatrist in the emergency services and intensive care units in pediatric, medical, and surgical wards, especially after suicide attempts, with patients suffering from anorexia or bulimia, children showing dangerous behavior, and medical or surgical complaints linked to difficulties in mood, behavior or cooperation. Liaison psychiatry may be described as the work of one person within the team and treatment net of a different speciality, which enables the efficacy of the existing treatment to be strengthened. There is an attempt to clarify the dynamics within the group of carers, so that the patient who is already in difficulties is not confronted with an unstructured bundle of relationships.

Inpatient services

Full-time hospitalization does become necessary for some children, especially in situations where the family can contribute nothing to counteract the child's pathological development, or when the family pathology makes outpatient treatment or stay in a day hospital impossible. Here too, the therapeutic milieu is central to the whole intervention. Daily activities are used for therapeutic purposes and represent a parallel to specific psychotherapeutic work with individuals, groups or families. To facilitate the child's later reintegration into the original environment, inpatient treatment always includes intensive contact and work with the family. After an initial period of hospitalization, the original arrangement can often be changed to a partial or complete outpatient set-up, depending on the development shown by the child and the family.

Due to the severity of certain pathologies, with their effects on the child's ability to learn and on social development, but also because of some children's very limited developmental resources or of very markedly disturbed families, outpatient treatment may be inadequate, and the use of a caring milieu, such as inpatient psychotherapeutic treatment, becomes unavoidable. For children with pervasive developmental disturbances, especially autistic children and those with psychosis of early childhood, prepsychosis or dysfunctional development, the aim is to provide impulses and further their psycho-physical development. There are, however, sometimes indications for other patients to be admitted, for example, in cases of severe depression, anxiety, compulsion, extreme difficulty in adapting, massively anti-social behavior, problems with eating etc. Such units have both educational and remedial pedagogic means of influence, which are all directed to the same, mutually agreed, psychotherapeutic goal.

Such centers were originally intended for crisis intervention or acute psychiatric situations, but they increasingly offered their help in long-term work, especially when there was an acute breakdown on the child's part or crisis within the family. Such units can also be used for preventive intervention, especially for children who encounter psychological difficulties because of a serious disturbance in their environment, children whose parents are themselves mentally ill, or who are at risk of physical or sexual abuse. Finally, observation or therapy may be carried out in complex psychopathological situations. The majority of independent psychiatric units for children or adolescents include an internal school, and in parallel with the treatment of patients with various severe disorders, there is also the possibility of long-term rehabilitation.

Severely disturbed children with psychiatric problems are often admitted to pediatric wards in psychological or social emergencies. A situation which might be perceived as stigmatization in the direction of psychiatry may thus be avoided, and a somatopsychic integration of both the psychiatrist for children and adolescents as of the pediatric specialist made possible. Departments for Child Psychiatry which are integrated into pediatric hospitals are favored for assessment and for introducing therapy in patients who are suffering from a psychotic breakdown, suicide attempts, severe somatopsychic problems or family breakdown.

Complementary services and rehabilitation

The number of suitable large families for the long-term care of small and school children, special classes for emotionally needy children and adolescents, and homes and communal dwellings for young people which have a child and adolescent psychiatric in-put is still inadequate.

Personnel

Psychiatric institutions for children and adolescents need more personnel than those for adults. There are no nationally binding regulations covering the amount of care needed. In day hospitals and residential hospital departments, social pedagogues, educators, and psychiatric nurses work together. In Switzerland there are still only the beginnings of a special training for the psychiatric nursing of children and adolescents.

Funding of services

In the first instance, the health and disability insurance are responsible for the costs of outpatient, day hospital, and hospital care. Health insurance is obligatory for everyone. In the case of the public institutions for children and adolescents, the cantons carry the deficit, since the insurance companies do not pay enough to cover the true costs. Recognized forms of psychotherapy and long-term supportive therapy have been so far accepted by these insurances, even if only for limited periods. The services of the school psychological services are free. Child guidance centers often ask for reduced fees.

Evaluation

There has not yet been a systematic evaluation of psychiatric care for children and adolescents in Switzerland. Guaranteeing quality, on the other hand, is part of the duty of evaluation falling on each service. This is mostly related to the evaluation of existing forms of organization and treatment. National and probably European systems of accreditation and certification with the corresponding evaluation are likely to be introduced in all hospitals and, thus, also in the psychiatric services for children and adolescents, in the coming years.

4. Cooperation with medical and non-medical disciplines

Cooperation with pediatrics

Recent years have seen an increase in the interventions by child and adolescent psychiatrists within children's hospitals, largely because many clinical areas require pediatric-psychiatric cooperation. Such liaison services provide multidisciplinary cooperation and therefore require scheduled interaction. If the differing points of view of pediatrics and of child and adolescent psychiatry in terms of treatment have been coherently integrated through regular teamwork, parallel and complementary psychiatric and somatic treatment is facilitated. Liaison psychiatry organized in this way simplifies the treatment of patients with certain kinds of disorders and also the establishment of research programs in the areas where the two disciplines meet. The goals of child and adolescent psychiatry in liaison activities are both preventive and therapeutic in nature. Intervention at the first signs of illness is thus possible, with a reduction in the risk of pathology developing later. Such cooperation is particularly indicated in the following areas: psychological reactions to somatic illness (psycho-oncology, psycho-neurology); psychological disorders linked to somatic problems (e.g., anorexia, bulimia, somatoform disorders, psychosomatic illness, suicide attempts); psychological disturbance after premature birth, in babies and small children (e.g., disturbed relationship between parent and child, deformities, chromosome abnormalities, genetic problems, problems with mourning a child's death, dialectic complementation of developmental pediatrics); physical or sexual abuse (multidisciplinary team for handling abuse). The liaison psychiatric activities may be directed toward the pediatric treatment team or directly toward the patient. They include not only case presentation and supervision, but also crisis intervention and focal therapy.

Cooperation with psychiatry

Admission to a psychiatric hospital for adults may be needed, in particular, for severely suicidal adolescents. Optimal treatment at the dividing line between adult and late or post-adolescent psychiatry in the common treatment of schizophrenic and depressive parents and their children and in the field of psychopharmacology demands close collaboration and consultation, which in turn often requires improved structural support. The developmental psychological aspects of nosology, i.e., the long-term course of disorders from earliest childhood to adulthood, are interesting both prospectively (i.e., from the point of view of the child and adolescent psychiatrist) and retrospectively (i.e., as seen by the adult psychiatrist). Cantonal and university services are usually organized in the same structure as the services for adults, with whom there are close professional contacts. To a lesser extent, children's and young people's medical services also have organizational links with pediatrics.

Cooperation with doctors in private practice

As Switzerland is small and densely populated, there are close contacts between the child and adolescent psychiatrists practising privately, pediatricians, general practitioners, and the cantonal and university services, both in terms of supervision, professional training, and planning, and through the national professional body. Private practitioners often use the specific diagnostic services of a psychiatric center for children and adolescents or of day and full-time hospitals; conversely, these services are often dependent on their privately practising colleagues for the care of those children, adolescents, and families who need long-term treatment. Private practice and the public services are seen as complementary parts of a single network of care reflected in the payment structure which is practically identical for both, though it varies from canton to canton. In the area of scientific research however, the experience of private practitioners is under-utilized in Switzerland.

Cooperation with non-medical institutions and professionals

In some cantons the child guidance services are well established and closely connected, including geographically, to the psychiatric services for children and adolescents (e.g., in Bern); but in the majority there are fewer centers for advice or much less direct cooperation. However, there is regular cooperation with the offices concerned with youth welfare (for example, guardianship, juvenile courts, probation and welfare services, etc.) whose organization varies greatly between the different cantons. This is both on the part of the psychiatric services for children and adolescents and, to a lesser extent, of their privately practising colleagues, and concerns assessment for both civil and criminal courts, implementing orders, shared care, placement, custodial rights, financial support, etc.

With regard to the question of schooling for children with psychological, emotional or learning difficulties, there is inevitably close cooperation with kindergartens, school psychological services, educational offices, and special schools.

In the areas of general child care (crèches, daycare, pedagogic assessment centers, boarding schools, children's homes and apprentices' lodgings, communal groups, etc.), there are more or less intensive contacts or even cooperation with the liaison psychiatric service. This may be because the institution wishes to have psychiatric assessment and treatment of the children and adolescents carried out or because the psychiatric services are looking for long-term placement with the possibility of psychotherapeutic treatment for appropriate patients. There is also a need for ongoing contact with educational authorities to ensure an optimum school curriculum for patients. For psychotherapy, cooperation is of great importance: on the applied side with occupational, art, music, psychomotor, and speech therapists as well as counsellors for parents and for actual psychotherapy with psychotherapists (e.g., psychologists) in private practice or in corresponding institutions. It can, thus, be seen that child and adolescent psychiatry in Switzerland is everywhere embedded in a net of youth welfare. Due to its bio-psycho-social basis, it holds a position with many valences.

5. Graduate/postgraduate training and continuing medical education

Graduate training: The role of medical faculties

The medical schools are part of the 5 universities. The title "psycho-social medicine" covers an area of study in the 1st, 2nd, and 3rd years, which is related to the patient's psychological position and needs, and to the doctor-patient relationship. Many students become interested in psychiatric issues as a result.

Child and adolescent psychiatry is taught as part of adult psychiatry and pediatrics (psychopathology, semiology, diagnosis, various forms of therapy). This comes in the 4–6th years, partly in the form of lectures, partly in small groups in personal contact with patients. Final assessment in child and adolescent psychiatry includes an interview with a patient and an examination of theoretical knowledge.

Postgraduate training, a joint effort

At present, with the agreement of the FMH, the professional societies of the corresponding specialists are responsible for both form and content of postgraduate training. The intention is, however, that this should be taken over by the universities and the FMH together. Postgraduate training is structured by a commission chosen by the professional society, and is continuously updated in content and form.

New regulations came into force on January 1, 1995. The contents (postgraduate training catalogue) are summarized in Table 2. They concern the following:

- The period of postgraduate study was increased from 5 to 6 years (of which 4 years should be in child and adolescent psychiatry), largely to give more time for training in psychotherapy.
- Theoretical postgraduate training was increased (according to the 4-year training in child and adolescent psychiatry) from 3 to 4 times 150 h in the year; the number of supervision hours increased to 160.
- Institutions for postgraduate training were divided according to exact criteria: Those of category A (see p. 368) must offer the candidate the opportunity to investigate patients of all ages and to attend a complete program of theoretical and practical instruction; there must be at least 3 senior post-holders with FMH title; and it must have one outpatient and at least two different day or full-time units (e.g., for children and adolescents). Other categories of institution offer only a part of these facilities.
- As before, the candidate must spend a year in adult psychiatry and a year in another clinical field (if possible pediatrics). Clinical research in child and adolescent psychiatry may be recognized as a part of the further training. The candidate has to produce a dissertation and demonstrate his or her ability and knowledge in an examination, which consists of three parts: written description of a clinical situation or a psychotherapy, discussion of a video, and a theoretical examination.

Continuing medical education in child and adolescent psychiatry and psychotherapy

The content and formal structure of this program are still being developed and tested. Its official introduction is planned for 1999 or 2000.

Table 2. Aims of training

Independent assessment and, when necessary, treatment, of children and adolescents with psychological problems and of their surroundings.
Working out a developmental diagnosis in multidisciplinary cooperation with doctors (pediatricians, neurologists, etc.) and others (psychologists, teachers, etc.).
Competent consultative work for child welfare agencies, schools, and courts.

Training programs for other disciplines

Institutions for further training are also concerned with the advanced training of clinical psychologists, nurses, and other paramedical workers and in addition give courses to teachers and those professionally concerned with the care of children.

6. Research

Research fields and strategies

Research is almost entirely confined to institutions attached to universities, which do however also show a high involvement in the services. Some psychology departments are doing research with children and adolescents, mostly in the area of cognition. Several of the cantonal university psychiatric services for children and adolescents are taking part in an international combined study. Unfortunately, there is yet no central coordination of national research in child and adolescent psychiatry. The following are at the center of current research: families and the development of relationships starting with pregnancy; parent-child relationship in the post-partum period; psychotherapy with mother and child in babyhood and toddler age; course of psychopathological phenomena from child- to adulthood; developmental psychopathology; disorders of brain function, partial disturbances in performance and the hyperkinetic syndrome; psychosomatics and eating disorders; epidemiological questions and results in psychological tests during school age and adolescence; problems of children and families in divorce; diagnosis and psychotherapy in adolescence; problems of children and young people whose parents are physically or mentally ill.

Research training and career development

Because of the inadequate number of positions for research and the relatively favorable situation for opening a private practice, too few graduates plan an academic career in research in the field of child and adolescent psychiatry in Switzerland. Nevertheless, in conjunction with adult psychiatry, there is a week-long seminar on research every 1–2 years, which receives good feedback and has a stimulating effect.

Funding

Most research activities are financed by outside resources (in the first instance the Swiss National Foundation). This means that a higher standard of research is achieved but also that continuity in research is made more difficult. There are various charities which support smaller research projects. As a non-EU country,

Switzerland can take only a small part in European research projects, including child and adolescent psychiatry.

7. Future perspectives

Research

The Swiss Society for Child and Adolescent Psychiatry represents the interests of colleagues in private practice, and has up to now shown little concern for research. This is an important new task, especially in evaluating the effectiveness of psychotherapy. It is, above all, necessary to organize interdisciplinary projects, but also intercantonal and interuniversity research, which in this small country must cross the language barrier, so that the few resources can be well utilized and expertise shared. Switzerland is also suitable for epidemiological long-term studies, since the population is relatively stationary. Among the most important tasks are increasing clinical research in the fields of prevention, diagnosis and therapy, encouraging the next generation and women, and informing the authorities and the public about new knowledge.

Training

Medical training – including the teaching of child and adolescent psychiatry – is currently undergoing revision at all Swiss universities. There have been huge increases in the demands made on postgraduate training, including in psycho-

Table 3. Content of further learning objectives

Basic Scientific Knowledge: Biological and developmental anthropology; general psychology and developmental psychology; development of personality; neuro-psychology; science of communication; sociogenesis.
Clinical Training: This is an important part of the further training. Particular weight is laid on the following aspects: Etiological pathogenesis; general and detailed psychopathology of children and adolescents.
Care Treatment and Prevention: Medical psychology; psycho-pharmacology; psychotherapy with different age groups and in different schools, with personal experience in the school chosen by the candidate; social and school psychiatry (including writing reports).

Table 4. Obligatory knowledge and abilities

Basic Scientific Knowledge: Psychological, somatic and social development of children and adolescents; clinical psychology (genetic, psychoanalytic, system theoretical and behavioral aspects); adult psychiatry, pediatrics (especially neurology and psychosomatics); pedagogics; social psychology.
Clinical Further Training: Diagnostics; knowledge in greater depth of etiopathogenesis and psychopathology; forensics, treatment; prevention.

therapy, which has been well organized for a number of decades and is tested by specialist examinations. The university hospitals will need more lecturers to meet the demands of undergraduate and postgraduate teaching and further training, and to increase the volume of research. It will be necessary to include more the privately practising colleagues for these various activities.

Improvement of services and care systems

There are major tasks in the realm of prevention: for example, suitable measures to reduce violence in schools; prevention of marginalization; more opportunities for children and young people, making towns less inhospitable; increased support for young couples on the way to parenthood; teaching that encourages development and creativity; improvement of emotional and cognitive communication and tolerance in a multicultural society (Bürgin 1997). In addition to psychodynamic methods more standardized interview techniques are needed to enable international comparisons to be made in the field of diagnostics. It is likely that test methods supported by computer, with increased quality controls, will become essential. After a long period of separate development, closer cooperation between child and adolescent psychiatry and neurology must be sought.

In the field of therapy, considerations of cost will make it unavoidable to question the necessity and efficacy of long-term care and to develop screening techniques to identify where short interventions will assist recovery in the less severely disturbed development of children, young people, and their families.

The proportion of research in relation to service in university hospitals and clinics must be improved. It is also of the utmost urgency to establish a national pool of expertise, to oppose any petty particularization, and to deepen the research culture in the field of child and adolescent psychiatry. This could probably be in cooperation with adult psychiatry, developmental psychology and neurology, on a biological, psychological-psychodynamic and also psycho-social level, and would lead to the creation of regional foci of research.

With regard to health care and organization of the services, it is necessary both to establish child and adolescent psychiatric services in all cantons and to increase the facilities of the existing institutions, since roughly 20–25 % of all school children show disturbances requiring help (Bettschart et al. 1980). In addition, there should be an attempt to distribute the services of child and adolescent psychiatrists in private practice more evenly throughout the country. Special clinics in university centers, on the one hand, and mobile teams, on the other, who can offer help in rural areas will meet a current need.

Selected references

Aichhorn A (1951) Verwahrloste Jugend. Internationaler Psychoanalytischer Verlag, Wien 1925. 6. Aufl.: Huber, Bern

Ajuriaguerra J de (1970) Manuel de Psychiatrie de l'Enfant. Masson, Paris

Arbeitskreis OPD (Hrsg.) (1996) OPD, Operationalisierte psychodynamische Diagnostik. Huber, Bern

Bettschart W, et al. (1980) L'enfant de 9 ans. Etude épidemiologique. Psychiatrie de l'Enfant 23, 2: 637–684
Bovet L (1951) Les aspects psychiatriques de la délinquance juvenile. Monographie No 1. OMS, Genève
Bürgin D (1980) Über einige „Grenzfunktionen" der Kinder- und Jugendpsychiatrie. Schweiz. Ärztezeitung, 61/42: 2729–2731
Bürgin D, Dudé R (1986) Ambulante Kinder- und Jugendpsychiatrie. Therapeutische Umschau 43/1: 63–68
Bürgin D (1990) Anmerkungen zu einigen Aspekten der Kinder- und Jugendpsychiatrie. Therapeutische Umschau 47/3: 193–200
Bürgin D (1997) Die Zukunft der Kinder- und Jugendpsychiatrie/-Psychotherapie. Schweiz. Arch. Neurol. Psychiat. 148, Suppl. III: 34–37
Claparède E (1926) Psychologie de l'enfant et Pédagogie expérimentale. Kündig, Genève
Duché DJ (1990) Histoire de la Psychiatrie de l'Enfant. PUF, Paris
Emminghaus H (1887) Die psychischen Störungen des Kindesalters. Laupp, Tübingen
Freud A (1980) Die Schriften der Anna Freud. Kindler, München
Freud S (1909) Analyse der Phobie eines fünfjährigen Knaben. Jahrbuch für psychoanalytische Forschung, Band 1. Franz Deuticke, Leipzig
Herzka H-St (1981) Kinderpsychopathologie. Schwabe, Basel
Hurni A (1990) Die Kinder- und Jugendpsychiatrischen Dienste der Schweiz. Diss. Basel
Itard JMG (1980) Victor d'Aveyron. In: Gineste Th, Postel J (eds) J. M. G. Itard de l'enfant connu sous le nom de "Sauvage de l'Aveyron". Psychiatrie de l'enfant, 23 (1): 251–307
Klein M (1932) Die Psychoanalyse des Kindes. Internationaler Psychoanalytischer Verlag, Wien
Lutz J (1937) Über die Schizophrenie im Kindesalter. Dissertation, Zürich
Lutz J (1961) Kinderpsychiatrie. Rotapfel, Zürich
Lutz J, Corboz RJ (1992) In: Steinhausen H-Chr (ed) Festschrift 70 Jahre Kinder- und Jugendpsychiatrischer Dienst des Kantons Zürich (1921–1991). Eigenverlag, Zürich
Meng H (1958) Psychohygienische Vorlesungen. Schwabe, Basel/Stuttgart
Misès R, Fortineau J, Jeammet P, Lane IL, Mazet P, Plantade A, Quémada N (1988) Classification francaise des troubles menteaux de l'enfant et de l'adolescent. Psychiatrie de l'Enfant 31: 67–134
Manheimer N (1899) Les troubles mentaux de l'Enfance. Société d'Editions Scientifiques, Paris
Moreau de Tours P (1888) La folie chez l'enfant. Baillière, Paris
Remschmidt H, Schmidt HM (1994) Multiaxiales Klassifikationsschema für psychische Störungen des Kindes- und Jugendalters nach ICD-10 der WHO. Huber, Bern
Rorschach H (1921) Psychodiagnostik. Huber, Bern
Séguin E (1883) Traitement moral des enfants arrierés. Baillière, Paris
Tramer M (1938) Allgemeine Kinderpsychiatrie. Schwabe, Bern
Züblin W (1967) Das schwierige Kind. Thieme, Stuttgart
Zulliger H (1954) Der Tafeln-Z-Test. Huber, Bern
Zulliger H (1957) Bausteine zur Kinderpsychotherapie und Kindertiefenpsychologie. Huber, Bern

Child and adolescent psychiatry in Ukraine

M. Levinsky and S. Aksentyev

1. Definition, historical development, and current situation

Definition

It is traditional in the Ukraine to understand child psychiatry as a subdivision of general psychiatry which studies the peculiarities of etiology, pathogenesis, epidemiology, clinical picture, and the course and outcome of mental dysfunctions in children, as well as the peculiarities of their treatment, disease prevention, and organization of psychiatric help to children.

Adolescent psychiatry is a subdivision of general psychiatry that deals with specific manifestation, course, causes, and mechanisms in mental disturbance development in the period of sexual maturation, as well as the peculiarities of their treatment and prevention at that age and basics of psychiatric help organization for adolescents.

Child psychiatry in this country formed itself into a separate field of general psychiatry only in the 1920s, while adolescent psychiatry developed into a separate field as child and adult psychiatry only in the 1970s. Before that time the younger adolescents were supervised by child psychiatrists and the older ones by those who dealt with the adult patients.

In accordance with the existing laws and regulations in the Ukraine at present (1995) the following professions are singled out: a child psychiatrist and adolescent psychiatrist. However, such specializations as child or adolescent psychotherapy are not singled out separately. This kind of psychiatric activity is taken up either by child and adolescent psychiatrists who get additional training in psychotherapy, or by psychotherapists dealing with adults.

Historical development

Child and adolescent psychiatry in the Ukraine is closely connected with the development of these disciplines in Russia. The reason lies in the fact that the Ukraine was incorporated early into the Russian Empire (1654–1917) and later into the USSR (1918–1991). That is why it is quite difficult to single out independent stages of development of the child and adolescent psychiatry in the Ukraine.

From historical manuscripts, it is known that in the times of Kievan Rus (9th–13th centuries) mental patients and feeble-minded individuals were rendered primitive types of help at monasteries. The monks at the Kievo-Pechersky Monastery (Kiev) had started caring after such patients. In medieval times Russia had religious and mystic notions of the mental illness, but the attitude toward the mentally ill was milder and more tolerant than in Western Europe at that time. In 1554, Ivan the Terrible, the Russian csar, issued a statute where he demanded that the monasteries should treat carefully the feeble-minded. Such help was provided for the mental patients up to the 18th century. In 1669, a law was passed in Russia which concerned the irresponsibility of the mentally ill and feeble-minded.

The first psychiatric department in Russia was opened in Moscow in 1776 at the Ekaterininskaya Hospital; it had 26 beds. The first psychiatric departments in Ukraine were organized in Kiev in 1786, then in Kharkiv (1796), Poltava (1803), Kamenets-Podolsky (1835), Odessa (1840), and Kherson (1852). The Maksakovsky Monastery in Chernigiv was turned into an institution for the mental patients in 1776.

At the beginning, psychiatry was not singled out from somatic medicine and was taught by the same professors who were teaching surgery and therapy. In 1834, Kharkiv University undertook the teaching of psychiatry as a separate discipline for the first time in Russia. The teaching was performed by Prof. P A. Butkovsky. The same year he published the first textbook in psychiatry in Russia.

In 1836, Prof. Butkovsky organized the first special school for mentally retarded children in Russia. This school was named the "School at the Hospital Gate". A similar school was organized in Paris in 1839 by E. Séguin.

The first Medical Institution for treating mentally retarded children and epileptics with recurrent psychomotor excitement was established in 1854 in Riga by Dr. Plats; it housed 30 children.

In 1863 a plan to create a wide network of institutions for retarded children in the Russian Empire was developed. This was done on the initiative of the Chief Administration for the Military Education Establishments. In 1865, all the military secondary schools (gymnasiums) had special "repeating forms" for those who could not cope with the curriculum of the previous academic year and also for those who did not master the curricula of the earlier years. In 1867, all those children who could not progress at the military secondary schools were placed into the special institution called a "progymnasium". Such progymnasiums were created in many larger cities. In 1873, G. P. Stepanov published a handbook called "Teaching the Dumb and Deaf, Blind, and Mentally Retarded".

Starting in 1868, a number of cities in the Russian Empire opened "Corrective Educational Establishments", where children with psychopathological personalities received education.

Due to the change in the political climate in Russia and to the reaction gaining strength in the 1890s, the progymnasiums and some other corrective establishments for children and adolescents were closed.

However, the necessity of educating and caring for mental patients and retarded children became socially meaningful. Thus, according to a 1893 survey of the mentally ill patients in the Moscow Gubernia (administrative unit), there were 3.53 mental patients (mostly oligophrenics and epileptics) per 1,000 children 0–10 years of age.

The end of 1890s and the beginning of the 1900s saw closer attention being given to the items concerning child and adolescent mental health in Russia. Child psychiatric departments were opened in the psychiatric hospitals. The first child psychiatric department with 25 beds was opened in Kherson, Ukraine, in 1899. Once again the medical training institutions, where combined corrective educational and psychological measures were undertaken, were opened. On the initiative of some religious public figures, a number of medical educative institutions, asylums, and agricultural colonies were organized for mentally retarded and epileptic children and adolescents. These institutions had a philanthropic character, which is reflected in their names, such as "Brotherhood of the Celestial Queen Asylum", "St. Emmanuel's Asylum", "St. Mary's Asylum".

Research studies in child psychiatry in the Russian Empire were started at the Department of Psychiatry of the Military Medical Academy (St. Petersburg) in the 1870s, which at that time was headed by Prof. I. P. Merzheyevsky. From 1872–1880 he performed morphological studies on the brains of several patients with congenital mental retardation and microcephaly; he managed to show that the reason for this basically lies in retarded development which is due to a intrauterine lesion.

Dr. I. A. Sikorsky worked at the department, which was headed by Prof. Merzheyevsky and in 1881 he published his research on stuttering and dyslalia in children. It was published in Germany in 1895 with some additional material in a translated version ("Über das Stottern", Berlin, 1895). The "Medico-pedagogical Herald" was started in St. Petersburg in 1885 by Dr. I. V. Molyarevsky, a pupil of Prof. Merzheyevsky. The journal printed psychological studies and observations made in the family and at school, clinical case histories of children, and reviews of books on medicine, psychiatry, psychology, hygiene, and pedagogic.

It was Dr. I. A. Sikorsky who was the first to raise in 1882 the problem of psychopathological examination of difficult children and consideration of their specific personality in developing the educative plan; this was done addressing the 4th International Congress on Hygiene. His monograph "Bringing-up in the Age of Primary Childhood" appeared in 1884. Later, in 1885, having the position of a Professor, I. A. Sikorsky headed the Psychiatry Department of Kiev University for more than 20 years. Here he continued to investigate the mental diseases of children and the medical and pedagogical correction of mentally retarded children. In 1906, Prof. Sikorsky opened a medico-pedagogical institution for retarded children in Kiev.

It is quite indicative of the then attitude toward the mental problems of children and adolescents that the first issue of one of the first psychiatric journals in Russia (edited by Prof. Merzheyevsky from 1883) opened with a paper by M. Y. Droznes, a psychiatrist from Kherson, called "Materials for the psychopathology of adolescents".

The department, headed by Merzheyevsky, also issued the works by S. N. Danillo "On Child Catatonia" (1886), "On the Theory of Mental Diseases in the Second Childhood Period" (1892), and others.

An original psychiatric school was formed in Kharkiv by Prof. Kovalevsky in the 1880s–1890s. It worked on the issues of child and adolescent psychiatry, and A. I. Yuschenko described adolescent progressive paralyses in 1893, which was the first time in history. It was in Kharkiv that a pedagogue was invited to work with children in a psychiatric hospital in 1912, which was for the first time in the Russian Empire.

In 1905 on the initiative of Prof. V. M. Dukhosky the first Department of Medical Pedagogic was created in St. Petersburg. In 1907 on the initiative of Prof. V. M.

Bekhterev the Pedagogical Institute was organized at the Psychoneurological Institute in St. Petersburg. This institute studied psychic development of children since its founding.

In 1911 in Moscow, Prof. G. I. Rossolimo started the Institute of Child Neurology and Psychology and funded it from his own means. Prof. G. I. Rossolimo suggested his own method of psychological examination of a child in 1910. This type of method received the name of "Psychological Profile of Rossolimo".

At the beginning of the 1900s, auxiliary classes and schools were created for mentally retarded children in a number of Ukrainian cities, such as Kharkiv, Dnepropetrovsk, Odessa, Balta, etc. Agricultural colonies were also organized for mentally retarded adolescents.

After a lengthy period, where there was no attention to the issues of psychiatry, which was connected with World War I, the October Revolution, and the Civil War, a wide network of psychiatric and social-pedagogical institutions for children was organized in the 1920s–1930s.

In the 1930s, Ukraine already had 13 psychiatric hospitals and 2 departments as part of general hospitals. In the town of Romny in the Sumskaya Region, the Ukrainian Central Psychoneurological Hospital having 250 beds was organized for children. The plan for decentralization of psychiatric aid was under development. In 1934, Ukraine had 29 pedagogic and psychoneurological offices at children's medical institutions. In those cities and district towns where there were no such offices for specialized help, the adult psychiatrists rendered these services to children.

The 1920s–1930s saw the organization of some research institutions in psychiatry and neurology in Kiev, Kharkiv, and Odessa. They had child psychiatry and neurology departments or research groups.

In 1924, one of USSR's first psychiatric and neurological journals "Modern Psychoneurology" was issued in Kiev. In 1931, its publication was given over to the Ukrainian Psychoneurological Academy (Kharkiv) where it was published through 1941, and its name was changed to "Soviet Psychology". This journal published many papers dealing with psychic pathology in childhood.

In the 1930s, a number of Medical Institutes in the Ukraine created Departments of Child Neurology and Psychiatry to study the specificity of childhood pathology and for a deeper teaching of those disciplines.

The development of child psychiatry in USSR was connected with the name Prof. G. E. Sukhareva. She contributed greatly to the development of child psychiatry in USSR. After graduating from the Medical Faculty she began her career as a psychiatrist in the Kiev psychiatric hospital and worked there from 1919–1931. From 1933–1935 she was the head of the Department of Psychiatry at the Kharkiv Medical Institute. In 1935 G. E. Sukhareva created the first Department of Child Psychiatry for postgraduate education in Moscow. She published the first monograph in USSR about schizophrenia in children and adolescents in 1937 in Kharkiv. Starting in 1938, Sukhareva was at the same time the head of the Child Psychoses Department at the Moscow Research Institute for Psychiatry.

In the prewar years, psychiatry in USSR developed and formed a preventive principle in this field, which determined the further development of child psychiatry. The attention of child psychiatrists was directed at detection of early forms of psychic dysfunctions and their timely treatment as well as their psychological and pedagogical correction at the phase when psychopathological dysfunctions could be fully leveled to normal. While developing the preventive trend, child psychiatrists concentrated on the issues of work in a dispensary and dynamic observation of the patients.

During World War II, many psychiatric hospitals in the Ukraine were either fully or partially destroyed. After the end of the war, gradual restoration of the psychiatric hospitals was started, and the building of the new ones began. The characteristic trait of the post-war stage was a review of the old, existing structure of hospitals, making smaller and creating specialized departments and services alongside the general psychiatric hospitals, reorganizing the diagnostic and therapeutic work using the latest preparation and introducing modern medical and diagnostic equipment. In relation to child psychiatry the following were done: organization of departments for smaller children and adolescents and for psychotic and borderline dysfunctions, creating a broader network of outpatient services, specialized kindergartens and schools, and psychoneurological sanatoriums. The education of medical staff for child psychiatry was also improving.

The former USSR had an All-Union Scientific Society of Neurologists and Psychiatrists which had a subdivision of child neurology and psychiatry. With the disintegration of USSR, Ukraine has formed the Ukrainian Scientific Society of Neurologists and Psychiatrists and an Association of Psychiatrists of Ukraine. These organizations discuss further prospects of development in psychiatry as a whole and in child and adolescent psychiatry in particular.

Current situation

Children and adolescents comprise 1/4 of the 50.5 million population of Ukraine. Help is rendered in outpatient conditions by 369 child and 69 adolescent psychiatrists (V. N. Kuznetsov, 1996). At the present, all the regions of the Ukraine have child and adolescent psychiatric departments in regional psychiatric hospitals and psychoneurological dispensaries*.

The department of Psychiatry at the Medical Universities have no clinics of their own, but are located on the premises of psychiatric hospitals. Thus, the clinical bases are being formed for the department. At such clinical bases, the academic staff of the department supervise patients and also counsel practicing physicians. The clinical bases have some additional funding.

The change in the state of the country, its jumping rhythm of life, breakdown of traditional psychological traditions, the change in the demands to the coming generation, and the complicated social and economic situation in the Ukraine have all led to a decline in general health and mental health in particular, especially for the child and adolescent population.

* Historically such medical institutions as psychoneurological dispensaries appeared in Russia at the beginning of the 20th century. Traditionally they include outpatient departments and inpatient departments for the non-psychotic forms of mental dysfunctions. At some dispensaries besides rendering help to mental patients the patients with neurological problems are also serviced. Besides medical help, those dispensaries also render social help to those who have mental problems.

To protect child and adolescent mental health in the Ukraine, for the early detection and more accurate diagnosis, and to improve the quality of restorative treatment of mental dysfunctions in children and adolescents, it is necessary not only to solve the socio-economic tasks, but also to reform the judicial basis of laws and regulations for psychiatric help and protection of mental health of the child and adolescent population of the Ukraine.

2. Classification systems, diagnostic and therapeutic methods

Classification systems

From the beginning of 1999 Ukraine use ICD-10, which was adapted to local clinical needs. For clinical purposes, traditional local psychiatric classification terms are also being widely used to describe mental dysfunctions.

Some psychiatric institutions use DSM-IV for research purposes. All psychiatric institutions of the Ukraine use uniform documentation for clinical purposes.

Diagnostic methods

At present a whole combination of clinical, psychodiagnostic, neurological, functional (X-ray, EEG, CT, MRI, etc.), biochemical, and several genetic methods are being used in the Ukraine. There is wide cooperation between the clinicians of different specializations when examining the mental patients of child and adolescent groups.

Some tests for psychological diagnosis of mental development and mental retardation have been worked out in the Ukraine, and a large number of foreign psychological tests have been adapted to the needs of the local population.

Therapeutic methods

A large number of therapeutic methods for the treatment of psychic dysfunctions are used in the Ukraine. As a rule, treatment is performed in combination with chemotherapeutical and non-chemotherapeutical means. In psychopharmatherapy, nootropic drugs, anxiolytics, antidepressants, antipsychotics, and anticonvulsants are used. Compared to the countries of Western Europe and America the psychostimulants are practically not used. Among the non-chemotherapeutical methods, physiotherapy is widely used (electrophoresis with some drugs, the use of various electric impulse action with the aim of sedation, balneotherapy, etc.).

In the last two decades, various methods of psychotherapy and psychocorrection have been used widely, and recently family counseling, family psychotherapy, play therapy, and different new psychological techniques based on psychodynamic or behavioral theories have been introduced.

3. Structure and organization of services in child and adolescent psychiatry

Guidelines for psychiatric services for children and adolescents with psychiatric disorders

The main principles of organizing the psychiatric services in the Ukraine for the population, children and adolescents included, are:

- differentiated character of these services for various patient groups. This principle is realized taking into consideration the character and the severity of the psychotic or non-psychotic dysfunctions in the children and adolescents;
- continuity in the rendering of services at different psychiatric institutions. This principle is realized by close functional communication between the psychiatric institutions of various levels, which is regulated by the rules of their interaction, documentation requirements, and their transferring to other institutions, continuous observation, and treatment of the patients;
- gradual steps in services. This principle is defined by different levels of inpatient and outpatient (outpatient department, daypatient department, etc.) psychiatric services, which form an entire system. This system includes primary mental institutions which are the closest to the population; they are psychiatric offices in the district outpatient departments for children, psychoneurological dispensaries which have the possibility to render inpatient and outpatient services, inpatient psychiatric services in the conditions of psychiatric hospitals or psychiatric departments in general profile hospitals, and rehabilitation services (vocational treatment workshops at psychiatric hospitals or psychoneurological dispensaries, special shops at industrial enterprises). All psychiatric help to different age groups is organized based on the territorial principle;
- dispenserial-dynamic care for mental patients. This principle is implemented in accordance with the five subsequent levels of the treatment and restorative process: the psychohygienic, corrective and educative, general rehabilitating, psychiatric treatment, and social aid levels. According to the system of dynamic dispensary registration and care by the child and adolescent psychiatrists such patients as those having a psychotic level of mental diseases with the corresponding character of social dysadaptation are obligatorily liable to dispensary supervision and care. On the other hand, patients having non-psychotic mental dysfunctions are not entitled to obligatory registration, supervision, and care and can be serviced in the so-called counseling group.

Types of services

At present, the Ukraine has the following treatment establishments for children and adolescents with mental dysfunctions:

- Inpatient services are rendered in child and adolescent departments of mental hospitals or psychoneurological dispensaries. Each region of Ukraine has 1–3 child and 1–2 adolescent psychiatric departments. There are special adolescent departments for drug-dependent and sniffing adolescents. The psychiatric beds in the Ukraine at present are 3.0 beds for children and 14.8 beds for adolescents per 10,000 of the corresponding population age group (V. N. Kuznetsov. 1996).
- For the last 15–20 years, help has been available to children and adolescents with mental diseases at institutions of the daypatient services. This type of treatment is given for two categories of patients:
  - the patients who underwent a course of intensive inpatient treatment and necessitate gradual integration into the usual social surroundings;
  - the patients who need psychiatric treatment, but do not necessitate inpatient care as to their mental state.
- The outpatient psychiatric services for the child and adolescent population are offered at the regional centers in the outpatient departments of psychoneurological dispensaries. In smaller towns and rural areas, there are child psychiatric offices organized at child polyclinics. Some psychiatric hospitals have outpatient departments with child psychiatrists on the staff. According to the existing normative regulations in the Ukraine, one child psychiatrist position is envisioned per 20,000 children 0–15 years of age for an outpatient network unit and one position for an adolescent psychiatrist per 20,000 adolescents of the 15–18 age group. While in rural areas, there is one general psychiatrist position per 50,000 of the population of all age groups but not less than one district psychiatrist for a rural district.

It should be stressed that both inpatient and outpatient psychiatric help in the Ukraine is offered mainly in medical institutions owned by the state (such as hospitals, outpatient departments, etc.). It is only in recent years that private psychiatrists began appearing, child and adolescent psychiatrists including. They are working within the structure of some private medical institutions and render help to outpatients. In accordance of acting within the Ukrainian regulations (1995) at present, lawful private practice may be the occupation only of such professionals who had special training in the institutions belonging to the Ministry of Health of the Ukraine and the certificate should state they are allowed to render medical and preventive care and have a license allowing them to establish medical services. In addition, it is forbidden to privately treat those patients who need urgent hospitalization for mental help. Drug addiction is also not allowed to be treated in private institutions.

Complementary services and rehabilitation

The main task of the complementary and rehabilitation services is aiding children and adolescents having lengthy and chronic mental dysfunctions. The need of different types of such services in the Ukraine is quite high, especially for those patients who cannot be integrated into common life conditions and medical institutions.

At present, the following types of such medical institutions are

- specialized "child homes" for children from 0–4 years of age with organic lesions of the CNS and dysfunctions. Twenty such institutions were organized within the framework of the Ministry of Health. Usually these "child homes" are homes for the children who have been abandoned by their parents due to different reasons or such children whose parents were deprived of their parental rights by the court. Furthermore, depending on the character of the mental defect, these children can be integrated into general or specialized boarding schools;
- within the system of the Ministry of Social Security, 63 specialized child boarding school houses have been organized. Such boarding schools have children from 4–18 years of age. The boarding school houses are specialized for different groups of children as those with moderate mental retardation, those with severe and profound mental retardation, and those with a combination of mental retardation and movement dysfunctions (like cerebral palsy, etc.);
- in recent years a number of cities in the Ukraine (Donetsk, Kiev, Krivoy Rog, Lviv, Mykolayiv, Odessa, Sumy, etc.) have created municipal rehabilitation centers for disabled children. They are funded by local budgets or have mixed funding (local budget and charity funds, local budget and parental fees). A number of these centers are specialized in rehabilitation of children with moderate and severe mental retardation, others in rehabilitation of children with cerebral palsy. All centers are concentrating their attention on medical rehabilitation, education and teaching work skills, and social rehabilitation.

Funding of services

Nowadays in the Ukraine, a state funding system of health services exists. The state took upon itself all the expenditure on medical servicing, child and adolescent mental diseases included, as they are rendered at the state-owned institutions. In private medicine, payment is made by the parents of the patients.

In some mental diseases, which have a chronic course, the patients are allotted a state subsidy as they are disabled from childhood. Disabled children needing lengthy medication (antipsychotics, anticonvulsants, etc.) receive them free. However, in connection with the complicated economical situation lately the amount of free medication for the given category of patients has decreased.

When a child stays at a special boarding institutions all the costs are absorbed by the state.

4. Cooperation with medical and non-medical disciplines

Cooperation with pediatrics

Child psychiatrists work very closely with pediatricians and child neurologists. Special explanatory work is conducted among pediatritians concerning the necessity of preventive work on mental dysfunctions and discovering the psychosomatic and psychic diseases in children at the earliest stages of the disease.

Cooperation between child psychiatrists and child neurologists is in the sphere of mutual management of patients with epilepsy, cerebral trauma, metabolic and other inherited diseases of CNS, the aftereffects of CNS infectious diseases, aftereffects of perinatal brain lesions, and in a number of other dysfunctions.

Cooperation with psychiatry

Child and adolescent psychiatric departments were traditionally developed within the structure of psychiatric hospitals and psychoneurological dispensaries. Child and adolescent psychiatry uses the same criteria for lengthy and dynamic supervision and treatment as general psychiatry. There is also close cooperation between the child and general psychiatrists when supervising the children who have parents with mental dysfunctions.

Cooperation with general psychiatrists is also observed when longitudinal prospective studies are performed for the children and adolescents for the sake of research.

Cooperation with non-medical institutions and professionals

As the most vivid example of cooperation between child psychiatrists and non-medical institutions, we point out the specialized pedagogical institutions. The Ukraine has a wide network of specialized institutions in the school education system for children with various psychic dysfunctions: 264 boarding schools for children with mild mental retardation, 19 schools for children with learning disorders, 17 schools for children with severe speech dysfunctions, 5 sanatorium schools of boarding type for children with borderline psychoneurologic diseases, and 12 boarding schools for cerebral palsy children; there are also boarding schools for children and adolescents with behavioral and conduct disorders (V. N. Kuznetsov 1996). In a number of cities, additional grades (forms) for children with learning disorders were created at local primary schools on the initiative of the local educational authorities. In addition, there are specialized kindergartens for children with speech disorders, mental retardation, cerebral palsy, and hearing and vision disorders. Most of those institutions have a staff child psychiatrist position.

There is also close cooperation of the child and adolescent psychiatrists with the psychologists of ordinary schools so as to prevent and discover mental disorders at an early stage.

Starting in 1992, social services have begun to appear for the youth in the Ukraine. Nowadays, they exist in practically all the towns and cities of district significance. Hot lines for confident conversations and psychological support exist for the youth. These services also cooperate with child and adolescent psychiatrists.

5. Graduate/postgraduate training and continuing medical education

The present-day Ukraine has no special department or courses on child and adolescent psychiatry and psychotherapy at the medical university or medical institute. The teaching of peculiarities of mental dysfunctions in children and adolescents is conducted for the university students at the Department of general psychiatry.

The training of a professional in child and adolescent psychiatry is realized during a specialized one-year internship after graduating from the medical university. The internship includes a 5-month lecture and seminar course directly at the Department of Psychiatry and 7-month practical work under the guidance of qualified doctors at the psychiatric institutions with a subsequent taking and passing of an examination.

It is necessary for all the doctors in the Ukraine in all professions to go through refresher courses once every five years. A Department of Child Psychoneurology was formed in 1966 at the Kiev Medical Academy of Postgraduate Education. This department conducts a cycle of studies in refresher courses in child and adolescent psychiatry and child neurology. The cycle usually lasts 1–3 months. It includes lectures, seminars, and practical workshops. The refresher courses are also conducted on general issues and on separate sections of child and adolescent psychiatry.

From 1985–1992, Odessa Medical Institute had a Department of Child and Adolescent Psychoneurology where postgraduate studies were also conducted in the line of child and adolescent psychiatry and psychotherapy. However, because of economic changes in the country the department was combined with the general psychiatry department and the refresher courses are conducted only 2–3 times during the academic year.

It should be stressed that teaching of mental dysfunctions in children and adolescents is included in the curriculum of training nurses, psychologists, speech therapists, teachers for special needs, and social workers.

6. Research

Research fields and strategies

During the last 2–3 decades, three leading schools in the Ukraine with respect to research in child and adolescent psychiatry and psychotherapy were formed: Kiev, Kharkiv, and Odessa research schools. The main research in Kiev is developed on the Department of Child Psychoneurology at the Kiev Medical Academy of Postgraduate Education. The main research trends are: psychic and neurologic dysfunctions in hereditary diseases, genetic aspects in psychiatry of childhood, neuroses and neurosis-like states in children and adolescents, neuropsychological and neurophysiological aspects of mental disturbances in children and adolescents, dysadaptation in children and adolescents at school, epilepsy and its treatment in children and adolescents, etc.

The main research in Kharkiv is developed on the basis of the Ukrainian Research Institute of Experimental and Clinical Neurology and Psychiatry. The main trends here are: dysadaptation in children and adolescents at school, conduct and personality disorders in adolescents, alcoholism and drug addiction in adolescents, stuttering and other speech disorders in children, neuroses and neurosis-like states in children, depressive states in children and adolescents, psychotherapy in psychosomatic disturbances in children, etc.

The main research trends in Odessa are developed at the Departments of General Psychiatry and Child and Adolescent Psychoneurology and at the Ukrainian Research Institute of Medical Rehabilitation and Resort Therapy. The main research trends are: vascular and autonomic nervous system dysfunctions in some mental disorders in children, specificity of mental disorders in children with cerebral palsy, epilepsy and its treatment in children and adolescents, tic disorders in children, conduct and personality disorders in adolescents and an inclination towards alcoholism, fetal alcohol syndrome, drug addiction in adolescents, suicidal behavior in adolescents, psychiatry of early childhood, etc.

Research on different aspects of child and adolescent psychiatry is also conducted at other medical institutions, but they do not have such a systematic character.

Research training and career development

There is a system of training the research and teaching staff in the Ukraine concerning the higher medical education, child and adolescent psychiatry included. All those students who express interest in research and teaching activities in the field of psychiatry can continue their education after graduating from the medical faculty taking a postgraduate course for 2 years for a master's degree at the department of psychiatry. The staff for research and teaching can also be trained in general and child psychiatry at a postgraduate school (3 years or extramurally 4 years), which are offered by the department of Psychiatry.

Funding

In general the funding of research projects in child psychiatry is provided from the state budget on the basis of competition. However, the volume of funding has decreased considerably in recent years due to the existing economic situation.

7. Future perspectives

The future development of psychiatry more than any other field of medicine cannot be analyzed separately from the socioeconomic development of the country and society in general. That is why it is quite difficult to clearly see the stages of the further development of child and adolescent psychiatry at the existing stage of socioeconomic development in the Ukraine. However, we can attempt to define the main trends in improving the care for the mental health of children and adolescents:

- reorganization of the structure for different types of psychiatric aid in accordance with the existing conditions in each region of the Ukraine, paying special attention to outpatient services;
- stimulating the development of new types of services for children and adolescents with mental disorders in the state health care system and in the other forms of property (public, charity, private, etc.);
- spreading the network of specialized medical, pedagogical, and restorative institutions for children and adolescents with different forms of mental disturbances within the system of education and social security;
- improvement of the vocational and social orientation for children and adolescents with chronic mental disturbances;
- development of preventive measures in the work trends in discovery and correction of premorbid and borderline mental disturbances in children and adolescents;
- enhancing the stimuli for clinical and theoretical research in the field of child and adolescent psychiatry, as many issues concerning the pathogenesis, etiology, clinical variants of the course, and rational management of mental disturbances in children and adolescents are inadequately studied;
- improvement of graduate and postgraduate training of physicians of various profiles, especially of family doctors in child and adolescent psychiatry;
- improvement of postgraduate training of physicians specializing in child and adolescent psychiatry and psychotherapy;
- improvement and enlargement of university training and postgraduate training of clinical psychologists, taking into consideration the lack of various field professionals in the Ukraine.

References

available upon request from the author

Child and adolescent psychiatry in the United Kingdom

P. Hill

1. Definition, historical development, and current situation

Child and adolescent psychiatry is recognised by the governmental Department of Health as a specialty of psychiatry but the boundaries of its responsibilities are vague as far as its interface with adult psychiatry is concerned. The most usual interpretation is that it addresses pre-school and school-age children (which could take it up to the age of 19 for some children) though some services use a cut-off of age 16 which is the age at which children can legally leave school.

Its historical roots are twofold: child guidance and hospital psychiatry. The child guidance movement which had started in the USA in 1921 spread to London in 1927. It was based on the idea of a psychiatrist, a psychologist and a social worker working as a team in a community clinic with close ties to education services. Child guidance clinics were subsequently gradually established throughout all parts of the UK, usually funded by local authorities (town or county councils) and sometimes by voluntary funds. In parallel with this specialised clinics in hospitals were also established, rather more slowly, within health services, which in 1948 became the unified National Health Service (NHS). Children with psychiatric disorders had been seen in psychiatric hospitals in the 19th century but there was little attempt to formalise this until 1939 when a national inquiry (The Feversham Committee) recommended that psychiatric services for children be separate from adult services.

Specialism began within the medical profession, too. By the 1950s a number of specialist child and adolescent psychiatrists had made their mark in the UK: John Bowlby, Mildred Creak, Kenneth Cameron, Emanuel Miller, James Anthony and Wilfrid Warren among others. Most were from the hospital clinic tradition. Alongside them was a paediatrician who had become a psychoanalyst, Donald Winnicott, and a number of other psychoanalysts, including two who had made the study and treatment of children their own major interest, Anna Freud and Melanie Klein.

Since the 1950s the development of child and adolescent psychiatry has been progressive, fuelled by the emergence of it as an academic discipline and the formation of the Royal College of Psychiatrists as a politically influential body. The two strands – community and hospital – have continued to be somewhat separate until the last decade and the separation from paediatrics has continued (see below). One result of this has been a lasting emphasis on social factors in formulation and in treatment.

The current situation is that child and adolescent psychiatry as a medical specialty is a rather small discipline, spread across community and hospital services. There are, based on the Royal College of Psychiatrists' 1997 census, 547

Table 1. Number of consultant child and adolescent psychiatrists in the UK

England	461
Scotland	46
Wales	27
Northern Ireland	12
Channel Islands	1

consultant child and adolescent psychiatrists in the UK (Table 1). Not all are on full-time NHS contracts but most are. Private clinical practice is virtually non-existent.

Child and adolescent psychiatry is numerically small and would be quite unable to take referrals of all children with psychiatric disorder. In the last few years in the UK it has become increasingly common to describe child and adolescent psychiatry in the setting of a wider concept of a child and adolescent mental health service or CAMHS for short. This idea includes three main concepts:

- a broad definition of child and adolescent mental health
- interdisciplinary and interagency cooperation
- several levels (tiers) of service

Mental health in the young is defined in developmental terms. For example, in two very influential documents – the Department of Health Handbook on Child and Adolescent Mental Health (Department of Health 1995) and the Health Advisory Service's publication "Together We Stand" (NHS Health Advisory Service 1995) – a definition of child and adolescent mental health (generously attributed to me in the second document but actually drawn up by a group of mental health professionals which I was chairing) is put forward:

- a capacity to enter into and sustain mutually satisfying personal relationships
- continuing progression of personal development
- an ability to play and learn so that attainments are appropriate for age and intellectual level
- a developing sense of moral right and wrong
- the degree of psychological distress and maladaptive behaviour being within normal limits for the child's age and context.

This is obviously influenced by the concept of health promoted by the World Health Organisation and is more than the absence of psychiatric disorder. It can easily be criticised, particularly for being too idealistic and for including a moral dimension, but seems to be generally acceptable to all the UK agencies concerned with child and adolescent mental health and this is politically important. An alternative view identifies child and adolescent mental health as a commodity – something which a young person should have enough of, cognitively and emotionally, in order to be able to cope constructively with adversity (Earle and Hill 1998). This has an advantage of broadening the concept beyond the individual to include family and social support but has unfashionably commercial overtones.

What follows from such definitions is that child and adolescent mental health is not just the responsibility of doctors, psychologists, nor of the Health Service as a whole. It necessarily involves parents, schools, social services, the criminal justice system, religious organisations and so on. Anyone or any agency who has influence on children's psychological maturation can contribute. At a service level, the primary agencies are Health, Education and Social Services. Within health services, psychiatry, psychology, pediatrics, psychotherapy, and psychiatric nursing are primary. In the UK there is a range of special provision in mainstream (ordinary) and special schools which assist the education of children whose learning is affected by mental health problems. Social Services are responsible for children's physical and emotional and moral safety as well as promoting parents' ability to cope with childcare. A full CAMHS therefore needs to involve and coordinate contributions from all these disciplines and agencies. This is in line with the strong social tradition in UK child and adolescent psychiatry. A complete child and adolescent mental health strategy for a local population will take into account how cuts or developments in one agency will have mental health implications for other involved agencies. If, as has been the case in recent years, social services withdraw social workers from child psychiatric clinics in order to focus on statutory child protection work, it needs to be recognised across agencies that there has been a reduction of resource and waiting times for first appointments in the NHS will therefore increase.

The third component of a CAMHS is organisation into layers, levels or "tiers" (the preferred term). The reasons for this are firstly to prevent duplication of services and secondly to increase efficiency. The written origin of the concept in the early 1990s lies in a privately circulated Royal College of Psychiatrists' conference document (Caring for a Community), but comparable ideas were being considered at the same time in Guys Hospital and Nottingham. In 1995 two documents with national impact were produced; a short "handbook" prepared by the Department of Health and a more substantial work by the Health Advisory Service: "Together We Stand", which provided expert advice for health commissioners. A

Table 2. The tiered system for child and adolescent mental health within the Health Service

Tier 4
• Highly specialised outpatient services, e.g. gender identity clinics, Tourette's clinics, sexual offender clinics • Inpatient units for children or adolescents
Tier 3
• Multi-disciplinary child and adolescent mental health teams typically containing some/all of: child and adolescent psychiatrists, clinical child psychologists, child psychotherapists, clinical nurse specialists, social workers, family therapists
Tier 2
• Mental health professionals working solo, e.g. clinical psychologists, clinical nurse specialists, primary child mental health workers
Tier 1
• Health professionals with some training in child mental health but whose responsibilities are wider: e.g. general practitioners, paediatricians, health visitors, school nurses

network of people in small groups maintained contact with each other in order to prepare these. It was an idea whose time had come.

There can be any number of tiers but the most popular model uses four (Table 2).

Taking things from the bottom up, within *tier 1* there are the professionals who are the front line or first point of contact that any child or family make with any service. Within the Health Service, for example, general practitioners (family doctors), health visitors (who must visit all mothers with new babies) and community paediatricians (who work in well-baby clinics and schools as part of their job) would be examples. From a Health Service perspective, most children with mental health problems will be dealt with at this level. This particularly applies to behaviour, sleep and feeding problems in pre-school children, enuresis, lesser degrees of hyperactivity in school children and minor somatising symptoms. Another way of conceptualising tier 1 work is to suggest that this is the appropriate tier for cases exposed to only a small number of psychosocial risk factors (Wallace et al. 1997). There is also a potentially valuable opportunity to prevent mental health problems arising or worsening, particularly through the work of health visitors. Cases that cannot be managed at tier 1 are referred on to higher tiers.

At *tier 2* level there are professionals whose primary task is within child and adolescent mental health and some (such as hospital paediatricians) who have some training in child mental health problems but who apply their skills working solo or within a unidisciplinary framework. Outpatient clinic psychiatrists will do some of their clinical work in this way but generally speaking this is the tier in which clinical psychology and clinical nurse specialists in child and adolescent psychiatry are, or should be, the most numerous disciplines. Ideally, professionals at tier 2 should be able to support tier 1 workers and to link into tier 3, either by referral or by taking their cases with them and joining tier 3 professionals in multi-disciplinary teams. There are various ways of organising such arrangements. Cases seen at tier 2 are numerous and can be affected by any form of child and adolescent psychiatric disorder or child and adolescent mental health problem so long as the clinician is satisfied that he or she can handle it alone or with minimal support. Generally speaking, most tier 2 cases will have several psychosocial risk factors. Mental health consultation to other workers or agencies, offering advice without taking clinical responsibility for the case, is usually a solo activity for mental health professionals and is characteristically a tier 2 activity.

One consequence of the tiered system has been the development of the concept of the primary child mental health worker, drawn from several disciplines and equipped with medium-level skills in assessment and psychological interventions, particularly behavioural and counselling (Hall & Hill 1994). These are now being employed in a number of child and adolescent mental health services, usually working from a clinic base and liaising with general practitioners and health visitors, occasionally with schools and social services, in other words as a tier 2 professional working at the interface with tier 1.

At *tier 3*, there are multi-disciplinary teams. These have been the traditional form of clinical organisation within child and adolescent psychiatric services for decades but are expensive and often slow. By confining them to tier 3, the idea is that their work can be focussed upon a relatively small number of severe or difficult cases that have high degrees of complexity and comorbidity or a number of adverse psychosocial risk factors. Historically, a typical team would have contained a child and adolescent psychiatrist, a psychologist (educational or clinical), several social workers and, especially in the London area, a child psychotherapist. Nowadays the pattern is more fluid. Virtually all teams contain senior (consultant) child and adolescent psychiatrists as team leaders. Nurses are now present in a large number of teams, working as community psychiatric nurses (clinical nurse specialists) with an emphasis on outreach work. Child psychotherapists who are non-medical and have a long training in psychoanalytic therapy have become more widespread, though still mainly found in south-east England. Family therapists, drawn from various disciplines but particularly social work and nursing, have become established. Educational psychologists have become preoccupied with special educational needs and have been replaced almost completely by clinical psychologists (who have a different training) as far as clinical work is concerned. A few teams have community paediatricians, occupational therapists, remedial teachers or speech and language therapists. Teams may take general cases from their local district or specialise within the district by taking, for example, ADHD or sexual abuse cases. Referrals can be made directly to tier 3 from tier 1 or 2 but a single case may start at tier 3 and after assessment be handled by a solo professional in tier 2 manner.

Highly specialised services, not required to be established in all localities but available at a distance, are at *tier 4*. This level includes all inpatient services for child and adolescent psychiatry. Few localities within the UK are large enough to need their own inpatient unit, either for children or adolescents as not many young people are referred to them. Quite often, then, an inpatient unit will serve a number of localities. On the other hand, a particular locality or district would often have enough appropriate clinical cases for a day unit but for one reason or another, day units have not become well established, been slow to develop and remain few in number. Some highly specialised outpatient services can be regarded as tier 4: gender identity clinics, trauma psychology, neuropsychology, some neuropsychiatry, sleep disorder clinics, sexual offender or autism services are typical examples. Whether tier 4 services only take referrals from tier 3 or whether they can take referrals from any tier is not fixed as policy but in practice most cases have already been assessed at tier 3. In contrast to so-called tertiary care in paediatrics (the same level of super-specialisation), the concept of tier 4 is poorly developed, there having been an apparent assumption that nearly all child mental health cases can be dealt with by local general teams. Under current financial arrangements within the NHS a referral to a specialised outpatient clinic has to be paid for specially (an extra-contractual referral) and agreed by the local Health Authority. The degree of resistance to this (Health Authorities refusing to fund) is quite extraordinary, especially as the decision not to fund seems often to be made by a non-medical official with no special knowledge of child and adolescent mental health acting in accordance with "policy". This causes considerable distress to families.

The tiered concept can be extended across agencies. Thus special educational needs coordinators, educational social workers (education welfare officers) and school nurses (NHS employed) in schools can undertake a considerable amount of work with children who have mental health needs, as do ordinary (field) social

Table 3. A typical mental health contributions grid across agencies

	Health Service	Education	Social Services	Youth justice
Tier 4	In-Patient Units	School for autistic children	Secure unit	Unit for mentally disordered offenders
Tier 3	Multi disciplinary CAMH Team	Pupil referral unit	Specialist foster care team for disturbed adolescents	
Tier 2	Clinical psychology service	Educational psychology service	Specialist social worker	
Tier 1	General practitioner	Pastoral care teacher	Field social worker	Probation officers

workers in social services and probation officers in the youth justice system. All are in the position of being able to make referrals to child and adolescent mental health services directly, in parallel with general practitioners from a health service base. All are then in tier 1.

In inter-agency work at tier 2, such professionals as educational social workers, specialist social workers in adolescent drug misuse work, school counsellors, or psychotherapists in voluntary organisations can be seen to be the equivalent of NHS mental health professionals working solo. It is less easy to draw close parallels with tier 3 though social services for adolescents and pupil referral units for disruptive children in schools manage correspondingly complex cases. At tier 4 the closest parallel are the highly specialised schools, residential units for mentally disordered young offenders and the specialist social services or independent sector units for adolescents needing secure accommodation.

For a community of local families and children, a two-dimensional grid can be drawn of relevant services from several involved agencies, taking note of agency boundaries and arranging services in a hierarchy of complexity in tiers. This makes clear the different contributions made by various agencies and should make clear overlaps and gaps (see Table 3).

The CAMHS concept is relatively new and is still evolving. It is widely supported. The House of Commons in the UK Parliament has an influential Health Committee which, when it examined child and adolescent mental health services recently, said "We congratulate those involved in drawing up the model and the Department of Health for recognising its importance" (House of Commons 1997a). The hope is that it will prove fruitful though as yet it is untested scientifically, and is not yet fully implemented.

CAMHS within the Health Service are not generously funded. According to current estimates most Health Authorities commit less than 6 % of their total spend on mental health on child and adolescent services. This is in spite of children under the age of 18 constituting 22–25 % of the local population.

The description of service structure above makes little mention of *day units*. These are not widely used and there are only some 30 such units in the UK. They are structured on different models: regular daily attendance in some, but attendance for one or two days a week in others.

2. Classification systems, diagnostic and therapeutic methods

Classification systems

One of the early problems to emerge from inter-agency CAMHS development has been the use of terminology. Medical diagnostic categories are not universally welcomed in a multi-agency CAMHS, neither is the use of psychometrics. The distinction between a mental health problem and a social problem is understandably difficult to draw yet this becomes crucial when expensive problems like self-harming or fire-setting adolescents with no family care are concerned.

Even within the Health Service the value of the ICD-10 classification is disputed. Managers like it as do some doctors. Non-medical professions often find it rigid and reductionist. Training in its use is less rigorous than in some other European countries. As an alternative, the Association for Child Psychology and Psychiatry (ACPP) (Berger et al. 1993) drew up a series of problem-based terms which have been generally welcomed and form the basis of a number of computerised databases. This is politically important as there is a tension between service managers who, for reasons of uniformity, usually want the database to be an extension of adult mental illness or hospital services and clinicians who want something more relevant to clinical needs. Many services use extensions of adult mental health databases though there are specialised computerised databases for CAMHS such as P-CARD and MAISY which are powerful tools but involve expenditure in information technology that not all services have been able to provide.

The ACPP database contains some measures of outcome and the topic was addressed by a paper by Berger, Hill and Walk (1993) which drew attention to the complexity of the issue. The Department of Health and Manchester University have developed a series of outcome measures known as HONOSCA (Health of the Nation Outcome Scales for Children) which are being piloted. They are included in a current exercise being carried out by the Audit Commission which will describe activity in a large number of CAMHS.

One well-recognised trap in measuring outcome is that a proportion of referrals will be for assessment only, no improvement as a result of treatment being intended. The aims of the referral may be met but there is no change in the child's condition. There is also a difficulty in evaluating the outcome of inter-professional consultation; workers may be satisfied at the discussion of a case with a mental health professional but it has been impossible to show whether this was ultimately beneficial to the child.

Diagnostic and therapeutic methods

Exactly what UK consultants in child and adolescent psychiatry do is an interesting question. Most lead multidisciplinary teams in outpatient clinics. Their reputation for relying predominantly on family therapy is probably unjustified. In an unpublished survey of 100 consecutive cases seen at two clinics which I carried out with colleagues five years ago, the most popular assessment and intervention method was indeed interviews with several family members all present (not usually the entire family, often mother and child) but this was the least likely to involve consultants. They were more likely to be involved in carrying out mental state examinations, prescribing medication, arranging treatment to be carried out by others, offering consultation to other professionals in the patient's absence, chairing discussions among staff, or going to management and academic meetings. The situation is changing rapidly. In 1994 it was possible for a leading child and adolescent psychiatrist to say of child mental health services "Compared to other health services, we have no drugs, no beds, no complicated equipment: we just need ourselves, our patients, time and space" (Kraemer 1994). Yet a survey by James (1996) demonstrated that 87 % of all the child and adolescent psychiatrist in the Oxford region were actively prescribing medication for their patients. A year later, half of 100 predominantly non-academic consultants and trainees were actively prescribing stimulants and half of the remainder intended to (Bramble 1997). A show of hands at a large academic meeting of most consultants in the UK in 1997 revealed the majority to be actively prescribing medication. Yet it is still the case that many are practising in premises remote from other medicine with few facilities for physical examination or investigation. The social tradition is strong and there are still those who maintain stoutly that ADHD is simply the result of inadequate parenting though they are likely to be in a minority (see, e.g. Bramble 1997).

What cases are seen?

About half of all cases referred to child and adolescent psychiatry teams (tier 3) have antisocial behaviour as a reason for referral or as a prominent part of the child's psychopathology (see e.g. Hoare et al. 1995). By and large neuropsychological problems, particularly epilepsy and learning disability, are likely to be managed by paediatricians. There is a sharp recent increase in the number of children with ADHD referred, one index of this being that the prescription of stimulant medication has increased dramatically since 1993. There is also a marked increase in the number of referrals of younger children with eating disorders (House of Commons 1997b).

One of the burdens for consultant child and adolescent psychiatrists is the number of expert witness reports required by Social Services Departments and the courts. These arise in connection with child protection cases, particularly sexual abuse, going through the legal system. A given local authority may need 20–30 reports a year, each demanding 20 or more hours or so of assessment and court attendance.

It is still the case that the vast majority of children and adolescents seen will receive psychological treatments as outpatients. Variations of family therapy and supportive psychotherapy or counselling with individuals are the most common. Focussed psychological treatments such as cognitive behavioural therapy, expert individual psychodynamic therapy, or parent training classes are less prevalent and most likely to be used in better-resourced centres. Recommendations to other agencies such as Education or Social Services take up a fair amount of time. Medication is increasingly used but still for a minority and almost always as a component of a total treatment programme. Manualised treatments, structured programmes and the extensive use of rating scales are generally confined to specialist centres associated with academic units.

What happens to referred cases?

A young person referred to a CAMHS at tier 2 or 3 can expect to have their problem characterised in psychological terms and placed within a family context. He or she (usually he) and his mother will be seen for several outpatient sessions in a clinic, the target problem discussed so that it can be understood and suggestions made for its management. Improvement is common but sustained follow-up not especially systematic. Roughly one in five referrals do not attend a first appointment for a variety of reasons. One of these is that parents do not always agree with a referrer that their child needs to be seen by a mental health professional. Stigma is still a problem in spite of clinics and services choosing titles for themselves which avoid the term "psychiatry". Unfortunately the more recent term "mental health" is still unpopular with the young and their parents. Nevertheless, recent audit surveys carried out by staff not directly connected with clinics, indicate that among those families seen, the service is appreciated by a high majority and improvements in target problems are reported by parents (Bendle et al. 1993). Medical referrers are generally satisfied but this is less true of educational referrers, perhaps because they want assessment and treatment of academic and behaviour problems in school and clinic-based mental health professionals are more used to working in a family context in the clinic or the home.

3. Structure and organization of services

The placement of child and adolescent psychiatry within a tiered structure which can be extended across agencies has been referred to above.

There is very little private practice in child and adolescent psychiatry in the UK. Virtually all psychiatric and psychology services are provided by the NHS. This offers healthcare to the whole UK population. There are small, standard charges for adult medicine prescriptions, vision testing and for adult dentistry but otherwise the service is free at the point of use. Apart from general practitioner services, it is separated into purchasers or commissioners (Health Authorities and some general practitioners) and providers (clinical services in hospitals and the community). Central government provides money to purchasers who then buy services for the local population through financial contracts with provider organisations such as a hospital. They can also purchase services from independent or voluntary organizations but this is not central.

The previous Conservative government made much play of this purchaser-provider split, hoping that market forces would reduce costs and increase efficiency. It was imagined that providers would compete with each other for contracts with providers. This ignored geography. Outside large cities there is often only one provider unit for each purchaser. Disillusionment with the new system set in quickly and it is not clear that any costs were saved since the new arrangements placed a heavy demand on managerial and administrative staff who increased in number dramatically. The current New Labour government is finding ways for purchasers and providers to co-operate with an emphasis on the views of general practitioners but it is too soon to know what this means in detail. More importantly a series of deaths caused by poor cardiac surgery technique at a children's hospital in Bristol has been one of the elements that have led to an insistence that managers of health services are responsible for the quality of clinical practice. This places clinicians in a stronger position.

One recent consequence of the new view of purchasing is a governmental direction that inpatient child and adolescent psychiatry will be commissioned centrally. This is welcome as there has been a fall in the volume of NHS provision and a slight increase in private units who tend to specialise in eating disorders or psychosomatic conditions, so-called "cherry-picking" of the more respectable cases, leaving the NHS units to deal with less amenable patients. At the other end of the spectrum, a few private units are taking the most behaviourally difficult but at a high price. The fragmentation of planning which the purchaser-provider split produced allowed this to develop since individual purchaser units could not afford to finance an entire inpatient unit.

In general, adolescent inpatient units are separate from children's inpatient units. The former need close nursing links with adult psychiatry, the latter with children's nursing. Neither are very numerous. It is surprisingly difficult to be precise about numbers but approximately 75 units provide residential treatment for children and adolescents in the UK. Most of these also provide day care but the number of specialist day hospitals or day units is much smaller. It can be very difficult to obtain the admission of a child or adolescent to an inpatient unit – there is a serious insufficiency of places. Turnover is rapid in order to free up beds. In general the cases referred will be psychotic, suicidal, starving or impossible to contain in outpatient practice.

The vast majority of children seen specifically by child and adolescent psychiatry services or child psychology services will be as outpatients (i.e. at tiers 2 and 3). These are outnumbered by the volume of children with mental health needs seen by community paediatricians and primary care teams (general practitioners and health visitors). In turn these are complemented by the work of teachers, education welfare officers (education social workers) and educational psychologists in the education system, social workers in social services, and voluntary workers and counsellors in a number of specialist areas. For instance, many children who need residential provision are managed in boarding special schools, and adolescents with extreme behaviour may be looked after by social services in secure units which are part of the social care system rather than the health system.

The tiered system mentioned above seeks to coordinate all this work.

4. Cooperation with medical and non-medical disciplines

One of the consequences of the child guidance system was the isolation of psychiatrists from their medical colleagues since they were initially employed by the local authorities rather than the NHS. Even when they were taken into the NHS they continued to be geographically separate in community clinics. Their hospital clinic colleagues often had links with adult psychiatry but close working links with pediatrics were somewhat unusual. This is still the case, with honourable exceptions. Quite often paediatric services (both hospital and community) are in different organisations (NHS Trust). The Royal College of Psychiatrists and the Royal College of Paediatrics and Child Health are two different bodies though some child psychiatrists belong to both. There are working links between the two and the Royal College of Paediatrics has a special interest group in psychology and psychiatry.

Cooperation with adult psychiatry is closer. At a national level this has been achieved through the Royal College of Psychiatrists which has responsibility for standards in training and clinical practice. It contains a faculty of child and adolescent psychiatry which is on equal standing with general psychiatry, medical psychotherapy, forensic, old age and mental handicap psychiatry. At the level of an individual service, links may be tenuous and there is a long-standing problem about who cares for 16–19 year-olds. Liaison between adult and child psychiatrists over cases in this range is often reactive rather than proactive. Nor is there an agreed national policy as to who, child psychiatrists or mental handicap (disability) psychiatrists, should look after the mental health needs of children with mental handicap; arrangements are left to local services and vary accordingly.

Links with non-medical disciplines are sometimes warm, occasionally competitive. The national Association for Child Psychiatry and Psychology and its journal have done much to maintain collaboration. The same is true for multi-disciplinary groups such as the Association for Family Therapy and the Association for the Professional Study of Adolescence. Nevertheless there are several services across the UK where psychiatrists and psychologists have little helpful to say to each other, each claiming primacy or supremacy. The multi-agency tiered model is intended to prevent the unnecessary duplication of services which this kind of rivalry has brought about.

5. Graduate/postgraduate training and continuing medical education

There are 23 medical schools in the UK, a smaller number than previously because of mergers of schools within London University. Sixteen of these schools have an academic child and adolescent psychiatrist, not always a professor. There are 18 professors in the UK generally (Table 4), three of which are within the two relevant postgraduate institutions, the Institutes of Psychiatry and Child Health. There are plans to establish three others.

Table 4. Number of professors in the various universities

London	8	Leeds	1
Liverpool	2	Leicester	1
Cambridge	1	Manchester	1
Cardiff	1	Newcastle	1
Glasgow	1	Nottingham	1

Child and adolescent psychiatry is a required subject in undergraduate medical training, examined at medical finals, and is taught in all medical schools though there is no agreed core or minimal time. Sometimes it is taught within psychiatry generally, sometimes within paediatrics. Undergraduate curricula are being reviewed in all medical schools and some have taken a curriculum framework such as human development in which child psychiatry has become more prominent because of the requirement that new curricula take a greater family perspective than previously.

Psychiatrists train in two stages in the first place. General professional training lasts three to three and a half years and usually includes six or seven placements in various psychiatric specialties, organised within a training scheme approved (and visited to ensure standards) by the Royal College of Psychiatrists. At the end of this they take the second part of the Royal College of Psychiatrists' membership exam. All psychiatrists in training now have to have supervised clinical experience of either child and adolescent psychiatry or mental handicap psychiatry. They are examined on theoretical knowledge of clinical child and adolescent psychiatry and child psychological development.

If they pass their examination trainees become members of the Royal College of Psychiatrists (MRCPsych), can apply for a post as a specialist registrar and enter higher specialist training in any of six specialties of psychiatry of which child and adolescent psychiatry is one. This emphasizes clinical supervision and seminar teaching while in a clinical post, is fairly rigorous. It is overseen by a Royal College of Psychiatrists committee (CAPSAC) which visits higher training schemes and approves higher training schemes and individual specialist training, awarding a certificate of completion of specialist training (CCST) if there has been satisfactory training for three years. Psychiatrists wanting to train part-time can do so according to a separately funded scheme. There is no final examination; appointment to a consultant position is by competition for an advertised and funded post. A CCST is essential for this.

Higher specialist training in child and adolescent psychiatry has been a success story. It has transformed the consultant ranks.

Continuing medical education is preferably known as continuing professional development (CPD). There is a Royal College scheme but it is generic across the specialties of psychiatry. It cannot be said that it is favourable to child and adolescent psychiatrists and appears to their eyes to be biased towards adult general psychiatrists. A number of child and adult psychiatrists work single-handed so that it is difficult to obtain cover on order to attend meetings away from base. There is also virtually no arrangement by which conferences and their fees are funded by pharmaceutical companies, unlike the situation in general psychiatry.

6. Research

All higher trainees are expected to carry out a piece of personal research and most do. These studies are mainly for training purposes. In parallel with this there has been a national drive to promote medical or clinical audit. An awareness of the need to predict, measure or review is now widespread and there is a more generally positive attitude towards research than in the past. Within the Health Service, a national programme of research and development, promoted by directors at regional level has been helpful to clinicians who want to carry out medium-sized clinical projects. Nevertheless, nearly all scientific research leading to scientific advances is carried out in academic departments. That at the Institute of Psychiatry in London, developed by Michael Rutter, is internationally recognised as especially productive. The pressures on UK universities are leading to greater investment in research effort and the funding policies of the major research-funding bodies are creating specialist centres. Cambridge and Manchester have well-developed programmes in depression, for instance. But collaboration across disciplines and between institutions, as in genetic research or studies in hyperkinesis, is vigorous so that it becomes less easy to say which department is leading or where a particular collaboration is centred. One of the great strengths of UK research in child psychiatry has been the active involvement of psychologists so that a developmental psychopathological perspective is usual.

Generally speaking, the research field is in good condition though there are some worries that there are not quite enough young researchers coming through. There are research training programmes which try to address these. An active Child Psychiatry Research Society meets to review studies which are at an early stage. Most current work is concerned with aetiology, particularly social and genetic influences. Intervention studies are less prevalent and there is little in psychopharmacology.

7. Future perspectives

Many commissioners of services have recently come to insist that their providers meet health care needs defined epidemiologically in the local population. Earlier work by Pearce and Holmes (1995) and the survey by Kurtz, Thornes and Wolkind (1994) laid the basis for this so that it is now not possible to evaluate a service without addressing this issue. The old Health Advisory Service which wrote "Together We Stand" is now re-born as HAS 2000; a body which has among other commitments, a distinct role in evaluating CAMHS and helping their development. They are developing standards for services by drawing on influential policy documents. The first standard on the list for child and adolescent mental health services is "there is a local child and adolescent mental health needs assessment". All else flows from this.

The need for treatment interventions to be justified by scientific evidence is now accepted. Treatment within a CAMHS needs to be evidence-based just as in the

Health Service generally. Sifting the published evidence on effectiveness is difficult. The national Cochrane database exercise is assembling published evidence relevant to all branches of medicine. The component for child and adolescent mental health has begun but will take some time to deliver. In the meantime, the Department of Health in England has commissioned evidence in the form of less formal reviews and two chapters have been published for the guidance of commissioners (Hall & Hill 1994; Wallace et al. 1997). A body within the Royal College of Psychiatrists called Focus aims to develop and disseminate evidence-based practice for all disciplines in a CAMHS and is therefore aimed at providers. It has established a forum of interested people, an e-mail discussion list and is currently carrying out systematic reviews of published evidence in order to answer issues raised by forum members about the management of ADHD.

A national body, the Audit Commission is currently carrying out a huge survey of child and adolescent mental health services. This will be published in 1999 and will contain a wealth of information. The first results appear to indicate an uneven distribution of resources across the UK. If this is confirmed, then it is probable that the government will need to do something about this to ensure that all children have equal access to services. Quite how this might be achieved is now being discussed.

Selected references

Bendle S, Hill P, Byrne P (1993) Audit of two child mental health services. Paper presented at SW Thames Audit Conference, Redhill, Surrey

Berger M, Hill P, Sein E, Thompson M, Verduyn C (1993) A Proposed Core Dataset for Child and Adolescent Psychology and Psychiatry Services. London: Association for Child Psychology and Psychiatry

Berger M, Hill P, Walk D (1993) Considerations in measuring outcome. In: Berger M et al. (eds) op cit. Reprinted in NHS Health Advisory Services Together We Stand. London: HMSO 1995, pp 183–192

Bramble D (1997) Psychostimulants and British child psychiatrists. Child Psychology and Psychiatry Review 2: 159–162

Davis H, Spurr P (1998) Parent counselling: an evaluation of a community child mental health service. Journal of Child Psychology and Psychiatry 39: 365–376

Department of Health (1995) A Handbook on Child and Adolescent Mental Health. London: HMSO

Earle J, Hill P (1998) Research into Practice, A Distance Learning Pack on Child Mental Health for Health Visitors. London, St. George's Hospital Medical School, Department of Psychiatry

Goodman R (1997) Child and Adolescent Mental Health services: Reasoned Advice to Commissioners and Providers. London, Maudsley Hospital

Hall D, Hill P (1994) Community Child Health Services. In: Stevens A, Raftery J (eds) Health Care Needs Assessment. Oxford: NHSME/Radcliffe Medical Press

Hoare P, Scarth L, Forbes F (1995) Audit of the Edinburgh Child Psychiatry Out-Patient Service. ACPP Review and Newsletter 17: 139–148

House of Commons (1997a) Session 1996-97. Health Committee, Fourth Report. Child and Adolescent Mental Health Services. Report together with the Proceedings of the Committee. London, The Stationery Office

House of Commons (1997b) Session 1996-97. Health Committee, Fourth Report. Child and Adolescent Mental Health Services. Volume II Minutes of Evidence and Appendices. London, The Stationery Office

James AC (1996) A survey of the prescribing practices of child and adolescent psychiatrists. Child Psychology and Psychiatry Review 1: 94–97

Kraemer S (1994) On working together in a changing world: dilemmas for the trainer. ACPP Review & Newsletter 16: 120–129

Kurtz Z, Thornes R, Wolkind S (1994) Services for the Mental Health of Children and Young People in England. A National Review. London: Public Health Directorate, South Thames Regional Health Authority
NHS Health Advisory Service (1995) Together We Stand: The Commissioning, Role and Management of Child and Adolescent Mental Health Services. London: HMSO
Pearce J, Holmes S (1995) Health Gain Investment Programme: People with Mental Health Problems, Part 4. Child and Adolescent Mental Health. Sheffield: Trent Regional Health Authority
Wallace SA, Crown JM, Cox AD, Berger M (1997) Child and Adolescent Mental Health. In: Stevens A, Raftery J (eds) Health Care Needs Assessment. Oxford: NHSME/Radcliffe Medical Press

MIX
Papier aus verantwortungsvollen Quellen
Paper from responsible sources
FSC® C105338

If you have any concerns about our products,
you can contact us on
ProductSafety@springernature.com

In case Publisher is established outside the EU,
the EU authorized representative is:
Springer Nature Customer Service Center GmbH
Europaplatz 3, 69115 Heidelberg, Germany

Printed by Libri Plureos GmbH
in Hamburg, Germany